BIPOLAR DISORDERS

CLINICAL COURSE AND OUTCOME

CLINICAL

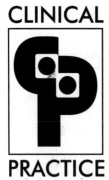

PRACTICE

Judith H. Gold, M.D., F.R.C.P.C.
Elissa P. Benedek, M.D.
Series Editors

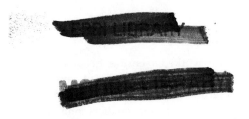

BIPOLAR DISORDERS

CLINICAL COURSE AND OUTCOME

Edited by

Joseph F. Goldberg, M.D., and
Martin Harrow, Ph.D.

Washington, DC
London, England

Note: The authors have worked to ensure that all information in this book concerning drug dosages, schedules, and routes of administration is accurate as of the time of publication and consistent with standards set by the U.S. Food and Drug Administration and the general medical community. As medical research and practice advance, however, therapeutic standards may change. For this reason and because human and mechanical errors sometimes occur, we recommend that readers follow the advice of a physician who is directly involved in their care or the care of a member of their family.

Books published by the American Psychiatric Press, Inc., represent the views and opinions of the individual authors and do not necessarily represent the policies and opinions of the Press or the American Psychiatric Association.

Copyright © 1999 American Psychiatric Press, Inc.
ALL RIGHTS RESERVED
Manufactured in the United States of America on acid-free paper **WM**
First Edition **207**
02 01 00 99 4 3 2 1 **B6165**
American Psychiatric Press, Inc. **1999**
1400 K Street, N.W.
Washington, DC 20005
www.appi.org

Library of Congress Cataloging-in-Publication Data
Bipolar disorders : clinical course and outcome / edited by Joseph F. Goldberg and Martin Harrow. — 1st ed.
    p. cm. — (Clinical practice)
    Includes bibliographical references and index.
    ISBN 0-88048-768-2
    1. Manic-depressive illness. I. Goldberg, Joseph F., 1963– .
II. Harrow, Martin. III. Series.
    [DNLM: 1. Bipolar Disorder—diagnosis. 2. Bipolar Disorder—
therapy.   WM 207 B6165 1998]
RC516.B528 1999
616.89'5—dc21
DNLM/DLC
for Library of Congress   98-22295
                                        CIP

British Library Cataloguing in Publication Data
A CIP record is available from the British Library.

Contents

Contributors

Robert J. Boland, M.D.
Assistant Professor, Department of Psychiatry and Human Behavior, Brown University; and Director, Consultation-Liaison Psychiatry, Department of Psychiatry, Miriam Hospital, Providence, Rhode Island

Charles L. Bowden, M.D.
Nancy U. Karren Professor of Psychiatry and Pharmacology and Chairman, Department of Psychiatry, The University of Texas Health Science Center at San Antonio

Gabriela Cora-Locatelli, M.D.
Clinical Associate, Biological Psychiatry Branch, National Institute of Mental Health, Bethesda, Maryland

William Coryell, M.D.
Professor of Psychiatry, The University of Iowa College of Medicine, Iowa City

Kirk D. Denicoff, M.D.
Clinical Associate, Biological Psychiatry Branch, National Institute of Mental Health, Bethesda, Maryland

Lisa B. Dixon, M.D., M.P.H.
Associate Professor and Director of Residency Training, Institute of Psychiatry and Human Behavior, University of Maryland School of Medicine

David L. Dunner, M.D.
Professor and Director, Center for Anxiety and Depression, Department of Psychiatry and Behavioral Sciences, University of Washington, Seattle

Ellen Frank, Ph.D.
Professor of Psychiatry and Psychology, University of Pittsburgh
School of Medicine, Department of Psychiatry; Western
Psychiatric Institute and Clinic, Pittsburgh, Pennsylvania

Mark A. Frye, M.D.
Assistant Professor of Psychiatry and Associate Director, Mood
Disorders Research Program, UCLA Neuropsychiatric Institute
and Hospital and West Los Angeles VA Medical Center, Los
Angeles, California

Michael J. Gitlin, M.D.
Clinical Professor of Psychiatry, University of California, Los
Angeles, School of Medicine; and Director, Affective Disorders
Clinic, University of California, Los Angeles, Neuropsychiatric
Hospital

Joseph F. Goldberg, M.D.
Assistant Professor of Psychiatry, The Joan and Sanford I. Weill
Medical College of Cornell University; and Director, Bipolar
Disorders Research Clinic, Payne Whitney Clinic, The New York
and Presbyterian Hospital, New York City

Frederick K. Goodwin, M.D.
Director and Professor of Psychiatry, The George Washington
University Medical Center, Center on Neuroscience, Behavior and
Society, Washington, D.C.

Ann L. Hackman, M.D.
Medical Director, Mobile Treatment Unit, Division of Community
Psychiatry, Institute of Psychiatry and Human Behavior,
University of Maryland School of Medicine

Constance Hammen, Ph.D.
Professor of Psychology, University of California, Los Angeles,
Department of Psychology

Martin Harrow, Ph.D.
Professor and Director of Psychology, Department of Psychiatry,
University of Illinois–College of Medicine, Chicago

Jonathan M. Himmelhoch, M.D.
Professor of Psychiatry, University of Pittsburgh School of
Medicine; and Director of Research, Affective Disorders Program,
Western Psychiatric Institute and Clinic, Pittsburgh, Pennsylvania

Paul E. Keck Jr., M.D.
Professor and Vice Chairman for Research, Department of
Psychiatry, University of Cincinnati College of Medicine,
Cincinnati, Ohio

Martin B. Keller, M.D.
Mary E. Zucker Professor and Chairman, Department of
Psychiatry and Human Behavior, Brown University;
Psychiatrist-in-Chief, Butler Hospital; and Executive
Psychiatrist-in-Chief, Brown Affiliated Hospitals, Providence,
Rhode Island

Timothy A. Kimbrell, M.D.
Assistant Professor of Psychiatry, The University of Arkansas for
Medical Science, Little Rock

James H. Kocsis, M.D.
Professor of Psychiatry, The Joan and Sanford I. Weill Medical
College of Cornell University; Payne Whitney Clinic, The New
York and Presbyterian Hospital, New York City

Gabriele S. Leverich, M.S.W.
Director of Longitudinal Studies, Biological Psychiatry Branch,
National Institute of Mental Health, Bethesda, Maryland

Mario Maj, M.D., Ph.D.
Professor of Psychiatry and Chairman, Department of Psychiatry,
First Medical School, University of Naples, Naples, Italy

David J. Miklowitz, Ph.D.
Professor of Psychology, Department of Psychology, University of Colorado, Boulder

Robert M. Post, M.D.
Chief, Biological Psychiatry Branch, National Institute of Mental Health, Bethesda, Maryland

Ranga N. Ram, M.D.
Assistant Professor of Psychiatry, State University of New York at Buffalo; and Medical Director, Comprehensive Psychiatric Emergency Program (CPEP) and Ambulatory Services, Erie County Medical Center, Buffalo, New York

Mauricio Tohen, M.D., Dr.P.H.
Associate Clinical Professor of Psychiatry, Harvard Medical School; Medical Advisor, Lilly Research Laboratories, Indianapolis, Indiana

George Winokur, M.D.[1]
Professor of Psychiatry, The University of Iowa College of Medicine, Iowa City

Carlos A. Zarate Jr., M.D.
Assistant Professor of Psychiatry, Harvard Medical School; and Director, Bipolar and Psychotic Disorders Outpatient Services, McLean Hospital, Belmont, Massachusetts

---

[1]Dr. Winokur died October 12, 1996.

Introduction
to the Clinical Practice Series

O ver the years of its existence the series of monographs entitled *Clinical Insights* gradually became focused on providing current, factual, and theoretical material of interest to the clinician working outside of a hospital setting. To reflect this orientation, the name of the Series has been changed to *Clinical Practice.*

The Clinical Practice Series will provide books that give the mental health clinician a practical, clinical approach to a variety of psychiatric problems. These books will provide up-to-date literature reviews and emphasize the most recent treatment methods. Thus, the publications in the Series will interest clinicians working both in psychiatry and in the other mental health professions.

Each year a number of books will be published dealing with all aspects of clinical practice. In addition, from time to time when appropriate, the publications may be revised and updated. Thus, the Series will provide quick access to relevant and important areas of psychiatric practice. Some books in the Series will be authored by a person considered to be an expert in that particular area; others will be edited by such an expert, who will also draw together other knowledgeable authors to produce a comprehensive overview of that topic.

Some of the books in the Clinical Practice Series will have their foundation in presentations at an annual meeting of the American Psychiatric Association. All will contain the most recently available information on the subjects discussed. Theoretical and scientific data will be applied to clinical situations, and case illustrations will be utilized in order to make the material even more relevant for the practitioner. Thus, the Clinical Practice Series should provide educational reading in a compact format especially designed for the mental health clinician–psychiatrist.

Judith H. Gold, M.D., F.R.C.P.C.
Series Editor

Foreword

> The universal experience is striking, that the attacks of manic-depressive insanity . . . never lead to profound dementia, not even when they continue throughout the life almost without interruption. . . . As a rule the disease runs its course in isolated attacks more or less sharply defined from each other or from health, which are either like or unlike, or even very frequently are [the] perfect antithesis.
>
> Kraepelin 1921

Since the advent of the psychopharmacological revolution, manic-depressive illness (bipolar disorder) has served as a principal point of focus for modern psychiatric research. Today, although the accumulation of knowledge of this illness and its treatment constitutes one of the extraordinary success stories of modern biomedical science, it remains in many ways a paradox. A paradox because, despite all we know, the illness too often is unrecognized or misdiagnosed and inappropriately or ineffectively treated. This disparity between optimal care on the one hand, and what is routinely provided on the other hand, is perhaps nowhere larger than in manic-depressive illness; and its human and economic impact remains excessive.

This book deals with course and outcome among patients with bipolar disorder. Throughout medicine, course and outcome are basic to the very concept of a disease entity. Indeed, Kraepelin's central insight, which continues as an organizing principle in modern descriptive psychiatry, was to bring clarity to the nineteenth-century confusion of multiple and proliferating diagnostic entities. He achieved this remarkable synthesis by classifying essentially all of the apparently diverse psychotic disorders into two groups, a distinction based on course and outcome. He observed that *dementia praecox* (schizophrenia) tends to be chronic and follow a deteriorating course, whereas manic-depressive illness is episodic and ultimately exacts a less devastating toll on those affected.

Further, an understanding of the pathophysiology—and ultimately etiology—of illness requires understanding its natural course. Indeed, the contemporary development of pathophysiological models for bipolar disorder is increasingly focusing on the biology of recurrence. Thus, one group of hypotheses posits that the episodic nature of the illness reflects a disturbance in the regulation of biological rhythms, whereas another hypothesis (outlined by Post et al., Chapter 5, in this volume) is based on kindling/sensitization as a model both for the inherent cyclicity of the illness and for the observations that 1) as episodes recur, they tend to come closer together, and 2) the degree of environmental stress associated with recurrent episodes becomes progressively less intense over time. As per the kindling hypothesis, this process may involve intermittent (but not chronic) subthreshold stimuli, either electrical or chemical, eventually producing neuronal depolarization responses of increasing intensity, even though the size of the stimulus is held constant. When the repeated stimuli are applied to the limbic system, seizures eventually ensue and characteristically they continue indefinitely after the removal of the stimulus. Apparently permanent change has been introduced; it is as if the neuronal system has developed a molecular memory of the stimuli and responds accordingly.

Finally, the study of natural course is vital because both clinicians and those making decisions about access to treatment (i.e., insurance and managed care companies) must understand what happens to patients who have manic-depressive illness in the absence of adequate ongoing treatment.

Today we face a paradox. Although the discovery of the prophylactic potential of lithium and the anticonvulsants has revived interest in the natural course of bipolar disorder, widespread use of these agents has substantially altered that course. Investigators must confront the fact that "natural" course now includes the unquantified effects of prophylaxis.

This book is both timely and needed. Drs. Goldberg and Harrow have pulled together many of the major contributors in this field and asked them to focus on a wide range of complex issues that, in addition to their relevance to course and outcome, have this in common: their importance is both conceptual and practical.

The book focuses on bipolar disorder, but, classically, manic-depressive illness comprised all severe forms of recurrent affective illness. Severe unipolar illness shares characteristics (other than the tendency to recur) with bipolar disorder (e.g., prophylactic response to lithium). As we have argued elsewhere (Goodwin and Jamison 1990), separating bipolar and recurrent unipolar disorders in formal diagnostic systems prejudges the relation between them, giving priority to polarity and neglecting the cyclicity common to both forms. Thus, important questions are never asked.

Nevertheless, this volume's focus on bipolar disorder is understandable, particularly for investigators in the United States who have had to struggle with a very broad concept of "unipolar." Indeed, until its most recent revision, the unipolar category in the DSM system did not address the issue of recurrence, leaving unipolar to incorporate just about any depression other than bipolar.

One of the intriguing issues addressed in this book and elsewhere (Goodwin and Jamison 1990) is the apparent decline over the years in the prophylactic effectiveness of lithium. During the 1970s, most controlled studies of lithium were conducted in research centers. Investigators reported complete response as defined by the elimination of the need for hospitalization in 75%–80% of patients. However, not all of this response was complete, as some of the patients in these studies had a partial decrease in frequency, duration, and/or severity of episodes. The psychic pain component of the illness seemed most responsive to lithium, which is reflected in the finding of a six- to sevenfold decrease in completed suicides in patients taking lithium as compared with those whose manic-depressive illness was not treated with maintenance lithium.

As noted above, contemporary follow-up studies show apparent response rates to lithium that are substantially lower than those in the "classical" studies, both open and controlled. Several reasons may account for this difference. First, follow-up studies today reflect the results of treatment in the community, as opposed to carefully controlled medication trials in a research setting. This bias suggests that the "true" effectiveness of lithium "in the real world" is lower than what was achievable in the controlled trials. However, it can be argued that patients who respond well to outpatient treatment seldom volunteer for research studies; thus, many of the lithium-responsive patients are already filtered out of the research population. This is simply an instance of an old paradox in medicine: the longer a successful treatment is around, the more difficult it is to demonstrate its effectiveness. Based on this paradox, one might expect that in a sample not affected by adverse selection, lithium would still show response rates in the range of the classical studies. Some support for this expectation is offered by contemporary reports on large practice samples—for example, Page and colleagues (1987) in the United States and Kukopulos and colleagues (1980) in Italy—in which lithium response remained close to those response rates achieved in the classical studies. These samples may have benefited from the most difficult patients being selected out.

Second, in addition to the changes in diagnostic practices over the last two decades described by Drs. Goldberg and Harrow in the Preface (a shift to more bipolar and fewer schizophrenic diagnoses), some environmental changes may have contributed to lithium resistance among manic-depressive patients, such as the increased use of drugs and alcohol among the young. Also, the last generation has experienced other cultural changes—for example, a threefold increase in the mobility of the population and a doubling of the divorce rate —which could leave patients vulnerable to manic-depressive illness with fewer supports. Last, we know that effective antidepressants can activate and accelerate the illness in some cases; indeed, the frequency of episodes has increased over the same time frame during which the availability of effective antidepressants has increased.

Finally, one fascinating hypothesis suggests that a cross-generational shift to more malignant forms of the illness may reflect a genetic mechanism involving unstable DNA. Several genetic neurological illnesses, such as Huntington's disease, have been shown to be characterized by genetic mutations—trinucleotide repeat amplifications—which are inherited unstable DNA sequences that tend to produce repeated additions of amino acid triplets during mitosis. Trinucleotide repeats would increase the severity of the illness in succeeding generations, perhaps contributing to greater treatment resistance.

Finally, it is both remarkable and wholly appropriate that one-quarter of the chapters in this volume focus on psychosocial and psychotherapeutic aspects of bipolar disorder. The data reviewed in those chapters, while still somewhat preliminary, show a substantial advantage of combined psychosocial/pharmacological strategies over medication alone. Interestingly, the size of the reported effects of adjunctive psychosocial interventions is larger than that observed in studies in which psychotherapy alone was administered to "good" psychotherapeutic candidates, that is, patients whose overall functioning is reasonably intact. Clearly, the evolution of effective medications for this severe psychiatric disorder has opened up major new vistas for psychotherapy broadly defined. It will behoove the health insurance and managed care industries to consider these data carefully, rather than to continue to rely on antiquated "Woody Allen" images of psychotherapy.

Frederick K. Goodwin, M.D.

References

Goodwin FK, Jamison KR: Manic-Depressive Illness. New York, Oxford University Press, 1990

Kukopulos A, Reginaldi D, Laddomada P, et al: Course of the manic-depressive cycle and changes caused by treatments. Pharmakopsychiatrie Neuro-Psychopharmakologie 13:156–167, 1980

Page C, Benaim S, Lappin F: A long-term retrospective follow-up study of patients treated with prophylactic lithium carbonate. Br J Psychiatry 150:175–179, 1987

Preface

*T*his volume is a compendium of findings from several major research programs studying the naturalistic course of contemporary bipolar disorders. Based in part on a symposium titled "Modern-Day Bipolar Disorders: Course and Outcome," presented at the 148th annual meeting of the American Psychiatric Association in 1995, it relates empirical data on outcome with practical information on the prognosis, course, and potential complications of bipolar disorders in the modern era.

Early twentieth-century psychiatrists distinguished manic-depressive illness from other severe psychiatric disorders not only according to symptoms but also on the basis of longitudinal course of illness. In contrast to the frequent deterioration and pervasive disability often seen in schizophrenia, clinical investigators in Europe and the United States noted almost a century ago that manic disturbances were usually periodic and were followed by a return to normal functioning. Since then, even with advances in pharmacotherapy, data have begun to challenge beliefs about good outcome for most bipolar patients.

In the 1980s, naturalistic follow-up studies began to demonstrate that lithium, for a variety of reasons, often appears less effective under routine clinical conditions than in randomized controlled trials. At the same time, concepts about bipolar illness began to change dramatically: prognosis and treatment response has been shown to vary with manic subtypes (e.g., rapid cycling, mixed-affective states, hypomania); comorbid substance abuse today frequently complicates the course of manic episodes; ongoing psychosocial, occupational, and economic disability has led to chronic impairment for many bipolar patients; and the shortcomings of lithium have spurred the development of adjuvant or alternative antimanic regimens, such as the anticonvulsants carbamazepine and valproate (or its sodium valproate:valproic acid form, divalproex sodium).

Several considerations are noteworthy in assessing the course of bipolar disorders in a contemporary clinical context:

- In the past quarter century, a major shift occurred in diagnostic patterns among psychiatrists in the United States and Europe. A tendency for American psychiatrists to diagnose schizophrenia more often than bipolar disorder had, until recently, caused an underrecognition of mania and a narrowed concept of primary affective versus schizophrenic psychopathology.
- Relatedly, the diagnostic nomenclature has evolved for describing mania, depression, or schizoaffective disorders based on standardized classification systems. Formal clinical definitions of mania have undergone multiple revisions through successive editions of DSM, published by the American Psychiatric Association (e.g., DSM-IV now includes a separate category for hypomania). Other research definitions (e.g., Research Diagnostic Criteria) have led to diverse inclusion and exclusion criteria for mania over the past several decades. Thus, many patients with prominent psychoses who were at one time considered to have schizophrenia have been reconceptualized more recently as having a severe form of bipolar disorder.
- With regard to treatment outcome, research in the delivery of health care services has begun to differentiate *efficacy* (outcome under idealized, controlled clinical conditions) from *effectiveness* (outcome under ordinary circumstances, while accounting for parameters that can diminish an optimal response, such as comorbid illnesses, medication noncompliance, and poor social support). Many clinicians have come to assume that if an antimanic medication shows proven efficacy in randomized clinical trials, it should be no less effective under ordinary treatment conditions. This assumption, however, may not necessarily be true.
- In recent years, increasingly complex forms of mania have been described. These forms include mixed or rapid-cycling affective states, tricyclic- or other antidepressant-induced switches into mania, mania secondary to comorbid medical or neurological conditions (e.g., HIV), and manic disorders that appear refractory to multiple adequate pharmacotherapy trials. Mania with comorbid alcoholism or drug abuse accounts

for a disproportionately large number of bipolar patients now seen in routine clinical practice. Severe, treatment-resistant forms of mania often challenge the capabilities of current psychiatric services, particularly in a climate of limited health care resources.

These and other factors bear on the interpretation of clinical trials, follow-up investigations, and epidemiological surveys across diverse samples of bipolar patients. As reports on bipolar outcome continue to grow in the literature, this book presents a modern perspective on illness course during naturalistic treatment. In particular, at a time when longitudinal studies are rare in the psychiatric literature, this volume brings together a large number of authoritative presentations from many of today's leading investigators in the field.

The goal of this book is to provide a concise, up-to-date summary of current knowledge about affective relapse, comorbid psychopathology, functional disability, and psychosocial outcome in contemporary bipolar disorders. Focusing on affective relapse and psychosocial adjustment, the chapters herein interweave clinical material with empirical findings from a number of major academic research programs. We have attempted to provide a broad overview of course and outcome for bipolar patients treated under typical treatment conditions.

The effect of lithium and anticonvulsants on outcome during controlled and naturalistic treatment is discussed in Goldberg and Harrow (Chapter 1), Maj (Chapter 2), Gitlin and Hammen (Chapter 3), Post et al. (Chapter 5), and Bowden (Chapter 8). Manic outcome in relation to specific comorbidities or subtypes of illness is described for mixed mania (Boland and Keller, Chapter 6), bipolar depression (Goldberg and Kocsis, Chapter 7), alcoholism and other substance abuse (Tohen and Zarate, Chapter 9, and Winokur, Chapter 10), rapid-cycling bipolar disorders (Dunner, Chapter 11), hypomania (Coryell, Chapter 12, and Himmelhoch, Chapter 13), and comorbid anxiety disorders (Chapter 13). The effect of psychosocial treatments on outcome is discussed from two perspectives: individual psychotherapy and family psychoeducation are presented as mechanisms to foster medication compliance and coping skills and to address the interpersonal sequelae of bipolar episodes (Miklowitz and Frank,

Chapter 4); and the role of public sector psychiatry and community-based treatment programs is examined for chronic bipolar illness, using the intensive case management and Program for Assertive Community Treatment (PACT) models (Hackman et al., Chapter 14). Finally, issues regarding pharmacoeconomics and the burden of disease are discussed in Goldberg and Keck (Chapter 15), in conjunction with a discussion of mania through the life cycle and a summary of clinical and treatment implications based on previous chapters.

As part of the Clinical Practice Series of the American Psychiatric Press, this book is intended for a broad audience, including psychiatric residents and general practitioners, clinical researchers, psychiatric nurses, psychologists, social workers, and other mental health professionals involved with bipolar inpatients and outpatients. By aiming the book at both clinicians and investigators, we have sought to relate naturalistic follow-up studies in mania to the routine clinical management of bipolar disorders over time.

We wish to make special mention of the work of George Winokur, M.D., whose untimely death occurred during the preparation of this book. Dr. Winokur was a pioneer not only in the phenomenology of affective disorders, but in other areas of psychopathology including substance abuse, psychotic disorders, and the biology and natural course of other chronic psychiatric illness. His contributions influenced the work of many contemporary clinical investigators, and his death marks the passing of one of the leading twentieth-century figures in American psychiatry.

This book could not have been completed without the time and energy of our co-contributors, whose research efforts have been invaluable to clinicians, investigators, and patients. We also wish to thank Ms. Joyce Whiteside for her technical assistance with manuscript preparation. Finally, we wish to thank our wives, Amy-Louise Goldberg and Helen Harrow, for their support and encouragement during the completion of this work.

Joseph F. Goldberg, M.D.
Martin Harrow, Ph.D.

CHAPTER 1

Poor-Outcome Bipolar Disorders

Joseph F. Goldberg, M.D.
Martin Harrow, Ph.D.

*I*n this chapter, we review clinical and psychosocial factors that contribute to poor outcome in bipolar disorders under routine treatment conditions. In particular, we describe a profile of bipolar patients who are at high risk for poor long-term outcome, drawing on data from the Chicago Follow-up Study and other research programs studying the course of contemporary bipolar disorders.

Naturalistic follow-up studies provide a unique source of data for the practicing clinician and for the clinical investigator. Systematic studies of large patient groups receiving treatment under ordinary conditions help bridge the gap between outcome in randomized clinical trials (RCTs) (demonstrating a best-possible treatment response during optimally controlled, idealized conditions) and case studies or anecdotal experience during customary treatment. Data from RCTs generally reflect outcome for highly select patient samples (e.g., those who have strong motivation for receiving treatment, those who are free from medical or psychiatric comorbidity, and those who have relatively stable social or eco-

Research from the Chicago Follow-up Study was supported in part by National Institute of Mental Health (NIMH) Grant MH-26341.

nomic home environments). Bipolar patients culled from RCTs often may not represent the type of patient clinicians ordinarily encounter. Along these lines, outcome with lithium under routine treatment conditions is examined further in Maj, Chapter 2, and outcome in open versus blinded treatment studies is discussed in Bowden, Chapter 8, in this volume.

Many patients hospitalized for acute mania are not prototypical, exhibiting unusual or complex symptoms, concurrent substance abuse, severe personality disorders, and difficult psychosocial problems of far-reaching proportions. They often bear only a faint resemblance to the type of bipolar patient who meets the rigorous criteria for inclusion in an RCT.

In the era before modern pharmacotherapy, poor outcome in mania was considered a relatively rare occurrence. Seminal investigators such as Kraepelin (1913) noted that manic or depressive episodes were generally periodic in nature and, typically, were followed by a return to normal functioning. Similarly, in Rennie's (1942) study of 208 cases from 1913 to 1916, more than 90% of patients were reported to have recovered from an initial episode. More than half eventually had at least one affective recurrence, but chronic illness was infrequent (<10%), and remissions lasting from 10 to 20 years were described as commonplace.

Research designs and diagnostic criteria for mania and for relapse have become more standardized and codified. Diagnostic systems have shifted to include patients with more severe psychopathology and prominent psychosis as meeting the criteria for a diagnosis of bipolar disorder. Changes in research methodology over the years may partly account for higher rates of poor outcome now reported in mania. Additionally, the epidemiology and severity of manic subtypes may have changed markedly in the last several decades. For example, rapid-cycling and mixed-affective states may be more common today than was the case before the introduction and widespread use of tricyclic antidepressants (Wolpert et al. 1990). Increased rates of alcoholism and other substance abuse in the population may have further altered the course of bipolar illness. Other unidentified environmental and epigenetic factors could also contribute to changes in the phenotype and prognosis of bipolar disorder.

Effect of Lithium in Research and Clinical Practice

In the 1970s, a series of RCTs suggested that with lithium prophylaxis, sustained remission and favorable outcome may be possible for an even greater majority of bipolar patients (reviewed by Moncrieff 1995). Based on these original studies of maintenance treatment, many clinicians have come to regard lithium as the standard of care for the long-term management of bipolar disorders, expecting a marked improvement in up to 70% of cases. However, Moncrieff (1995) challenged such optimistic interpretations of these original trials, identifying previously underrecognized protocol biases: In some reports, patients assigned to the placebo group had discontinued their medication before entering a study, thus potentially inflating the relapse rates on the placebo. In other reports, medication was not assigned in double-blind fashion, diagnoses were not uniform, or efforts to prevent relapse (e.g., through increased social support) were not always similar for patients taking the active drug and for those taking the placebo.

Under more routine clinical conditions, many studies have reported relapse during the first 1–2 years of lithium treatment in nearly 50% or more of bipolar patients (Denicoff et al. 1994; Dickson and Kendell 1986; Goldberg et al. 1995a; Kocsis and Stokes 1979; Maj et al. 1989; O'Connell et al. 1991; Tohen et al. 1990). Coryell and colleagues (1997) observed over a 5-year follow-up that short-term relapse rates were lower among bipolar patients who took lithium than among those who did not, but the probability of an affective recurrence after the first 32 weeks of recovery was comparable for patients who were either taking or not taking lithium. Several factors have been identified to account for the generally higher relapse rates observed in natural history studies than in RCTs. These factors include poor medication compliance (Goodwin and Jamison 1990; Guscott and Taylor 1994; Kocsis and Stokes 1979; Strakowski et al. 1998); less frequent or rigorous monitoring of treatment (Masterton et al. 1988); underdosing of lithium and failure to achieve adequate serum drug levels (Guscott and Taylor 1994); abrupt discontinuation of lithium, which may accelerate relapses (Faedda et al. 1993; Suppes et al. 1991) and, potentially, also induce subsequent treatment-refractoriness according to some studies (Maj et al. 1995; Post et al. 1992) but not others (Coryell et al. 1998; Tondo et al. 1997); and poor family relationships or lack of social support (Miklowitz et al. 1988).

Affective Relapse and Functional Outcome

Psychosocial impairment appears to be closely related to affective relapse. Complex interrelationships may exist between syndromal relapse and functional outcome for bipolar patients (Coryell et al. 1993; Gitlin et al. 1995; Goldberg et al. 1995b). These interrelationships are discussed at greater length in Gitlin and Hammen, Chapter 3, and Coryell, Chapter 12, in this volume. An initial survey of the literature indicates a generally high correlation between frequent, severe affective relapse and poor psychosocial adjustment.

Table 1–1 presents major findings about outcome in mania from a series of naturalistic follow-up studies during the past two decades. In general, longer follow-up periods have been associated with higher rates of affective relapse, although even relatively short follow-up periods (<1-year duration) indicate a high percentage of patients with impairment in at least one major area of overall functioning. Notably, Tsuang et al. (1979) found that occupational impairment was common and persistent in up to one-quarter of the patients studied, even 30 years after an initial manic episode. Other investigators have documented ongoing problems in social or family relationships (Gitlin et al. 1995; Miklowitz et al. 1988) and difficulty sustaining economic independence or autonomous living arrangements (Dion et al. 1988; Tohen et al. 1990), despite the remission of acute affective symptoms with appropriate pharmacotherapy.

The Chicago Follow-up Study

Based at Michael Reese Hospital, the Illinois State Psychiatric Institute, the University of Chicago, and the University of Illinois–Chicago, the Chicago Follow-up Study began as a prospective, ongoing, long-term assessment of adults hospitalized in the 1970s and 1980s for acute bipolar-manic, unipolar-depressive, or psychotic episodes (Goldberg et al. 1995a, 1995b, 1996; Harrow et al. 1990). We followed up patients at approximately 2-year intervals, and a sub-

Table 1–1. Naturalistic outcome studies in bipolar disorders

Investigators	N	Follow-up period	Comment
Tsuang et al. (1979)	100	30 years	24% had poor work functioning; 29% had ratings of "poor" psychiatric symptoms
Dion et al. (1988)	67	6 months	67% had poor work functioning; those with multiple admissions had greatest impairment
Harrow et al. (1990)	73	1.7 years	34% had very poor global functioning; outcome was poorer for bipolar patients than for unipolar patients
Tohen et al. (1990)	75	4 years	28% were unable to work; 19% could not live independently at follow-up
O'Connell et al. (1991)	248	1 year	19% had very poor overall outcome
Coryell et al. (1993)	29	5 years	31% never achieved sustained recovery (≥ 8 weeks)
Goldberg et al. (1995a)	51	4.6 years	22% had poor outcome; 14% had persistent poor functioning at two follow-ups
Gitlin et al. (1995)	62	4.3 years	35% had poor occupational functioning; 61% had only fair or poor social functioning
Strakowski et al. (1998)	109	1 year	65% failed to achieve functional recovery; all subjects had no prior hospitalizations
Keck et al. (1998)	134	1 year	76% failed to achieve functional recovery; patients with mixed or manic episodes at index did not differ in recovery rates at follow-up

stantial database has accumulated for a large sample of former bipolar and unipolar-depressed inpatients. Using semistructured interviews and standardized instruments rated by trained research personnel, we have continued to collect longitudinal information on a series of measures over time, including psychiatric symptoms (affective, psychotic, and anxiety-neurotic) in the year prior to each follow-up, factors involved in thought disorder, negative symptoms, work functioning or role performance, family and social adjustment, rehospitalization, premorbid and family genetic histories, and subsequent treatment (including pharmacotherapy and psychotherapy) during the follow-up period.

We evaluated an original cohort of 73 bipolar-manic and 66 unipolar-depressed patients at index hospitalization and then reevaluated them approximately 1.7 years after index hospitalization. We followed up with these patients again approximately 4.6 years and approximately 8 years after they entered the research program.

At index, the cohort consisted mainly of young adult patients who were relatively free from the effects of chronic illness or long-term treatment. The mean age at entry into the study was 25.5 years. Senior research psychiatrists or psychologists used Research Diagnostic Criteria (RDC; Spitzer et al. 1978) and DSM-III (American Psychiatric Association 1980) to diagnose bipolar I disorder (or nonpsychotic, unipolar major depression for the comparison sample) in patients in the sample at the time of index hospitalization.

We rated psychotic symptoms (i.e., delusions or hallucinations) and manic or depressive symptoms at baseline and at follow-up with the Schedule for Affective Disorders and Schizophrenia (SADS; Endicott and Spitzer 1978). We evaluated overall psychosocial functioning at baseline and again for the year prior to each follow-up with the LKP Scale, a global index of overall functioning (Levenstein et al. 1966). This measure takes into account multiple areas of adjustment, including work and social adaptation, life disruptions, self-support, symptoms, relapse, and rehospitalization. This eight-point scale was standardized to reflect three broad categories of overall outcome, designated as good functioning (scores of 1 or 2), moderate impairment (scores of 3–6), or uniformly poor overall functioning (scores of 7 or 8). In addition, we rated individual areas of functioning (such as work performance and frequency of social interactions) with separate outcome scales developed by Strauss and Carpenter (1972).

Are There Subgroups of Bipolar Patients With Consistent Outcome Patterns?

Based on analyses from the first few follow-up assessments, some general findings are evident regarding prognosis and outcome in bipolar disorders. As shown in Table 1–2, distinct outcome clusters have emerged for patients whose functional outcome status at successive follow-ups has been consistently good, intermediate, or poor. Based on this matrix and other related data on relapse and rehospitalization over two successive follow-ups during a 4.5-year period, three major groupings of bipolar patients can be described:

1. The first subgroup (approximately 15%–20% of patients) appears to have *good overall functioning*, or complete remission, in a

Table 1–2.   Changes in outcome over time for bipolar and unipolar patients

Outcome at 4.5-year follow-up	Outcome at 2-year follow-up		
	Good functioning	Moderate impairment	Poor functioning
Bipolar-manic patients (*n* = 51)			
Good functioning	10	8	3
Moderate impairment	4	8	7
Poor functioning	0	4	7
Unipolar-depressed patients (*n* = 49)			
Good functioning	12	6	2
Moderate impairment	3	16	3
Poor functioning	1	1	5

Source.   Reprinted from Goldberg JF, Harrow M, Grossman LS: "Course and Outcome in Bipolar Affective Disorder: A Longitudinal Follow-up Study." *American Journal of Psychiatry* 152:379–384, 1995. Copyright 1995, American Psychiatric Association. Used with permission.

consistent manner at two or more successive follow-ups. Few if any of the patients in this group have manic or depressive recurrences that necessitate rehospitalization during this time, and many appear to have been stabilized on lithium prophylaxis during the first year after their index episode.

2. The second subgroup (approximately 10%–15% of patients) shows *consistently poor outcome at multiple follow-up assessments*. Patients in this category often have many recurrent affective episodes, frequent rehospitalizations, and very poor work performance at each follow-up. Many patients in this subgroup (one-third or more) appear unable to regain their highest levels of premorbid work or social functioning (Harrow et al. 1990).

3. The third subgroup (approximately 50%–60% of patients) encompasses a more heterogeneous patient population. *Outcome for this majority of bipolar patients appears variable;* many have a stable pattern of moderately impaired functioning over serial follow-up assessments (perhaps 15%–20% of all bipolar patients), and the remainder show greater or lesser degrees of remission and overall adjustment without a consistent trend. Thus, patients in this category may have some degree of work impairment, subsyndromal affective symptoms, or occasional rehospitalizations, but considerable potential exists for either improvement or decline.

Outcome appeared significantly less favorable for bipolar-manic patients than for unipolar-depressed patients. We found no gender differences in overall adjustment for the patient cohort at follow-up. We observed uniformly poor outcome (i.e., poor outcome in multiple areas of functioning) much less frequently in the unipolar-depressed sample than in the bipolar-manic sample across multiple follow-up assessments. In addition, the bipolar cohort as a collective group has shown significant overall improvement over time by the 4.5-year follow-up. Thus, a one-way repeated-measures analysis of variance (ANOVA) using the full eight-point overall outcome scale revealed a highly significant main effect when we analyzed the phase of disorder (or time period of assessment) ($F = 10.80$, df $= 1.98, P < .001$) (Goldberg et al. 1995a). This observation could suggest a capacity for resilience or adaptability in coping with the results of chronic or recurrent mental illness.

We assessed occupational impairment at each follow-up period using the four-point Strauss-Carpenter index of work performance (Strauss and Carpenter 1972). This scale reflects the amount of time subjects have been able to function effectively as workers, students, or homemakers during the year prior to each follow-up. At each follow-up assessment, fewer than half of the bipolar patients were able to maintain adequate role performance; moreover, when compared with unipolar-depressed patients, significantly fewer bipolar patients were able to work at least half of the time in the year preceding the first follow-up ($\chi^2 = 5.15$, df $= 1$, $P < .05$) (Goldberg et al. 1995a).

Affective Relapse and Overall Outcome

We observed a strong association between affective relapse and poor overall outcome in the bipolar sample. As indicated in Table 1–3 (Goldberg et al. 1995b), bipolar patients who had a full manic or depressive syndrome in the year prior to the first and/or second follow-ups had significantly or near-significantly higher rates of poor overall outcome than did those relatively few patients who had poor outcome and an absence of affective recurrence during the follow-up year. Affective relapse was not associated with poor outcome among the unipolar-depressed sample, although the overall rates of affective relapse in each follow-up year were similar in the bipolar and unipolar samples. This observation suggests that affective relapse disrupts global functioning more profoundly in bipolar disorders than in unipolar disorders, despite an equivalent frequency of recurrent syndromes within each diagnostic group.

Medication Use and Overall Outcome

We examined patterns of lithium and other medication use among our bipolar-manic and unipolar-depressed samples at each follow-up period. Approximately 60% of the bipolar-manic patients taking lithium had either uniformly poor outcome or moderately impaired functioning at each follow-up assessment (Goldberg et al.

Table 1–3. Relationship between affective syndromes at follow-up and overall outcome

Patient group	2-Year follow-up		4.5-Year follow-up	
	Good outcome or moderate impairment	Uniformly poor outcome	Good outcome or moderate impairment	Uniformly poor outcome
Bipolar with				
no manic syndrome	14[a]	4[a]	27[b]	2[b]
full manic syndrome	4[a]	5[a]	6[b]	7[b]
Unipolar with				
no depressive syndrome	14[c]	3[c]	22[d]	5[d]
full depressive syndrome	10[c]	3[c]	13[d]	2[d]

[a] $\chi^2 = 3.0$, df $= 1$, $P < .08$.
[b] $\chi^2 = 11.75$, df $= 1$, $P < .001$.
[c] $\chi^2 = 0.14$, df $= 1$, NS.
[d] $\chi^2 = 0.19$, df $= 1$, NS.

Source. Reprinted from Goldberg JF, Harrow M, Grossman LS: "Recurrent Affective Syndromes in Bipolar and Unipolar Mood Disorders at Follow-Up." *British Journal of Psychiatry* 166:382–385, 1995. Copyright 1995, The Royal College of Psychiatrists. Used with permission.

1995a). We then analyzed functioning scores after stratifying the scores by different medication subgroupings.

We compared overall outcome scores at the 2-year assessment for bipolar patients taking lithium alone ($n = 8$), those taking lithium plus neuroleptics with or without antidepressants ($n = 21$), those taking neuroleptics alone ($n = 4$), and those taking no medications ($n = 8$). Outcome was significantly better for the small subgroup of bipolar patients taking lithium alone than for the patients who were taking lithium plus other medications (Kruskal-Wallis $T = 9.35$, df = 3, $P = .025$). Similarly, at the second follow-up, outcome was again significantly better for the bipolar patients who were taking lithium alone ($n = 9$) than for those taking lithium plus neuroleptics with or without antidepressants ($n = 17$), those taking neuroleptics alone ($n = 4$), or those taking no medications ($n = 11$) (Kruskal-Wallis $T = 11.66$, df = 3, $P = .009$) (Goldberg et al. 1996). Work impairment and full manic or depressive syndromes in each follow-up year were also significantly less common among the bipolar patients who were taking lithium alone. Although relatively few bipolar patients were taking lithium alone at follow-up, more than 80% of them had no recurrent affective episode in the year prior to the first or second follow-ups (Goldberg et al. 1995b).

Other investigators have shown that lithium monotherapy is rarely prescribed during maintenance treatment of bipolar disorder (Sachs et al. 1994), and data are inconclusive as to whether patients who require multiple medications fare better than those taking lithium alone (Goldberg et al. 1996). Good outcome during lithium monotherapy may occur for only a small percentage of bipolar patients who do not require additional medications and are stabilized on a treatment regimen early in the course of their disorder.

Characteristics of Poor Outcome

Our research group reviewed clinical and narrative material obtained at each follow-up for the subsample of bipolar patients who had consistently poor outcome at two or more follow-up assessments. Following are several representative case vignettes:

> Mr. A, a 26-year-old single white man at index with no family history of affective illness, had been hospitalized twice for manic epi-

sodes since age 21, prior to the index admission. By the 8-year follow-up, he had shown a persistent pattern of rapid-cycling bipolar disorder, leading to multiple rehospitalizations. He had erratic work functioning and an unstable living situation at each assessment. Although he exhibited grandiose and paranoid delusions on interview, his manic symptoms did not appear to include formalized delusions. Throughout the year preceding the first follow-up, he took lithium, neuroleptics, and a tricyclic antidepressant; at the second and third follow-ups, he took lithium, neuroleptics, and carbamazepine (the latter was eventually changed to valproate) without improvement. Uniformly poor outcome was persistent at each follow-up.

Mr. B, a 25-year-old single white man at index with a family history of both affective and nonaffective psychosis, had five psychiatric hospitalizations since age 17, prior to the index admission. At follow-up, he reported distinct, severe high and low periods accompanied by grandiose and referential delusions, violent and agitated behavior, and 6- to 9-month rehospitalizations during each follow-up year. Despite having completed 1 year of college prior to index, he had poor work functioning in a variety of low-skill jobs. He had not complied with a stable regimen of lithium prophylaxis until after his fourth hospitalization for mania. Throughout the year prior to the first follow-up, he continued to take lithium in combination with neuroleptics. Carbamazepine augmentation was begun by the second follow-up assessment and continued intermittently at the third follow-up. At each assessment, we noted moderate-to-severe affective symptoms along with widespread impairment in role performance and family and social relationships.

Ms. C, an 18-year-old black woman at index, had a family history of major depression and alcoholism and was hospitalized once briefly in the year preceding the index admission. In the year prior to each follow-up, Ms. C. was rehospitalized for both manic and depressive episodes. Mixed manic and depressive symptoms were evident at follow-up interviews, as was moderate alcohol abuse. She completed eleventh grade but did not obtain her general equivalency diploma, and she was chronically unable to work throughout the 8-year follow-up period. Her medication regimen included lithium and neuroleptics, with which her compliance was poor. Indeed, she claimed to miss manic "highs" and reported deliberately stopping her lithium, invariably leading to affective relapse and rehospitalization. She had few lasting friendships and poor, unstable relationships with family members, whom she relied on for financial support. Refusing to attend Alcoholics Anonymous, she maintained a marginal lifestyle and was periodically homeless. We noted very poor outcome at each follow-up.

The preceding case vignettes typify some common features among bipolar patients who have poor treatment outcome. In the first vignette, rapid-cycling affective episodes were prevalent at each follow-up assessment. Originally described by Dunner and Fieve (1974), some evidence suggests that rapid cycling appears to be associated strongly with nonresponse to lithium and may be related to an increased risk for suicide in bipolar patients (Fawcett et al. 1987). The presence of rapid cycling may not always persist after the first few years of illness and in time may become a less robust predictor of long-term course and outcome (Coryell et al. 1992). Issues regarding rapid cycling and the course of bipolar disorder are discussed in greater detail in Dunner, Chapter 11, in this volume.

A negative family history of affective illness has been associated with poorer treatment outcome during lithium prophylaxis (e.g., Prien et al. 1974), but data in this area are inconclusive. Among the larger sample of bipolar patients in the Chicago Follow-up Study, the presence of mania or depression in a first-degree relative appears linked with higher relapse rates at follow-up.

The second vignette was remarkable for late initiation of lithium prophylaxis. Gelenberg et al. (1989), Tondo et al. (1998), and others have found evidence indicating that therapeutic serum lithium levels (0.8–1.0 mEq/L) confer less protection against a manic or depressive recurrence when patients have had multiple affective episodes before lithium maintenance is established. Some patients who have a psychotic illness—particularly when the symptoms are complex or unusual—may not be given a diagnosis of bipolar disorder until after two or more episodes have elapsed. A late diagnosis of bipolar illness often delays the start of treatment with a mood stabilizer, which may contribute to a poorer clinical course and outcome. Patients with nonprototypical psychotic illnesses may eventually receive a diagnosis of schizoaffective disorder or atypical psychosis (e.g., psychotic disorder not otherwise specified), although they may have only a severe form of bipolar illness.

The presence of delusions (and, less often, hallucinations) was common at index hospitalization for three-quarters of the original bipolar cohort in the Chicago Follow-up Study; however, less than one-quarter of the bipolar patients at each follow-up had prominent signs of psychosis (Goldberg et al. 1995; Prien et al. 1974). For both the bipolar and the unipolar samples, a strong association was found between the presence of psychosis at index hospitalization and subsequent psychosis at follow-up. This observation could suggest a specific vulnerability to recurrent psychotic symptoms during affective relapse for some patients with affective disorders. Bipolar patients who had grandiose, paranoid, or other delusions at follow-up did not have poor global functioning in all instances.

In the third vignette, multiple risk factors for poor outcome were apparent. First, bipolar illness with concurrent alcoholism has been linked to increased treatment resistance, more frequent rehospitalizations, and more severe functional disability. Epidemiological surveys suggest that rates of comorbid mania and substance abuse may be as high as 30%–60% (Brady and Sonne 1995). Substance abuse may predispose bipolar patients to mixed or dysphoric manic states, which present an additional risk factor for poor treatment outcome. Second, intense family discord has also been described as an important contributor to poor outcome during lithium treatment (e.g., Miklowitz et al. 1988; see also Miklowitz and Frank, Chapter 4, in this volume).

Finally, the issue of medication noncompliance poses an additional obstacle to sustained remission and stable life circumstances. Abrupt discontinuation of lithium may hasten relapse (Faedda et al. 1993; Suppes et al. 1991), and controversy exists about whether subsequent rechallenge trials of lithium may be less effective than before an abrupt discontinuation (Coryell et al. 1998; Maj et al. 1995; Post et al. 1992; Tondo et al. 1997). (This issue is examined in further detail by Maj, Chapter 2, and Post et al., Chapter 5, in this volume.) Augmentation of lithium with carbamazepine or valproate may improve outcome for some bipolar patients, although we did not observe such improvement when these agents were added for the

severely ill patients described earlier in this chapter. Early intervention with mood-stabilizing anticonvulsants may be as important as
is the early initiation of lithium in order to optimize treatment response.

Severe psychiatric illnesses such as bipolar disorder often manifest themselves during young adulthood, and the resultant disruption to educational, work, marital, and other pursuits can be both
devastating and long lasting. Good premorbid functioning may increase the probability of better psychosocial outcome for some patients; however, the cumulative effects of recurrent illness may
mitigate against this effect by facilitating or kindling later episodes.
Intense psychosocial support early in the course of illness, when the
disorder appears more modifiable and responsive to environmental
stresses, may be especially important to prevent poor outcome.

Summary

Poor outcome, or at least moderate impairment in psychosocial adjustment, is common in patients with bipolar disorder. Residual
symptoms, which are common for many bipolar patients between
episodes (see also Keller et al. 1992), and a lengthy duration of illness
prior to beginning an optimal treatment regimen are often significant determinants of good versus poor outcome. Many bipolar patients have some degree of improvement as the time from their index
episode increases, perhaps reflecting an improved adaptation to the
stresses of a chronic, recurrent illness. Nevertheless, more than
one-half of bipolar patients manifest some degree of functional disability after the onset of their illness, and a core subgroup of
10%–15% of patients show profound impairment in multiple areas,
with little improvement. Our evidence indicates that affective relapse is more detrimental to functional outcome in bipolar patients
than in unipolar-depressed patients.

Lithium prophylaxis under naturalistic conditions may be associated with good outcome for only a minority of bipolar patients receiving treatment under routine conditions. Patients who respond
to a treatment regimen in the first year may have a significantly
better prognosis than those who are not stabilized during this period. Patients who are not effectively stabilized shortly after an ini-

tial manic or depressive episode may be more likely to receive subsequent adjunctive pharmacotherapy. However, that initial period of poorly controlled psychopathology may predispose patients to a more malignant course of illness.

Alternatively, some patients who have complex affective and psychotic symptoms, and in whom the diagnosis may be unclear or is made late, could have an unusually severe variant of bipolar illness with poor outcome. Such nosological distinctions challenge the current diagnostic classification system and require further study.

Prominent and common risk factors for poor outcome in mania include rapid-cycling and mixed-affective states, concurrent substance abuse, poor or erratic treatment compliance, inadequate medication dosing or follow-up, poor psychosocial support, and the late initiation of treatment. Gradual improvement is possible for many bipolar patients who receive standard treatment in the community. The factors we noted earlier in this chapter may decrease the likelihood of sustained remission and consistently good outcome, especially in patients who receive treatment, during the first year after their index episode, that does not produce a stable remission.

References

American Psychiatric Association: Diagnostic and Statistical Manual of Mental Disorders, 3rd Edition. Washington, DC, American Psychiatric Association, 1980

Brady KT, Sonne SC: The relationship between substance abuse and bipolar disorder. J Clin Psychiatry 56:19–24, 1995

Coryell W, Endicott J, Keller M: Rapidly cycling affective disorder. Arch Gen Psychiatry 49:126–131, 1992

Coryell W, Scheftner W, Keller M, et al: The enduring psychosocial consequences of mania and depression. Am J Psychiatry 150:720–727, 1993

Coryell W, Winokur G, Solomon D, et al: Lithium and recurrence in a long-term follow-up of bipolar affective disorder. Psychol Med 27:281–289, 1997

Coryell W, Solomon D, Leon AC, et al: Lithium discontinuation and subsequent effectiveness. Am J Psychiatry 155:895–898, 1998

Denicoff KD, Blake KD, Smith-Jackson EE, et al: Morbidity in treated bipolar disorder: a prospective study using daily life chart ratings. Depression 2:95–104, 1994

Dickson WE, Kendell RE: Does maintenance lithium therapy prevent recurrences of mania under ordinary clinical conditions? Psychol Med 16:521–530, 1986

Dion GL, Tohen M, Anthony WA, et al: Symptoms and functioning of patients with bipolar disorder six months after hospitalization. Hosp Community Psychiatry 39:652–657, 1988

Dunner DL, Fieve RR: Clinical factors in lithium carbonate prophylaxis failure. Arch Gen Psychiatry 30:229–233, 1974

Endicott J, Spitzer RL: A diagnostic interview: the Schedule for Affective Disorders and Schizophrenia. Arch Gen Psychiatry 35:837–844, 1978

Faedda GL, Tondo L, Baldessarini RJ, et al: Outcome after rapid vs. gradual discontinuation of lithium treatment in bipolar disorders. Arch Gen Psychiatry 50:448–455, 1993

Fawcett J, Scheftner W, Clark D, et al: Clinical predictors of suicide in patients with major affective disorders: a controlled prospective study. Am J Psychiatry 144:35–40, 1987

Gelenberg AJ, Kane JM, Keller MB, et al: Comparison of standard and low serum levels of lithium for maintenance treatment of bipolar disorder. N Engl J Med 3321:1489–1493, 1989

Gitlin MJ, Swendson J, Heller TL, et al: Relapse and impairment in bipolar disorder. Am J Psychiatry 152:1635–1640, 1995

Goldberg JF, Harrow M, Grossman LS: Course and outcome in bipolar affective disorder: a longitudinal follow-up study. Am J Psychiatry 152:379–384, 1995a

Goldberg JF, Harrow M, Grossman LS: Recurrent affective syndromes in bipolar and unipolar mood disorders at follow-up. Br J Psychiatry 166:382–385, 1995b

Goldberg JF, Harrow M, Leon AC: Lithium treatment of bipolar affective disorders under naturalistic follow-up conditions. Psychopharmacol Bull 32:47–54, 1996

Goodwin FK, Jamison KR: Manic-Depressive Illness. New York, Oxford University Press, 1990

Guscott R, Taylor L: Lithium prophylaxis in recurrent affective illness: efficacy, effectiveness and efficiency. Br J Psychiatry 164:741–746, 1994

Harrow M, Goldberg JF, Grossman LS, et al: Outcome in manic disorders: a naturalistic follow-up study. Arch Gen Psychiatry 47:665–671, 1990

Keck PE Jr, McElroy SL, Strakowski SM, et al: 12-Month outcome of patients with bipolar disorder following hospitalization for a manic or mixed episode. Am J Psychiatry 155:646–652, 1998

Keller MB, Lavori PW, Kane JM, et al: Subsyndromal symptoms in bipolar disorder: a comparison of standard and low serum levels of lithium. Arch Gen Psychiatry 49:371–376, 1992

Kocsis JH, Stokes PE: Lithium maintenance: factors affecting outcome. Am J Psychiatry 136:563–566, 1979

Kraepelin E: Psychiatrie. Leipzig, Germany, Verlag von Johann Ambrosius Barth, 1913

Levenstein S, Klein DF, Pollack M: Follow-up study of formerly hospitalized voluntary psychiatric patients: the first two years. Am J Psychiatry 122:1102–1109, 1966

Maj M, Pirozzi R, Kemali D: Long-term outcome of lithium prophylaxis in patients initially classified as complete responders. Psychopharmacology 98:535–538, 1989

Maj M, Pirozzi R, Magliano L: Nonresponse to reinstituted lithium prophylaxis in previously responsive bipolar patients: prevalence and predictors. Am J Psychiatry 152:1810–1811, 1995

Masterton G, Warner M, Roxburgh B: Supervising lithium—a comparison of a lithium clinic, psychiatric outpatient clinics and general practice. Br J Psychiatry 152:535–538, 1988

Miklowitz DJ, Goldstein MJ, Nuechterlein KH, et al: Family factors and the course of bipolar affective disorder. Arch Gen Psychiatry 45:225–231, 1988

Moncrieff J: Lithium revisited: a re-examination of the placebo-controlled trials of lithium prophylaxis in manic-depressive disorder. Br J Psychiatry 167:569–574, 1995

O'Connell RA, Mayo JA, Flatow L, et al: Outcome of bipolar disorder on long-term treatment with lithium. Br J Psychiatry 159:123–129, 1991

Post RM, Leverich GS, Altshuler L, et al: Lithium discontinuation-induced refractoriness: preliminary observations. Am J Psychiatry 149:1727–1729, 1992

Prien RF, Caffey FM, Klett CJ: Factors associated with treatment success in lithium carbonate prophylaxis. Arch Gen Psychiatry 31:189–192, 1974

Rennie TAC: Prognosis in manic-depressive psychoses. Am J Psychiatry 98:801–814, 1942

Sachs GS, Lafer B, Truman CJ, et al: Lithium monotherapy: miracle, myth and misunderstanding. Psychiatric Annals 24:299–306, 1994

Spitzer RL, Endicott J, Robins E: Research Diagnostic Criteria: rationale and reliability. Arch Gen Psychiatry 35:773–782, 1978

Strakowski SM, Keck PE Jr, McElroy SL, et al: Twelve-month outcome after a first hospitalization for affective psychosis. Arch Gen Psychiatry 55: 49–55, 1998

Strauss JS, Carpenter WT: The prediction of outcome in schizophrenia: characteristics of outcome. Arch Gen Psychiatry 27:739–746, 1972

Suppes T, Baldessarini RJ, Faedda GL, et al: Risk of recurrence following discontinuation of lithium treatment in bipolar disorder. Arch Gen Psychiatry 48:1082–1088, 1991

Tohen M, Waternaux CM, Tsuang MT: Outcome in mania: a 4-year prospective follow-up of 75 patients utilizing survival analysis. Arch Gen Psychiatry 47:1106–1111, 1990

Tondo L, Baldessarini RJ, Floris G, et al: Effectiveness of restarting lithium treatment after its discontinuation in bipolar I and bipolar II disorders. Am J Psychiatry 154:548–550, 1997

Tondo L, Baldessarini RJ, Hennen J, et al: Lithium maintenance treatment of depression and mania in bipolar I and bipolar II disorders. Am J Psychiatry 155:638–645, 1998

Tsuang MT, Woolson RF, Fleming JA: Long-term outcome of major psychoses; I: schizophrenia and affective disorders compared with psychiatrically symptom-free surgical controls. Arch Gen Psychiatry 39:1295–1301, 1979

Wolpert EA, Goldberg JF, Harrow M: Rapid cycling in unipolar and bipolar affective disorders. Am J Psychiatry 147:725–728, 1990

Lithium Prophylaxis of Bipolar Disorder in Ordinary Clinical Conditions: Patterns of Long-Term Outcome

Mario Maj, M.D., Ph.D.

*A*s Goldberg and Harrow noted in the Preface of this book, interest has increased recently in the *effectiveness* (i.e., outcome in ordinary clinical conditions), as opposed to the *efficacy* (i.e., potential usefulness as emerging from double-blind randomized clinical trials), of lithium prophylaxis in patients with bipolar affective disorder (Aagaard and Vestergaard 1990; Dickson and Kendell 1986; Gitlin et al. 1995; Guscott and Taylor 1994; Harrow et al. 1990; Keller et al. 1993; Kukopulos et al. 1995; Maj et al. 1989; Markar and Mander 1989; O'Connell et al. 1991; Schou 1993; Tohen et al. 1990). It has been pointed out that data on effectiveness may be more relevant to assessments of the economic benefits of lithium prophylaxis than to those of its efficacy (Guscott and Taylor 1994; see also Goldberg and Keck, Chapter 15, in this volume).

However, studies on the long-term outcome of lithium prophylaxis in routine clinical conditions are scarce and often suffer from multiple methodological flaws, including

The author would like to thank Drs. Raffaele Pirozzi and Lorenza Magliano for their collaboration in data collection and analysis and Dr. Luca Bartoli for his help in setting up the manuscript.

- An *observation period* that is too short (e.g., less than 2 years), or is not homogeneous among patients (which is illogical, unless survival analysis procedures are applied), or is not clearly specified (e.g., only the average duration is provided)
- A lack of information on *dropouts* (which are either ignored or mentioned without any detail on their characteristics)
- A lack of information on the *setting of treatment prescription and monitoring* (which obviously represents a crucial variable in determining the treatment outcome, but which is often ignored, in patent contrast to the careful description of the setting of patient assessment)

Moreover, researchers seldom realize that the assessment of a patient's "response" to lithium prophylaxis is a complex task, for several reasons, including the following:

- *The irregularity of the natural course of bipolar disorder.* Kraepelin (1909, p. 468) already pointed out that "the nature and duration of episodes and interepisodic intervals do not remain always the same in each case; on the contrary, there may be many changes, so that each case must be ascribed every time to new forms." An episode, or a cluster of episodes, may be followed unpredictably by a spontaneous free interval lasting many years. If lithium prophylaxis is implemented in coincidence with this interval, the patient may be incorrectly regarded as a responder to treatment, whereas he or she would have been free of recurrences even if not receiving treatment. On the other hand, in many patients the duration of interepisodic intervals decreases with the progression of illness (Angst 1981; Zis et al. 1979). This means that the effect of lithium on the frequency of affective episodes may be neutralized by a force pushing in the opposite direction, so that, even if the patient responds to the drug, the course of the disorder may remain unmodified (or an initial decrease in the frequency of episodes may be followed by the apparent development of tolerance to the drug).
- *The multiplicity of the dimensions on which response has to be evaluated.* The usual classification of bipolar patients as "non-

responders" or "responders" to lithium prophylaxis, based on the presence or absence of recurrences during the observation period, may be too simplistic. On the one hand, it disregards the crucial variable represented by time. For example, the risk of recurrence increases with the duration of the observation period, so that a patient may be classified as either a responder or a nonresponder, depending on the time frame taken into account; moreover, lithium may become effective after a latency period lasting several months, during which time the patient may have one or more recurrences. This classification also disregards those cases in which lithium apparently loses its effect with time.

On the other hand, the previously mentioned classification does not convey the variety of outcomes of lithium prophylaxis. For example, it does not encompass those cases in which recurrences do occur but with a decreased frequency, duration, and/or severity; or in which manic episodes do not occur but depressive episodes persist or even become longer; or in which—despite the absence of full affective episodes during treatment—the subthreshold affective morbidity remains so significant as to impair the patient's family, social, and/or occupational functioning.

- *The frequent inadequacy of exposure to lithium.* Incomplete compliance is the rule rather than the exception among bipolar patients taking lithium. An intermittent pattern of compliance is particularly common, in which periods during which the drug is taken more or less regularly (lasting several weeks or months and occurring especially after recurrences) alternate with other periods (usually longer) during which compliance is grossly irregular. Even if the 12-hour serum lithium levels (i.e., lithium levels measured on blood drawn 12 hours after the last ingestion of the drug) are constantly within the range believed to be useful for prophylactic purposes, the patient may not be taking the drug regularly. Some patients learn to deceive their physicians by concentrating lithium ingestion in the day(s) preceding the blood checks. Hence, many patients who are classified as nonresponders may actually be hidden noncompliers. On the other hand, if consumption of lithium

is regular and 12-hour serum lithium levels are within the prophylactic range, the patient's exposure to the drug may be
inadequate: in fact, because of the huge interindividual variability of the drug's half-life, 12-hour serum levels within the
useful range do not guarantee a constantly adequate serum
concentration across a 24-hour period (Amdisen 1987).

- *The influence of environmental factors.* The impact of external factors—both biological (e.g., sleep deprivation or abuse of caf-
feine) and psychosocial (e.g., stressful life events)—on the
course of bipolar disorder may be significant in some cases,
thus countervailing the effect of lithium prophylaxis. Therefore, assessment of a patient's response to the drug should
consider these factors.

Based on my group's 20 years of experience with lithium prophylaxis of bipolar disorder, I acknowledge in this chapter the
above-mentioned methodological problems by approaching the effectiveness of long-term lithium treatment in a descriptive and mul-
tidimensional way.

In the first section of the chapter, I focus on the outcome of lithium prophylaxis after 5 years. I aim to answer the following questions: 1) How many bipolar patients started on lithium prophylaxis
are still taking the medication after 5 years? 2) What are the most frequent causes of interruption of lithium prophylaxis before the term
of 5 years? 3) What patterns of outcome of lithium prophylaxis can
be identified after 5 years? 4) What are the most significant clinical
and demographic correlates of those patterns of outcome?

In the second section of the chapter, I deal systematically with a
phenomenon that my group first described in 1989 (Maj et al. 1989)
and that has been observed subsequently by at least two other
groups (Kukopulos et al. 1995; Post et al. 1993): the reappearance of
multiple affective episodes after 5 years or more of completely successful lithium prophylaxis, despite persistently adequate compliance (late nonresponse). We have assessed the prevalence and
predictors of this phenomenon, and I discuss here its possible interpretations.

In the third section of the chapter, I cover a phenomenon first
described by Post et al. (1992): refractoriness to reinstituted lithium

prophylaxis in bipolar patients who relapsed after discontinuation of successful lithium treatment (so-called lithium-discontinuation-induced refractoriness). I discuss here my group's data (Maj et al. 1995) on the prevalence and predictors of this phenomenon.

Outcome of Lithium Prophylaxis at 5 Years

We have collected historical cohort data on all patients who started lithium prophylaxis at the Center for Affective Disorders of the First Psychiatric Department of Naples University between January 1, 1975, and October 31, 1990, and who fulfilled at intake Research Diagnostic Criteria (RDC; Spitzer et al. 1975) for bipolar I affective disorder. The sample consisted of 375 patients (168 men and 207 women; age range 20–68 years; mean age ± SD, 41.1 ± 10.1 years). They were prescribed lithium carbonate, conventional form, at the initial dose of 600 mg/day, subsequently adjusted in order to obtain 12-hour serum lithium levels in the range of 0.5–1.0 mEq/L. At the time when lithium was started, 55 patients were taking neuroleptics, 131 were receiving benzodiazepines, and 13 were taking antidepressants. None was taking other mood stabilizers. Before treatment started, demographic and clinical data were collected for each patient from all available sources, and each patient's family history of bipolar illness in first-degree relatives was investigated using the Family History Research Diagnostic Criteria (FH-RDC; Endicott et al. 1975).

Since starting lithium treatment, each patient has been seen at least bimonthly. His or her psychopathological state has been evaluated at each visit, by clinical interview and, starting in 1978, by the Comprehensive Psychopathological Rating Scale (CPRS; Åsberg et al. 1978) and the Schedule for Affective Disorders and Schizophrenia (SADS; Endicott and Spitzer 1978). New affective episodes have been recorded, as well as 12-hour serum lithium levels and major intercurrent life events (i.e., death of a close family member, major financial or work difficulties, major physical illness, divorce or marital separation, or hospitalization of a family member for severe illness). The physician in charge of each patient has adjusted treatment according to clinical judgment.

At the beginning of lithium treatment, patients were provided with detailed information about bipolar affective disorder, the aims of lithium prophylaxis, and the possible side effects of treatment. On subsequent visits, patients have had the opportunity to discuss with a psychiatrist issues concerning treatment, its efficacy, and its side effects. Patients were informed at the outset that data concerning the outcome of their treatment would be used for research purposes but that they would not be personally identifiable in any report.

Of the initial sample of 375 patients, 337 (89.9%) could be interviewed 5 years after the beginning of prophylaxis. Of the other patients, 8 were dead and 30 could not be traced. No significant baseline difference was detected between patients who were available at follow-up and those who were not. At the follow-up visit, 228 patients (60.8% of the initial sample and 67.6% of those who were interviewed) were still taking lithium. The only significant baseline difference between patients who were taking lithium and those who were not at follow-up concerned the percentage of patients who had psychotic features in their index episode, which was higher in the latter group ($\chi^2 = 2.13$, df = 1, $P < .05$).

Of the 109 contacted patients who were not taking lithium at follow-up, 16 had interrupted prophylaxis after medical advice (because of an unsatisfactory balance between the benefits and the side effects of treatment), and 93 had done so by their own initiative. In the latter cases, the alleged main reason for interruption of treatment was perceived inefficacy in 35 cases, trouble related to side effects in 27, conviction of being cured and of not needing drugs in 15, hassle to take medicines in 11, and loss of energy or productivity in 5. Interruption of treatment was followed by a recurrence within 5 months in 40 (44.9%) of the 89 patients for whom reliable information could be obtained.

Of the 228 patients who were still taking lithium at follow-up, 90 (39.5%) had had no affective episode during the observation period (group A); 106 (46.5%) had had at least one affective episode but with a reduction of at least 50% of the mean annual morbidity (mean number of weeks of illness per year) during the observation period as compared with the 2-year period preceding the index episode and the start of lithium prophylaxis (group B); and 32 (14%) had had at least one affective episode, without the above-mentioned 50% reduction of the mean annual morbidity (group C). Of the 90 patients in group A, 35 (15.4% of the total sample) had had at least two symptoms listed in the RDC for either mania or major depression on the occasion of at least two visits during the observation period. Of the 106 patients in group B, 15 (6.6% of the total sample) had had affective episodes only during the first year of prophylaxis, and 22 (9.6% of the total sample) had had only major depressive episodes during the observation period.

As shown in Table 2–1, significant differences among the groups were found with respect to the prelithium number of affective episodes, number of hospitalizations, and frequency of rapid cycling (defined as the occurrence of at least four RDC affective episodes in the year preceding intake; see Maj et al. 1994 for further details). Groups B and C both differed significantly from group A on each of those variables. Moreover, group C differed significantly from group A with respect to the mean age at intake (significantly higher in the former group). Another difference between groups C and A, concerning the frequency of the depression-mania/hypomania-free interval (DMI) pattern of course before the start of prophylaxis, approximated statistical significance ($\chi^2 = 3.6$, df = 1, $P < .06$).

Late Nonresponse to Lithium Prophylaxis

We have collected historical cohort data on all group A patients (i.e., those who did not have any RDC affective episode during the first 5 years of lithium prophylaxis, subsequently called treatment period I) who have continued lithium treatment, with serum lithium levels in the range of 0.5–1.0 mEq/L, for another 5-year period or up to the second new affective episode (treatment period II). During treatment period II, these patients were evaluated bimonthly with the SADS. We defined as *late nonresponders* those patients who had at least two manic or major depressive episodes (defined according to RDC) during treatment period II and as *stable responders* those who did not present any major affective episodes during that period. We compared these two groups with respect to clinical and demographic variables (see Table 2–2) and performed a stepwise logistic regression analysis, using outcome of treatment as the dependent variable and the above-mentioned clinical and demographic items as independent variables.

Table 2–1. Demographic and clinical features of bipolar patients with different patterns of outcome of lithium prophylaxis

Variable	Pattern of outcome		
	A (n = 90)	B (n = 106)	C (n = 32)
Age at intake (years, mean ± SD)	39.5 ± 9.5	41.8 ± 10.2	43.5 ± 10.6+
Sex (% men)	43.3	47.2	40.6
Age at first psychiatric contact (years, mean ± SD)	29.7 ± 3.2	29.3 ± 4.0	29.1 ± 5.6
Time since first psychiatric contact (years, mean ± SD)	10.0 ± 6.6	12.2 ± 7.4	13.1 ± 8.0
No. affective episodes before start of prophylaxis (mean ± SD)*	5.9 ± 3.2	7.2 ± 3.3^	8.6 ± 2.9++
No. hospitalizations before start of prophylaxis (mean ± SD)**	3.6 ± 2.3	5.3 ± 2.7^^	5.9 ± 2.2++
Rapid-cycling pattern (%)*	0	27.3^^	28.1++
DMI pattern (%)	11.1	17.9	25.0
History of bipolar disorder in first-degree relatives (%)	28.9	18.9	15.6
Psychotic features in the index episode (%)	12.2	17.9	21.9
Mean serum lithium levels during observation period (mEq/L ± SD)	0.62 ± 0.05	0.65 ± 0.09	0.66 ± 0.09
Major life events during observation period (%)	22.2	28.3	34.4

Note. Patterns of outcome: A = no Research Diagnostic Criteria (RDC) affective episode during the observation period; B = at least one RDC affective episode during the observation period, reduction of at least 50% of the mean annual morbidity with respect to the 2-year period preceding the index episode and the start of lithium prophylaxis; C = at least one affective episode, without a reduction in mean annual morbidity. SD = standard deviation; DMI = depression-mania/hypomania-free interval. Significant differences among the three groups: $*P < .0001$, $**P < .00001$. Significant differences between groups A and B: $^P < .01$, $^^P < .00001$. Significant differences between groups A and C: $^+P < .05$, $^{++}P < .00001$.

Table 2–2. Demographic and clinical features of late nonresponders and stable responders to lithium prophylaxis

Variable	Late nonresponders (n = 8)	Stable responders (n = 48)
Age at intake (years, mean ± SD)	46.5 ± 8.5*	39.6 ± 8.4
Sex (% men)	37.5	47.9
Age at first psychiatric contact (years, mean ± SD)	29.5 ± 2.8	29.7 ± 5.9
Time since first psychiatric contact (years, mean ± SD)	17.0 ± 8.6**	10.2 ± 5.8
No. affective episodes before start of prophylaxis (mean ± SD)	8.7 ± 3.1*	5.7 ± 3.3
No. hospitalizations before start of prophylaxis (mean ± SD)	5.5 ± 2.1***	3.1 ± 2.1
Family history of major affective disorders (%)	25.0	27.1
Mean serum lithium levels during treatment period II (mEq/L, mean ± SD)	0.61 ± 0.03	0.62 ± 0.07
Major life events during treatment period II (%)	25.0	25.0
Menopause during treatment period II (%)	20.0	24.0

Note. SD = standard deviation.
*$P < .05$. **$P < .02$. ***$P < .01$.

Inclusion criteria were fulfilled by 67 patients (31 men and 36 women; mean age at intake, 40.1 ± 8.9 years), of whom 8 (11.9%) showed the pattern of late nonresponse and 48 (71.6%) that of stable response. The 11 patients who had just one affective episode during treatment period II were excluded from the analysis.

As shown in Table 2–2, late nonresponders were significantly older than stable responders and had a significantly longer duration of illness and higher number of previous affective episodes and hospitalizations. The mean serum lithium levels, the percentage of patients with major life events, and the proportion of female patients having menopause during treatment period II did not differ significantly between the two groups. Within the late nonresponders, the mean serum lithium levels during treatment period II did not differ significantly from those during treatment period I, nor did the mean values of red blood cell/serum lithium ratio (average of five determinations in each period). On stepwise logistic regression analysis, the number of hospitalizations before admission was the only variable entering the model (improvement χ^2 = 6.61, df = 1, P < .01).

Refractoriness to Reinstituted Lithium Prophylaxis in Previously Responsive Patients

We have followed up prospectively all patients who attended the previously mentioned Center for Affective Disorders between January 1, 1979, and December 31, 1992, who met the following five criteria: 1) diagnosis of bipolar I disorder, ascertained by the SADS; 2) absence of affective episodes during the 2 years preceding the index episode (i.e., the episode during or after which lithium prophylaxis was started); 3) absence of RDC affective episodes during at least 2 years of treatment with lithium carbonate (serum lithium levels in the range 0.5–1.0 mEq/L); 4) discontinuation of lithium treatment for reasons other than recurrence of illness or occurrence of serious side effects; and 5) reintroduction of lithium prophylaxis after one or more RDC major depressive or manic episodes following discontinuation. These criteria were fulfilled by 54 patients (24 men and 30 women; mean age, 42.7 ± 8.7 years).

We followed up these patients for 1 year after recovery from the episode during which lithium was resumed or up to the first recurrence with onset after lithium reintroduction. During the follow-up period, serum lithium levels were maintained in the range of 0.6–0.8 mEq/L. We interviewed patients at bimonthly intervals with the SADS. We defined as *nonrelapsers* those patients who did not present any RDC manic or major depressive episode in the year after recovery from the episode during which lithium was reintroduced, whereas *relapsers* were those patients who had at least one RDC manic or major depressive episode with onset after lithium reintroduction. We compared these two patient groups with respect to several demographic and clinical variables (see Table 2–3) and performed a stepwise logistic regression analysis, using relapse/nonrelapse on reintroduced lithium prophylaxis as the dependent variable, and the demographic and clinical items as independent variables.

Forty-four patients were identified as nonrelapsers and 10 as relapsers on reintroduced lithium prophylaxis. The only significant difference between the two patient groups concerned the duration of lithium treatment before discontinuation, which was longer in the latter group. Relapsers tended to be older and to have a longer duration of illness and a higher number of affective episodes before the start of the first lithium treatment period, but these differences were not statistically significant. On stepwise logistic regression analysis, the duration of lithium treatment before discontinuation was the only variable that entered the model (improvement $\chi^2 = 4.9$, df = 1, $P < .02$).

Among relapsers on reinstituted lithium prophylaxis, six (11.1% of the total sample) reproduced exactly the pattern described by Post et al. (1992); that is, they had been taking effective lithium treatment for at least 5 years before discontinuation. Two of the six, after having, respectively, three and four affective episodes after lithium reintroduction, remained on successful lithium prophylaxis for the subsequent 2 years.

Discussion

Our data on the outcome of lithium prophylaxis after 5 years confirm and extend those reported previously by our group (Maj et al. 1989), supported by analogous findings by several other groups (Aagaard

Table 2–3. Demographic and clinical features of nonrelapsers and relapsers on reinstituted lithium prophylaxis

Variable	Nonrelapsers (n = 44)	Relapsers (n = 10)
Age (years ± SD)[a]	42.0 ± 8.7	46.0 ± 7.2
Sex (% men)	45.5	40.0
Duration of illness (years, mean ± SD)[a]	11.1 ± 7.3	14.0 ± 6.6
No. affective episodes before first lithium treatment period (mean ± SD)	5.6 ± 3.7	7.4 ± 2.2
Duration of first treatment period (years, mean ± SD)	5.4 ± 3.1	8.4 ± 4.9*
Modality of lithium discontinuation (% abrupt)	79.5	80.0
Time to first recurrence after lithium discontinuation (months, mean ± SD)	11.6 ± 12.5	11.8 ± 9.8
Time between lithium discontinuation and reintroduction (months, mean ± SD)	13.5 ± 13.4	13.9 ± 9.7
Mean serum lithium levels during follow-up period (mEq/L, ± SD)	0.67 ± 0.05	0.67 ± 0.06

Note.   SD = standard deviation.
[a]At the time of lithium reintroduction.
*P < .05.

and Vestergaard 1990; Gitlin et al. 1995; Harrow et al. 1990; Keller et al. 1993; Kukopulos et al. 1995; Markar and Mander 1989; O'Connell et al. 1991; Tohen et al. 1990).

We suggest that the effect of lithium prophylaxis on the long-term course of bipolar disorder in ordinary clinical conditions be reconceptualized in the following terms:

- The drug, if taken regularly at adequate doses, competes vigorously, at least in some cases, with the biological mechanisms underlying the disorder. However, this competition results more frequently in reduced morbidity than in complete suppression of episodes (of those patients who completed a 5-year treatment period, more than 85% showed a reduction of at least 50% of the mean number of weeks of illness per year, but fewer than 40% were completely free of episodes).
- As implied by the image of "competition," the more virulent the illness, the less dramatic the likely effect of lithium: in patients with a high number of prelithium episodes and hospitalizations, the likelihood of complete suppression of morbidity is very low, and evidence that rapid cycling is a "predictor of nonresponse" probably should be interpreted in this framework. In other words, rapid cycling, as currently defined, may not be a qualitatively distinct subtype of the illness but simply a severe variant.
- The effect of lithium prophylaxis on the course of bipolar disorder in ordinary clinical conditions is influenced considerably by the poor acceptance of treatment by many patients.
- Only 60% of patients undergoing lithium prophylaxis were still attending the unit and on lithium treatment after 5 years, and in only a minority of these cases was treatment inefficacy (perceived by the patient or observed by the clinician) cited as the reason for discontinuation.
- Interruption of lithium prophylaxis is accompanied by a high risk of recurrence, and repeated short interruptions of treatment related to poor compliance may reduce considerably the effect of prophylaxis on the course of bipolar illness in ordinary clinical conditions.

- The gap between the efficacy (therapeutic potential as emerging from double-blind randomized clinical trials) and the effectiveness (outcome in ordinary clinical conditions) of lithium prophylaxis is related only in part to deficiencies in patient selection and treatment surveillance. Even in a specialized setting, that gap is conspicuous, suggesting that factors inherent in the relationship between the patient and the drug play a prominent role, independent of the treatment setting.

At least one of eight patients with bipolar disorder treated successfully with lithium for 5 years will have multiple late relapses (late nonresponse) despite persistently adequate compliance. The most likely explanation for this phenomenon is that the "driving force" of the illness (Post et al. 1993) finally overwhelms the drug's prophylactic effect. In fact, patients who eventually developed late nonresponse had a significantly higher number of previous affective episodes and hospitalizations and a significantly longer duration of illness as compared with stable responders. Although the older age of late nonresponders is likely to be simply an epiphenomenon of the longer duration of illness, a direct effect of aging on responsiveness to lithium prophylaxis cannot be excluded.

Our clinical impression is that late nonresponse to lithium may be counteracted in some cases by the addition of another mood stabilizer (e.g., carbamazepine or valproate) and that this phenomenon is one of the reasons that combinations of mood stabilizers are used so commonly in clinical practice. Systematic investigations supporting these views are clearly warranted.

Refractoriness to reinstituted lithium prophylaxis occurs in almost one of five bipolar patients who have a history of at least 2 years of successful lithium treatment and of at least one recurrence after treatment discontinuation.[1] The risk of this refractoriness seems to increase with the length of the prediscontinuation lithium treatment period. Although systematic information about the duration

---

[1] Editor's note: See also Post et al., Chapter 5, in this volume for further discussion of lithium discontinuation–induced refractoriness.

of refractoriness is now unavailable, preliminary evidence suggests that the refractory state may be reversible in some cases.

Present knowledge of the biological mechanisms behind the prophylactic effect of lithium is so modest that any attempt to interpret lithium-discontinuation-induced refractoriness remains largely speculative. Lithium's prolonged mood-stabilizing activity, once interrupted, may in some cases rebound in a period of instability that makes the patient unresponsive to reintroduced lithium prophylaxis. However, our findings do not rule out the alternative hypothesis that the addition of one or more episodes to the cumulative load alters the neurobiological substrates of mood dysfunction, so that the patient is no longer responsive to lithium (Post et al. 1993). Although the number of previous affective episodes was not significantly higher in our refractory patients, a definite trend was observed in that direction.

In conclusion, the limited effect of lithium prophylaxis on the long-term course of bipolar disorder in ordinary clinical conditions is likely to be the product of at least three factors: 1) poor acceptance of treatment by many patients; 2) the driving force of the illness, which may overwhelm the drug's prophylactic effect, at the outset or in the long term; and 3) the association of treatment interruption (including multiple short discontinuations because of poor compliance) with a high risk of relapse. These factors may be relevant to all long-term treatments with psychotropic drugs.

References

Aagaard J, Vestergaard P: Predictors of outcome in prophylactic lithium treatment: a 2-year prospective study. J Affect Disord 18:259–266, 1990

Amdisen A: The 12-hour standardized serum lithium (12h-st SLi), in Depression and Mania: Modern Lithium Therapy. Edited by Johnson FN. Oxford, England, IRL Press, 1987, pp 88–91

Angst J: Course of affective disorders, in Handbook of Biological Psychiatry. Edited by Van Praag HM, Lader MH, Rafaelsen OJ, et al. New York, Marcel Dekker, 1981, pp 225–242

Åsberg M, Perris C, Schalling D, et al: Comprehensive Psychopathological Rating Scale: CPRS. Acta Psychiatr Scand 27 (suppl):5–27, 1978

Dickson DE, Kendell RE: Does maintenance lithium therapy prevent recurrences of mania under clinical conditions? Psychol Med 16:521–530, 1986

Endicott J, Spitzer RL: A diagnostic interview: the Schedule for Affective Disorders and Schizophrenia. Arch Gen Psychiatry 35:837–844, 1978

Endicott J, Andreasen NC, Spitzer RL: Family History Research Diagnostic Criteria. New York, New York State Psychiatric Institute, Biometrics Research, 1975

Gitlin MJ, Swendsen J, Mueller TL, et al: Relapse and impairment in bipolar disorder. Am J Psychiatry 152:1635–1640, 1995

Guscott R, Taylor L: Lithium prophylaxis in recurrent affective illness: efficacy, effectiveness and efficiency. Br J Psychiatry 164:741–746, 1994

Harrow M, Goldberg JF, Grossman LS, et al: Outcome in manic disorders: a naturalistic follow-up study. Arch Gen Psychiatry 47:665–671, 1990

Keller MB, Lavori PW, Coryell W, et al: Bipolar I: a five-year prospective follow-up. J Nerv Ment Dis 181:238–245, 1993

Kraepelin E: Psychiatrie, 8 Aufl. Leipzig, Barth, 1909–1915

Kukopulos A, Reginaldi D, Minnai G, et al: The long term prophylaxis of affective disorders, in Advances in Biochemical Psychopharmacology, Vol 49. Edited by Gessa GL, Fratta W, Pani L, et al. New York, Raven, 1995, pp 127–147

Maj M, Pirozzi R, Kemali D: Long-term outcome of lithium prophylaxis in patients initially classified as complete responders. Psychopharmacology 98:535–538, 1989

Maj M, Magliano L, Pirozzi R, et al: Validity of rapid cycling as a course specifier for bipolar disorder. Am J Psychiatry 151:1015–1019, 1994

Maj M, Pirozzi R, Magliano L: Nonresponse to reinstituted lithium prophylaxis in previously responsive bipolar patients: prevalence and predictors. Am J Psychiatry 152:1810–1811, 1995

Markar HR, Mander AJ: Efficacy of lithium prophylaxis in clinical practice. Br J Psychiatry 155:496–500, 1989

O'Connell RA, Mayo JA, Flatow L, et al: Outcome of bipolar disorder on long-term treatment with lithium. Br J Psychiatry 159:123–129, 1991

Post RM, Leverich GS, Altshuler L, et al: Lithium-discontinuation-induced refractoriness: preliminary observations. Am J Psychiatry 149:1727–1729, 1992

Post RM, Leverich GS, Pazzaglia PJ, et al: Lithium tolerance and discontinuation as pathways to refractoriness, in Lithium in Medicine and Biology. Edited by Birch NJ, Padgham C, Hughes MS. Carnforth, Marius, Marius Press, 1993, pp 71–84

Schou M: Lithium prophylaxis: about "naturalistic" or "clinical practice" studies. Lithium 4:77–81, 1993

Spitzer RL, Endicott J, Robins E: Research Diagnostic Criteria (RDC) for a Selected Group of Functional Disorders, 2nd Edition. New York, New York State Psychiatric Institute, Biometrics Research, 1975

Tohen M, Waternaux CM, Tsuang MT, et al: Outcome in mania: a 4-year prospective follow-up of 75 patients utilizing survival analysis. Arch Gen Psychiatry 47:1106–1111, 1990

Zis AP, Graf P, Goodwin FK: The natural course of affective disorders: implications for lithium prophylaxis, in Lithium: Controversies and Unresolved Issues. Edited by Cooper TG, Gershon S, Kline NS, et al. Amsterdam, Excerpta Medica, 1979, pp 381–398

Syndromal and Psychosocial Outcome in Bipolar Disorder: A Complex and Circular Relationship

Michael J. Gitlin, M.D.
Constance Hammen, Ph.D.

Despite more than a century of careful observation by some of the most thoughtful clinical researchers in the field, it remains difficult to describe accurately the long-term outcome of bipolar disorder. Although bipolar disorder is often assumed to have a relatively benign outcome (especially in comparison to schizophrenia), studies published before the advent of maintenance pharmacotherapy as well as those published more recently have documented significant morbidity and dysfunction (Bratfos and Haug 1968; Carlson et al. 1974; Coryell et al. 1989, 1993; Goldberg et al. 1995a, 1995b; Harrow et al. 1990; Hastings 1958; Keller et al. 1993; Maj et al. 1998; Marker and Mander 1989; O'Connell et al. 1991; Sachs et al. 1994; Shobe and Brian 1971; Tohen et al. 1990; Tsuang et al. 1979; Winokur et al. 1993). The multiple definitions of outcome utilized across studies, however, have prevented simple generalizations. For each major domain of outcome—symptomatic/syndromal and psychosocial/functional—several methods exist for measuring outcome. In evaluating symptomatic/syndromal outcome, the most common method simply counts the number of episodes a bipolar patient has over a certain time period. Even this method can be used in a variety of ways. For example, Goodwin and Jamison (1990) noted that many early observers, including Kraepelin, counted as a single episode a 1-year-long hospitalization with multiple polarity switches. Alternatively, a second, less commonly used method of outcome measurement evaluates both episodes and subtle (subsyndromal) affective symptoms that might contribute to the disorder's overall morbidity.

Psychosocial/functional outcome uses a different set of observations and measures but typically evaluates patients in the major psychosocial domains that intuitively define normal function. Thus, the capacity to work, go to school, have romantic relationships and/or friends, and have reasonable relationships with family members defines outcome in a manner to which patients and their families have traditionally been more attuned than have researchers. Studies have documented significant psychosocial dysfunction among treated bipolar patients (Coryell et al. 1993; Dion et al. 1988; Goldberg et al. 1995b; Tohen et al. 1990).

In attempting to understand the relationship between these two domains, the most intuitive conclusion would be that poor syndromal outcome predicts poor psychosocial function. Some studies support this conclusion (Goldberg et al. 1995b; Harrow et al. 1990; O'Connell et al. 1991). Yet, this relationship is likely to be far more complicated than that. For example, Coryell et al. (1993) found that patients with syndromal recovery (from major depression, not bipolar disorder) sustained throughout a 2-year period still showed significant impairment in occupational and marital relations. Similarly, Mintz et al. (1992), examining occupational recovery after depressive episodes, noted that work restoration lagged behind symptom remission. Because bipolar patients are at risk for depressions of at least similar severity to those experienced by unipolar patients, they are likely to share the risk for similar residual effects beyond the destructive effects of manic episodes. Additionally, the relative roles of number of episodes versus a more cumulative measurement of global psychopathology in affecting psychosocial function have rarely been studied.

Any discussion of the relationship between syndromal and psychosocial outcome must also include the possibility of the inverse relationship—that psychosocial function and life stresses may provoke affective symptoms and syndromes. The affective syndromes are then likely to lead to further psychosocial dysfunction, creating a vicious cycle. In this chapter, we present data from our recent studies in support of a complex relationship between syndromes and functioning in bipolar individuals, in which dysfunction in one domain leads to poor outcome in the other.

Outcome of Treated Bipolar Patients: UCLA Sample

In the early 1980s, while observing patients in the UCLA Affective Disorders Clinic, an outpatient clinic specializing in the evaluation and long-term treatment of unipolar and bipolar disorders, we became aware of the number of patients who, despite vigorous pharmacotherapy, had poor syndromal and/or psychosocial outcomes. Because of these preliminary clinical observations, we began to study systematically both types of outcome and the relationship between the two (Gitlin et al. 1995).

During a 6-year period, 160 patients with DSM-IV (American Psychiatric Association 1994) bipolar I disorder were treated in the clinic for more than 3 months. Of these patients, 82 were treated for 2 years or more. This group constituted our study population. Their mean length of follow-up was 4.3 years (SD = 1.5, range = 2–6.5 years). The 82 patients had a mean age of 37 (SD = 11.7) and were generally well educated (44% had college degrees). Only 18% were married; 82% were either single or divorced. Mean age at onset of bipolar disorder was 24 years. The mean number of past manic episodes was 5.5 (SD = 4), and the mean number of past depressive episodes was 4.3 (SD = 3.7). These patients did not differ in clinical history—age at onset; numbers of manias, depressions, or hospitalizations—from those patients seen in the clinic who were followed up for less than 2 years.

After an extensive initial evaluation, patients were seen with variable frequency but averaged monthly visits. Treatment was prescribed in an uncontrolled manner but with the general philosophy that maintenance treatment was virtually always indicated, except possibly after a first episode.

At each clinic visit, the treating psychiatrist filled out a detailed symptom checklist covering all manic or depressive symptoms since the last visit. Dates for onset and end of these symptoms were also recorded. These data were then scored independently by research staff and plotted on a time line using the following scale: 0 = no symptoms, 1 = mild symptoms (no more than two total symptoms for mania or depression, including the mood symptom), 2 = moderate symptoms (diagnosed hypomania or dysthymia, or minor depression—i.e., exhibiting two to four of nine depressive symptoms for 2 weeks or more in contrast to the requisite five symptoms for a diagnosis of major depression), 3 = marked symptoms (diagnosed mania or major depression), and 4 = severe symptoms (mania requiring hospitalization or major depression requiring hospitalization or with serious suicide attempt).

We used the time lines to measure syndromal outcome over the follow-up period in two ways. First, we counted the number of manic and depressive episodes. Second, we developed an aggregate measure of cumulative symptoms called the Average Mood Symptom Scale (AMSS) score, which takes into account milder affective symptoms as well as the length and severity of episodes. The AMSS is defined as the average symptom level score per unit of time. For example, a patient with level 2 symptoms (minor depressive disorder or dysthymia) for 3 months followed by 3 months of a depressed mood without other depressive symptoms (level 1) would have an average mood symptom score of 1.5.

The psychiatrist measured psychosocial status at each visit with three separate four-point scales to evaluate job status, social functioning, and family interactions. On these four-point scales, 4 = full, stable, progressing employment; normal social functioning; and supportive relations with family; and 1 = sustained unemployment or dysfunctional at home or school, complete social withdrawal, and no family contact or chaotic contact. Scores of 2 and 3 in all three areas reflect more intermediate functioning.

Basic Outcome

Despite virtually continual pharmacotherapy, relapses and subsyndromal symptoms among patients were the rule rather than the exception. The likelihood of either a full manic or a full depressive episode within 5 years was 73%, with 37% of the relapses occurring within the first year. Furthermore, of those who relapsed, 70% had multiple episodes that were equally likely to be depressions or manias.

Only 17% of all patients were essentially euthymic with few to no consistent mood symptoms observed. Of those patients who did not relapse, almost half (46%) still showed significant symptoms such as hypomania or minor depressive disorder. Using the AMSS, our cumulative measure of psychopathology, we found that 26% of the patients had an average symptom score higher than 1.0, indicating substantial affective symptoms. Table 3–1 shows the distribution of patients who spent substantial amounts of time at an average AMSS level of 2.0 or greater (i.e., experiencing hypomania, mania, nearly major depression, or major depression). Thirty percent of the patients were significantly symptomatic for more than one-quarter of the entire follow-up time.

All patients received ongoing treatment during the observation period, and the vast majority had continuous treatment during both acute episodes and maintenance treatment. Because these data were collected between 1984 and 1990, most patients' disorders were treated with lithium and a smaller number with carbamazepine or valproate. A systematic evaluation of the aggressiveness of pharm-

Table 3–1. Percentage of follow-up period during which 82 bipolar patients experienced moderate, marked, or severe affective symptoms

Percent of follow-up period[a]	No. (%)
>50	12 (15)
25–49	12 (15)
10–24	16 (20)
1–9	28 (34)
0	14 (17)

[a]Mean = 4.3 years (SD = 1.5).

Source. Reprinted from Gitlin MJ, Swendsen J, Heller TL, et al: "Relapse and Impairment in Bipolar Disorder." *American Journal of Psychiatry* 152:1638–1640, 1995. Copyright 1995, American Psychiatric Association. Used with permission.

acotherapy (using a scheme in which all maintenance treatments were converted to a five-point scale, depending on doses and/or serum drug levels) indicated that more aggressive treatment was not associated with better outcome. Additionally, the median medication rating was a lithium level of 0.7–0.89 or 700–999 mg of carbamazepine or 1,250–1,499 mg of valproate. Therefore, the relatively poor syndromal outcome of our patients could not be explained by low levels of pharmacotherapy.

Psychosocial ratings also showed considerable dysfunction in this group of continually treated patients. Occupational outcome was worst; only 28% showed a good outcome and 35% a poor outcome. Social ratings showed a good outcome for 39%, whereas 7% had a poor outcome. Family interaction ratings indicated that 45% had a good outcome and 9% a poor outcome.

Relationship Between Syndromal and Psychosocial Outcome

As shown in Table 3–2, manias and depressions differed in their effect on specific psychosocial domains. The number of depressions was associated with family dysfunction more than was the number of manias ($t = 2.57, df = 78, P < .02$). Similarly, social maladjustment was associated with the number of depressions more than with ma-

Table 3–2. Correlation of symptomatic and psychosocial outcome in 82 bipolar patients

	Occupational	Social	Family
No. of manias	−.25	−.12	−.23
No. of depressions	−.20	−.31*	−.46**
Total no. of episodes	−.25	−.27	−.42**
Mean score on affective mood scale	−.52**	−.47**	−.60**

*$P < .01$.
**$P < .0001$.

Source. Reprinted from Gitlin MJ, Swendsen J, Heller TL, et al: "Relapse and Impairment in Bipolar Disorder." *American Journal of Psychiatry* 152:1638–1640, 1995. Copyright 1995, American Psychiatric Association. Used with permission.

nias at a trend level ($P < .10$). The number of manias was associated with occupational dysfunction more than was the number of depressions, but this result did not reach statistical significance.

Table 3–2 also shows that average mood symptom scores were more highly correlated with poor psychosocial outcome than were number of episodes. These results suggest that cumulative psychopathology may more accurately represent the destructive process by which bipolar disorder leads to poor psychosocial function. These effects were most clear in predicting occupational outcome. For family and social outcome (i.e., the ability to have friends, a primary romantic relationship, or a nonchaotic family life), both cumulative affective morbidity and depressive episodes played important roles.

As suggested earlier in this chapter, not only did syndromal outcome predict psychosocial dysfunction, but also psychosocial functioning independently predicted syndromal relapse. Bipolar patients with poorer functioning in social, family, and work domains when not having an acute episode tended to relapse faster than did those with better psychosocial function. When controlling for a history of past episodes, this relationship was statistically significant for occupational adjustment ($P = .05$). In other words, those with better work performance when not having an episode were less likely to relapse than were those with poor job function. Consistent with this observation, a hierarchical multiple regression analysis to predict time to first relapse showed that psychosocial function ratings independently contributed to the time to first relapse beyond that of number of manic and depressive episodes ($R^2 = 0.07$, $\Delta F = 5.38$, df $= 1.79$, $P = .0007$).

Life Events and Relapse

These findings—that psychosocial factors predict syndromal relapse—are consistent with a series of studies in which we examined the role of stressful life events in triggering relapse. Ellicott et al. (1990) found that bipolar patients with high levels of life stress (as determined by a validated interrater-reliable interview performed blind to symptom status) had a risk of relapse 4.53 times higher than patients without stress. These results could not be explained by differing levels of medication treatment or compliance as rated by the treating clinician. Of note, patients with low-to-moderate levels of stress were not at higher risk for relapse, implying a threshold effect for the impact of threatening events.

A related question is whether the effects of stress in predicting or triggering relapse apply to later as well as earlier episodes. Kraepelin initially suggested that precipitating events play a larger role in the first few episodes of the disorder but that, with an increasing number of episodes, later episodes are more likely to be autonomous in origin (Goodwin and Jamison 1990). Few studies have systematically examined this question, although it is both clinically satisfying and consistent with Post's influential hypothetical model of increasing sensitization to stressors resulting in more autonomous episodes (Post et al. 1986). We have explored this question in two ways. First, we examined only bipolar patients who had more than 12 episodes and found that high stress conditions still predicted a greater risk for relapse ($P < .008$) (Swendsen et al. 1995). Second, we divided patients who relapsed at the median number of manic and depressive episodes (Hammen and Gitlin 1997). Those with a greater number of episodes were more likely to have had a major event in the 6 months prior to relapse compared with those with fewer episodes (76% versus 40%, $P = .03$). Additionally, those with a greater number of prior episodes relapsed more rapidly after a major event compared with those with fewer prior episodes. As with our earlier analysis, the greater association of stressors and relapse risk for patients with many prior episodes held true only for the effect of severe and not minor stressors.

Overall, then, our findings consistently suggest that severe stressors are a significant risk factor for relapse in bipolar patients, regardless of the number of episodes. Furthermore, those with more prior episodes may be at increased risk for stress sensitivity. In this way, the relationship between syndromal and psychosocial outcome may function as a continuous cycle in which affective morbidity (measured by number of episodes or nature of subsyndromal symptoms) leads to poor functioning, which may in turn lead to greater risk of episodes, leading to poorer functioning, and so on. Also, in view of research on unipolar disorders implicating early childhood adversity and family disruption as risk factors for depression, studies of the childhood experiences of bipolar patients may be warranted as factors influencing vulnerability to stress.

Personality and Outcome in Bipolar Patients

Maladaptive personality traits constitute another dimension that may link psychosocial and syndromal outcomes. Unfortunately, the measurement of personality traits and disorders has been marred by significant problems in reliability and validity (Zimmerman 1994). Even without these methodological problems, few studies have examined the relationship between personality traits in bipolar patients and their effects on outcome.

As previously suggested, the interaction of personality factors and the course of bipolar disorder may be understood in a variety of ways (Akiskal et al. 1983). In general, personality can be conceptualized either as an independent series of psychological traits or as subsyndromal manifestations of the mood disorder. Based on Akiskal et al.'s subsyndromal model, temperamental aspects of personality (e.g., impulsiveness, moodiness, emotional reactivity) would be considered trait (or chronic) aspects of the mood disorders, not separate influences on the course of the classic Axis I disorder.

Some personality traits (e.g., Cluster B traits) may increase the likelihood of the types of psychosocial stressors that then trigger episodes, thereby functioning as a stress generator. In another study from our group, more than 60% of bipolar patients' stresses were partly or entirely the result of their own behaviors or characteristics (Hammen 1995). Our data do not allow us to better characterize these traits as independent psychopathological phenomena, as resulting from incipient manic or depressive episode, or as related to the temperamental aspects of mood disorders.

Personality factors may also modify the effects of stress in triggering affective episodes. Using a variety of personality inventories, including the Eysenck scale for extroversion-introversion (Eysenck and Eysenck 1978) and the Lazare-Klerman-Armor scale for obsessionality (Hirschfeld et al. 1983), we found that personality variables predicted both relapse and stress sensitivity (Swendsen et al. 1995). Specifically, bipolar individuals who are introverted and obsessional were more likely to relapse, but extroversion and low obsessionality provided some protection from relapse, even under highly stressful conditions. Introversion presumably reflects less access to the type of social network that might buffer the negative effects of stress, whereas obsessional individuals might worry excessively about a stressor's potential effect. With the recent finding of increased neuroticism along with lower ego resiliency and emotional stability in euthymic bipolar patients compared with nonbipolar control subjects (Solomon et al. 1996), the results of both studies suggest that bipolar individuals may be especially vulnerable to the untoward effects of stressors that might trigger relapse.

Finally, some personality traits may be exaggerated or emerge de novo as complications of multiple affective episodes. For example, a patient with mild preexisting narcissistic personality traits might be at higher risk for a more pervasive demoralization after a series of virulent manic episodes, with subsequent feelings of shame and social withdrawal. Similarly, dependent traits might emerge or be accentuated as a result of feelings of fearfulness and helplessness in the face of multiple hospitalized affective episodes. In these ways, multiple destructive affective episodes could function as severe stressful events, with bipolar patients developing certain personality characteristics as a consequence of these episodes.

Case Vignettes

Mr. A, a bright 59-year-old college graduate, has a history of bipolar I disorder since age 28. His initial psychotic manic episode, which resulted in a 1-month hospitalization, was characterized by grandiosity, paranoid delusions, and frenzied activity. During the postmanic depression that lasted 4 months, Mr. A quit his job. His marriage dissolved soon thereafter, although he and his ex-wife remained in contact as friends for many years. Even two decades later, Mr. A cannot explain why the marriage broke up, attributing it simply to the manic and depressive episodes.

After being supported by his family for a year, Mr. A found new work and eventually remarried. He had two more manic episodes over the next decade, each of which required hospitalization. He was able to continue working between episodes, but after the third episode, his second wife left him, and he has never remarried.

Since the third episode, Mr. A has been taking maintenance mood stabilizers, initially lithium and later lithium and carbamazepine in combination. However, he has been unemployed for the last 20 years, supported by Social Security and a small trust fund left to him by his parents.

Although Mr. A's family and personal background for the first 35 years of his life was middle class, he has lived on the periphery of society for the last two decades. His only history of drug abuse (except in the midst of a manic episode) has been daily marijuana smoking for the last 15 years. He has had only one manic episode in the last 10 years. Over the last decade, however, he has had multiple brief and mild mood swings, both hypomanic and depressed, each lasting no more than a few days. In his mind, these subsyndromal episodes remind Mr. A of the ever-present danger of relapse.

When asked about his life path, Mr. A acknowledges a deep fear of the effects of his manias, preferring not to start relationships when they will be destroyed during the next episode. His usual mood is dysphoric but without vegetative features. He is deeply cynical about political leaders and frequently dabbles in extremist political groups, although he stays on the fringe of these groups. Regarding his lack of employment, he simply rails against the capitalist world, alternating with a feeling that he is too smart and too educated for the types of jobs he would be offered.

Ms. B is a 41-year-old woman with a history of bipolar disorder and borderline and dependent personality disorders. After a depressive episode during her teens, she was in individual psychotherapy for many years, focusing on the chaotic and enmeshed relationships in her family. At age 24, she had a clear manic episode that resulted in a brief hospitalization. She has been taking maintenance mood stabilizers since then. After the initial manic episode, Ms. B worked at low-level sales jobs for the next few years. During this time, she had two moderate depressive episodes and one brief mania requiring hospitalization. When Ms. B was 30, her mother, on whom she had been profoundly dependent, died.

For the next 7 years, Ms. B's mood disorder and life were unmanageable. Most of the time, she showed an admixture of depressive traits, helpless dependency, a complete lack of confidence, and an inability to function. Her siblings, although angry and exhausted by her demands, helped support her financially. She generally exhibited a childish manner with a sense of such cognitive perplexity and inability to follow instructions that neuropsychological tests were performed. However, no deficits other than those consistent with moderate depression were found. Multiple antidepressants and one course of electroconvulsive therapy were unhelpful. Eventually, Ms. B entered into a romantic relationship, got married, and improved somewhat, being able to work at low-level sales jobs again. She continues to show mild depressive symptoms, marked dependency traits, and an odd cognitive style.

Clinical Implications

How should clinicians interpret the information just presented in their work with bipolar patients? First, our syndromal outcome data are consistent with many other studies published over the last few years demonstrating that even in treated bipolar populations, relapse and/or subsyndromal symptoms are common (Coryell et al. 1989, 1993; Goldberg et al. 1995a; Goodwin and Jamison 1990; Harrow et al. 1990; Keck et al. 1998; Keller et al. 1993; O'Connell et al. 1991; Sachs et al. 1994; Strakowski et al. 1998; Tohen et al. 1990; Winokur et al. 1993). Therefore, patients and families should not expect a complete amelioration of affective symptoms simply because pharmacotherapy has been instituted. Clinicians must tread a fine line between unrealistic optimism and nihilistic pessimism, reminding those they treat that, although treatments are far from perfect, evidence is still overwhelming that they greatly improve outcome.

Second, the significant relationship between cumulative affective morbidity—which includes both the length of episodes and the nature of subsyndromal symptoms—and psychosocial outcome suggests the importance of chronic low-level symptoms in predicting functional outcome. Therefore, clinicians need to consider more vigorously treating mild symptoms that extend for weeks to months in patients with bipolar disorder. Notably, Keller and colleagues (1992) found that more than one-half of bipolar patients who were maintained on low serum lithium levels (0.4–0.6 mEq/L) had subsyndromal affective symptoms, and the emergence of subsyndromal symptoms was associated with a fourfold risk of developing a full major affective relapse.

Third, clinicians should be mindful of the complex relationship between psychosocial factors and syndromal outcome. The likely scenario of the vicious cycle noted above—in which disturbances in one sphere lead to dysfunction in the other with further disruption in the first arena—implies that intervention in any area of the cycle might be beneficial. Thus, both pharmacological intervention (with the goal of diminishing symptoms and syndromes) *and* psychosocial intervention might each independently improve outcome. Given our consistent data on the effects of life events and psychosocial stressors in triggering relapses in both early and later episodes, any clinical intervention that can prevent or ameliorate certain stressors (e.g., couples therapy that might improve a marital relationship and prevent a marital separation) could improve syndromal outcome. This suggestion is consistent with the findings of Miklowitz et al. (1988) and others that the quality of family relationships, such as the presence of high expressed emotion characterized by criticism, hostility, and emotional overinvolvement, is associated with higher relapse rates in bipolar patients. Preliminary data also suggest the efficacy of behavioral family management in reducing relapse (Miklowitz and Goldstein 1990). Such psychosocial treatments are discussed in greater detail in Miklowitz and Frank, Chapter 4, in this volume.

Similarly, if poor occupational function predicts a shorter time to relapse (as it did in our study), more vigorous attention to patients' vocational life—through social service agencies, job retraining, or simply encouraging patients to look for work—might also be a factor in preventing relapse and improving the long-term course of the disorder.

A final link between psychosocial variables and syndromal outcome reflects the potential effect of education and compliance on long-term outcome. In our study, clinician-rated compliance did not predict outcome; however, a previous study from our group showed a strong positive effect of a brief compliance-based intervention on outcome (Cochran 1984). In that study, new bipolar patients in the Affective Disorders Clinic were assigned randomly to either standard medication management or standard care plus six sessions with a psychology graduate student. The sessions focused on altering cognitions and behaviors that interfere with compliance, such as concerns about the medication and the nature of bipolar disorder. At 6-month follow-up, the brief cognitive/educational intervention resulted in significantly greater compliance, less medication discontinuation, fewer episodes, and a 75% reduction in rehospitalizations. Although this study did not evaluate the effect of compliance-enhancing therapy on functional outcome, it is reasonable to assume that given the more benign syndromal outcome, greater attention to compliance through education and cognitive techniques would retard the psychosocial deterioration caused by the disorder.

Clinical Research Implications

The two major areas needing further work are in 1) further characterizing the relationship between syndromal and psychosocial outcome and 2) designing and then validating psychosocial treatment approaches to improve outcome. In the first area, it is still unclear why functional recovery lags behind syndromal recovery in so many patients. Although this phenomenon has been best studied in unipolar patients (Coryell et al. 1993; Mintz et al. 1992), clinical observations suggest this same phenomenon exists with bipolar patients (M. Goldstein, personal communication, June 1996). Some of the clinical factors suggested above that should be explored further include subtle, subclinical symptoms that are not easily rated on symptom checklists; diagnostic comorbidities such as substance abuse (Black et al. 1988; Tohen et al. 1990; see also Tohen and Zarate, Chapter 9, and Winokur, Chapter 10, in this volume); and personality traits. Psychotherapeutic strategies would follow the identification of risk factors—for example, family therapy, vocational approaches, or psychotherapy to enhance coping capacities in the presence of stressors.

Conclusion

Converging evidence suggests that the psychosocial outcome of treated bipolar patients is not nearly as optimistic as expected given the increasing number of effective pharmacotherapeutic options. Although the number of relapses probably predicts poor functional recovery, our data suggest that cumulative psychopathology, which includes both the length of episodes and the nature of subsyndromal symptoms, more strongly predicts poor psychosocial outcome than does the number of episodes.

In understanding the long-term outcome of bipolar disorder, psychosocial dysfunction should not simply be considered a result of affective symptoms and episodes. Rather, psychosocial problems—whether measured in occupational status, extent of social life, quality of family relationships, or simply external stresses—may affect the course of bipolar disorder by contributing to the development of further episodes. In this way, a cycle of poor function–syndromal exacerbation–poorer function may describe a path to chronic disability. Another factor that must be considered is personality, both as a potential protective factor that might diminish the number of life events that increase the chance for relapse and as a source of resilience in the recovery from affective episodes. The challenge for the next decade will be to more clearly characterize risk factors and protective factors and to design interventions to enhance psychosocial outcome.

References

Akiskal HS, Hirschfeld RMA, Yerevanian BI: The relationship of personality to affective disorders: a critical review. Arch Gen Psychiatry 40: 801–810, 1983

American Psychiatric Association: Diagnostic and Statistical Manual of Mental Disorders, 4th Edition. Washington, DC, American Psychiatric Association, 1994

Black DW, Winokur G, Hubert J, et al: Predictors of immediate response in the treatment of mania: the importance of comorbidity. Biol Psychiatry 24:191–198, 1988

Bratfos O, Haug JO: The course of manic-depressive psychosis: a follow up investigation of 215 patients. Acta Psychiatr Scand 44:89–112, 1968

Carlson GA, Kotin J, Davenport YB, et al: Follow-up of 53 bipolar manic-depressive patients. Br J Psychiatry 124:134–139, 1974

Cochran SD: Preventing medical noncompliance in the outpatient treatment of bipolar affective disorders. J Consult Clin Psychol 52:873–878, 1984

Coryell W, Keller M, Endicott J, et al: Bipolar II illness: course and outcome over a five-year period. Psychol Med 19:129–141, 1989

Coryell W, Scheftner W, Keller M, et al: The enduring psychosocial consequences of mania and depression. Am J Psychiatry 150:720–727, 1993

Dion GL, Tohen M, Anthony WA, et al: Symptoms and functioning of patients with bipolar disorder six months after hospitalization. Hosp Community Psychiatry 39:652–657, 1988

Ellicott A, Hammen C, Gitlin M, et al: Life events and the course of bipolar disorder. Am J Psychiatry 147:1194–1198, 1990

Eysenck H, Eysenck S: Manual of the Eysenck Personality Inventory. San Diego, CA, Educational and Industial Testing Service, 1978

Gitlin MJ, Swendsen J, Heller TL, et al: Relapse and impairment in bipolar disorder. Am J Psychiatry 152:1638–1640, 1995

Goldberg JF, Harrow M, Grossman LS: Course and outcome in bipolar affective disorder: a longitudinal follow-up study. Am J Psychiatry 152: 379–384, 1995a

Goldberg JF, Harrow M, Grossman LS: Recurrent affective syndromes in bipolar and unipolar mood disorders at follow-up. Br J Psychiatry 166: 382–385, 1995b

Goodwin FK, Jamison KR: Manic-Depressive Illness. New York, Oxford University Press, 1990

Hammen C: Stress and the course of unipolar and bipolar disorder, in Anxiety and Depression in Adults and Children. Edited by Mazure C. Washington, DC, American Psychiatric Press, 1995, pp 82–96

Hammen C, Gitlin M: Stress reactivity in bipolar patients and its relation to prior history of disorder. Am J Psychiatry 154:856–857, 1997

Harrow M, Goldberg JF, Grossman LS, et al: Outcome in manic disorders: a naturalistic follow-up study. Arch Gen Psychiatry 47:665–671, 1990

Hastings DW: Follow-up-results in psychiatric illness. Am J Psychiatry 114: 1057–1060, 1958

Hirschfeld R, Klerman G, Clayton P: Personality and depression: empirical findings. Arch Gen Psychiatry 40:993–998, 1983

Keck PE Jr, McElroy SL, Strakowski SM, et al: 12-Month outcome of patients with bipolar disorder following hospitalization for a manic or mixed episode. Am J Psychiatry 155:646–652, 1998

Keller MB, Lavori PW, Kane JM, et al: Subsyndromal symptoms in bipolar disorder: a comparison of standard and low serum levels of lithium. Arch Gen Psychiatry 49:371–376, 1992

Keller MB, Lavori PW, Coryell W, et al: Bipolar I: a five-year prospective follow-up. J Nerv Ment Dis 181:238–245, 1993

Maj M, Pirozzi R, Magliano L, et al: Long-term outcome of lithium prophylaxis in bipolar disorder: a 5-year prospective study of 402 patients at a lithium clinic. Am J Psychiatry 155:30–35, 1998

Marker HR, Mander AJ: Efficacy of lithium prophylaxis in clinical practice. Br J Psychiatry 155:496–500, 1989

Miklowitz DJ, Goldstein MJ: Behavioral family treatment for patients with bipolar affective disorder. Behav Modif 14:457–489, 1990

Miklowitz DJ, Goldstein MJ, Nuechterlein KH, et al: Family factors and the course of bipolar affective disorders. Arch Gen Psychiatry 45:225–231, 1988

Mintz J, Mintz LI, Arruda MJ, et al: Treatment of depression and the functional capacity to work. Arch Gen Psychiatry 49:761–768, 1992

O'Connell RA, Mayo JA, Flatow L, et al: Outcome of bipolar disorder on long-term treatment with lithium. Br J Psychiatry 159:123–129, 1991

Post RM, Rubinow DR, Ballenger JC: Conditioning and sensitization in the longitudinal course of affective illness. Br J Psychiatry 149:191–201, 1986

Sachs GS, Lafer B, Truman CJ, et al: Lithium monotherapy: miracle, myth and misunderstanding. Psychiatric Annals 24:299–306, 1994

Shobe FO, Brian P: Long-term prognosis in manic-depressive illness. Arch Gen Psychiatry 25:334–337, 1971

Solomon DA, Shea MT, Leon AC, et al: Personality traits in subjects with bipolar I disorder in remission. J Affect Disord 40:41–48, 1996

Strakowski SM, Keck PE Jr, McElroy SL, et al: Twelve-month outcome after a first hospitalization for affective psychosis. Arch Gen Psychiatry 55:49–55, 1998

Swendsen J, Hammen C, Heller T, et al: Correlates of stress reactivity in patients with bipolar disorder. Am J Psychiatry 152:795–797, 1995

Tohen M, Waternaux CM, Tsuang MT: Outcome in mania: a 4-year prospective follow-up of 75 patients utilizing survival analysis. Arch Gen Psychiatry 47:1106–1111, 1990

Tsuang MT, Woolson RF, Fleming AJ: Long-term outcome of major psychoses: schizophrenia and affective disorders compared with psychiatrically symptom-free surgical conditions. Arch Gen Psychiatry 36:1295–1301, 1979

Winokur G, Coryell W, Keller M, et al: A prospective follow-up of patients with bipolar and primary unipolar affective disorder. Arch Gen Psychiatry 50:457–465, 1993

Zimmerman M: Diagnosing personality disorders. Arch Gen Psychiatry 51:225–245, 1994

CHAPTER 4

New Psychotherapies for Bipolar Disorder

David J. Miklowitz, Ph.D.
Ellen Frank, Ph.D.

*B*ipolar disorder is unquestionably an illness with genetic and biological underpinnings. Abundant evidence indicates that bipolar disorder runs in families; that concordance for the disorder is higher among monozygotic than dizygotic twin pairs (Gershon 1990); and that dopamine, catecholamine, serotonin, γ-aminobutyric acid (GABA), and neuroendocrine systems appear to function irregularly in patients who have the disorder (Silverstone and Romans-Clarkson 1989). Furthermore, pharmacological agents such as lithium carbonate and anticonvulsants (i.e., valproate, carbamazepine) provide significant protection against recurrences of the illness. In contrast to the situation with many other psychiatric disorders, strong consensus exists regarding optimal drug regimens and dosages for acute, continuation, and long-term outpatient maintenance of bipolar disorder (Hirschfeld et al. 1994).

Preparation of this chapter was supported in part by National Institute of Mental Health Grants MH-43931, MH-42556, MH-29618, and MH-55101; a grant from the John D. and Catherine T. MacArthur Foundation Network on the Psychobiology of Depression; and a Faculty Fellowship from the University of Colorado at Boulder. The authors wish to express special thanks to David Kupfer, Cindy Ehlers, and Michael Goldstein for their role in the development of these psychosocial treatment models and to John Clarkin, Ivan Miller, Gabor Keitner, and Steve Carter for their conceptual input.

What role could psychosocial therapies play in the treatment of this disorder? Why would a clinician prescribe an adjunctive psychotherapy for a recently ill bipolar patient when optimizing the patient's drug regimen may be all that is required? Isn't psychotherapy in the context of bipolar disorder an outmoded intervention based on disproved theories of psychosocial etiology?

In this chapter, we address developments in the psychosocial treatment of bipolar disorder. First we provide a rationale for the role of psychotherapy in the overall treatment of the illness. Then we examine the ways in which psychotherapy may augment the efficacy of drug regimens by encouraging pharmacological adherence, addressing psychosocial provoking factors, and modifying the patient's modes of coping with environmental provoking agents.

We describe several newly developed, manual-based psychosocial treatment models, which are being evaluated in randomized, controlled clinical trials. Our primary focus is on two treatments: family-focused treatment of bipolar disorder (Miklowitz and Goldstein 1990, 1997), a psychoeducational family or marital intervention, and interpersonal and social rhythm therapy (Frank et al. 1994), an individual psychotherapy based on the interpersonal therapy of depression (Klerman et al. 1984). Both interventions are designed to be adjunctive to optimal, well-controlled pharmacotherapy regimens.

Limitations of Pharmacotherapy for Bipolar Disorder

Ceilings appear to exist on the effectiveness of standard drug regimens for bipolar disorder when these drugs are administered alone. Controlled maintenance trials of lithium consistently indicate that only about 40% of patients remain well, without an illness recurrence over 2- to 3-year periods, when maintained on standard dosages (Markar and Mander 1989; Prien et al. 1984; Shapiro et al. 1989; Small et al. 1988). The survival rate increases to 60% over 3 years when higher dosages are prescribed (i.e., those that target serum lithium concentrations of 0.8–1.0 mEq/L), although higher dosages increase the frequency of side effects and the likelihood of withdrawal from maintenance therapy (Gelenberg et al. 1989). Only about 60% of bipolar patients respond to lithium alone (Goodwin and Zis 1979), and about 60% respond to carbamazepine alone (Stromgren and Boller 1985). Thus, the pharmacotherapy of bipolar disorder, although arguably more advanced than the corresponding treatments for any other psychiatric disorder, has limited effectiveness in delaying recurrences over the long-term course of the illness.

Bipolar disorder is often difficult to treat pharmacologically because these patients have high rates of nonadherence to medication. Estimates of the number of patients who discontinue lithium against medical advice are 32%–45% in empirical studies (Jamison et al. 1979; Shaw 1986); however, true rates are suspected to be much higher. Patients give various reasons for discontinuing their medications, such as experiencing negative feelings about having their moods controlled, missing their high periods, and experiencing side effects (Jamison and Akiskal 1983; Jamison et al. 1979). The short- and long-term negative effects of medication nonadherence can be considerable (e.g., Jamison and Akiskal 1983; Post 1993; Strober et al. 1990).

Bipolar disorder also has a host of social and occupational complications that appear only modestly related to its symptomatic manifestations, as noted in Goldberg and Harrow, Chapter 1, and Gitlin and Hammen, Chapter 3, in this volume (see also Coryell et al. 1993; Harrow et al. 1990). For the 6 months after an acute manic or depressive episode, 57% of patients cannot maintain employment, and only 21% work at their expected level of employment, even when they are relatively symptom free and maintained on standard drug regimens (Dion et al. 1988). The likelihood of maintaining employment decreases as the patient's disorder becomes more chronic (Dion et al. 1988). Finally, other types of social dysfunction—such as marital conflict, separation, and divorce—are very high among patients with this disorder (Coryell et al. 1993; Silverstone and Romans-Clarkson 1989).

Thus, significant reasons exist to consider adding a well-planned, carefully conceptualized psychotherapy to the outpatient drug regimen of the recurrently ill bipolar patient. In support of this argument, the National Institute of Mental Health (NIMH) Workshop on the Treatment of Bipolar Disorder (Potter and Prien 1990) listed psychosocial interventions as a key area needing further development in the next decade of research on bipolar disorder. The primary objective of psychosocial interventions with bipolar patients is to address risk factors and associated features of the disorder that are difficult to address with pharmacotherapy alone (i.e., management of life stress, noncompliance, and social-occupational dysfunction).

A Model for Understanding Recurrences of Bipolar Disorder

In order to further understand the assumptions behind current psychotherapies for bipolar disorder, we describe here the bidirectional interplay that may occur between biological vulnerability and psychosocial stress in evoking symptoms of bipolar disorder. Goodwin and Jamison (1990) have articulated an *instability model,* which we have modified (see Figure 4–1) to include specific stress components (i.e., family versus other life stress) and mediating mechanisms (i.e., social rhythm dysregulation) that we believe to be "key players" in the onset of affective episodes. This model has several assumptions.

First, bipolar disorder is a genetically based illness with correlated dysregulations in the production or actions of certain neurotransmitter or neuroendocrine pathways. Second, stressful life events may elicit the expression of these vulnerabilities by disrupting the patient's daily routines, which disrupts circadian rhythms.

A major life event, one of either a positive nature (e.g., getting married) or a negative nature (e.g., losing a job) may act as a *zeitstorer* (Ehlers et al. 1993) that disrupts well-established social, and then circadian, rhythms. Stated differently, major life events can result in the sudden loss of social *zeitgebers* (Ehlers et al. 1988) that maintain the stability of biological or social rhythms (e.g., regular working hours, the consistent presence of family members). Thus, for example, the death of a spouse may precipitate mania through the pathway of changes in social routines (e.g., when one eats, exercises, or socializes), which may disrupt circadian sleep-wake cycles. Data suggest that life event–precipitated disruptions in daily rhythms

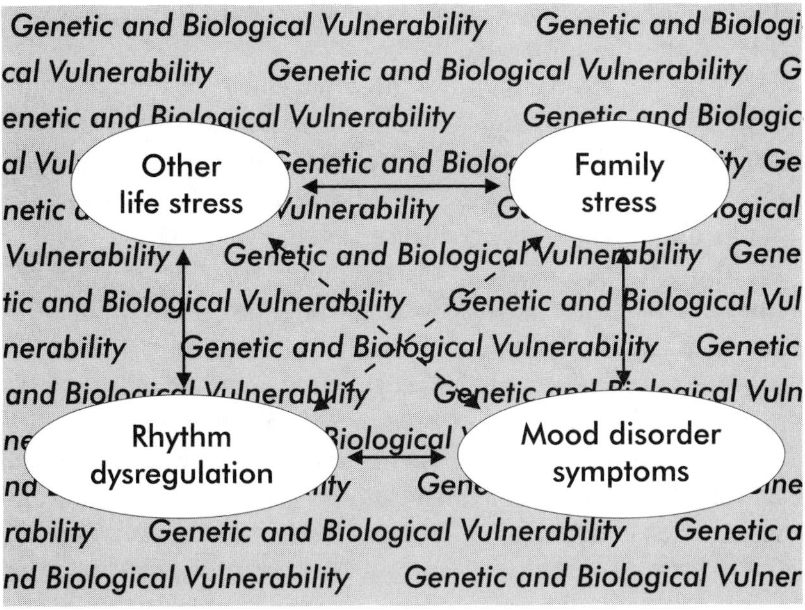

Genetic and Biological Vulnerability   Genetic and Biologi
cal Vulnerability   Genetic and Biological Vulnerability   G
enetic and Biological Vulnerability   Genetic and Biologic
al Vul   **Other**   Genetic and Biolor   **Family**   ity Ge
netic (**life stress**   ulnerability   G   **stress**   ogical
Vulnerability   Genetic and Biological Vulnerability   Gene
tic and Biological Vulnerability   Genetic and Biological Vul
nerability   Genetic and Biological Vulnerability   Genetic
and Biological Vulnerability   Genetic and Biological Vuln
ne   **Rhythm**   Biological   **Mood disorder**
na   **dysregulation**   ity   Gen   **symptoms**   ine
rability   Genetic and Biological Vulnerability   Genetic a
nd Biological Vulnerability   Genetic and Biological Vulner

Figure 4–1. A vulnerability-stress/instability model of bipolar episodes. *Source.* Reprinted from Miklowitz DJ, Goldstein MJ: *Bipolar Disorder: A Family Focused Treatment Approach.* New York, Guilford, 1997. Copyright 1997, Guilford Press. Used with permission.

precede episodes of affective disorder (Ehlers et al. 1993; Johnson and Roberts 1995; Malkoff-Schwartz et al. 1998). Of course, major life events also have significant psychological consequences (i.e., grief, loss of self-esteem) independent of their effects on daily rhythms.

Third, family stress can trigger genetic or biological vulnerabilities to mood disorders when it reaches a certain threshold of psychological aversiveness that patients or family members can no longer tolerate (Miklowitz 1994). Ongoing family stress is suspected to accelerate the onset of manic or depressive recurrences in a vulnerable family member and/or increase the severity of these recurrences. Several studies have found that in short-term follow-ups (9 months to 1 year), high levels of family *expressed emotion* (critical, hostile, and/or emotionally overinvolved attitudes among parents or spouses) predict a greater likelihood of recurrences of bipolar (Miklowitz et al. 1988, 1996; O'Connell et al. 1991; Priebe et al. 1989) and unipolar depressive disorders (Hooley et al. 1986; Vaughn and Leff 1976) among vulnerable patients.

This model predicts that acutely stressful life events, more chronic forms of family stress, and associated social (followed by circadian) rhythm dysregulation serve as additive or interactive *non-specific liability factors* (Fowles 1992) that conjointly contribute to a patient's likelihood of mood disorder recurrences. These stress factors, although not specific to the lives of bipolar patients, operate against the background of disorder-specific genetic and neurophysiological vulnerabilities. Thus, the addition of a psychosocial treatment to a proper pharmacotherapy regimen may provide enhanced protection against recurrences, particularly if the psychosocial treatment 1) helps patients to cope with the destabilizing effects and 2) reduces the aversive effects of the social-familial environment and/or increases its protective effects.

Goals of Psychotherapy With Bipolar Patients

Before describing specific psychosocial approaches, we list the goals that underlie current methods:

1. The therapist, using his or her alliance with the patient, encourages adherence to drug regimens. This may be the most direct benefit of adding psychotherapy to pharmacological maintenance. By educating the patient or the family about bipolar disorder, addressing concerns about side effects, exploring resistances to accepting the illness, determining the symbolic meaning of medication-taking, and addressing worries about the future, the therapist enhances the likelihood of treatment adherence.

2. The therapist attempts to enhance the patient's social and occupational functioning and the patient's capacities to manage stressors within the social-occupational environment. To address these goals, the therapist helps the patient explore ways to cope with stressors in the interpersonal, occupational, or family environment.

3. The therapist attempts to enhance the protective effects of the social-familial environment. As discussed earlier in this chapter,

chronic family stress and acutely stressful life events are associated with an increased likelihood of mood disorder recurrences (for reviews, see Johnson and Roberts 1995; Post 1992; Silverstone and Romans-Clarkson 1989). Psychotherapies can be used to directly modify environmental stress, for example, by training family members to use effective communication strategies to avoid aversive family interactions.

4. Standard pharmacological maintenance approaches often overlook efforts to decrease the trauma associated with the disorder. An episode of mania or depression, particularly one that involves hospitalization, is difficult for the patient and/or family to accept. Fears that the symptoms will recur, intrusive recollections of events leading up to or co-occurring with the episode (e.g., being held in hospital restraints), and emotional numbing can all follow an acute episode, in patients or their family members. Exploring and evaluating emotional reactions to the events that occurred during the illness, providing explanations for treatment decisions made during the episode, and empathizing with and normalizing the patient's or family's post-traumatic stress symptoms can be quite powerful interventions after an index episode.

A Family Psychoeducational Model

Our observation that levels of family expressed emotion (EE) are key predictors of relapses of bipolar disorder over short-term periods of follow-up (Miklowitz et al. 1988), and the voluminous literature linking family EE to relapses of schizophrenia and depression (for a review, see Kavanagh 1992), led us to develop a family psychoeducational treatment for bipolar disorder (Miklowitz and Goldstein 1990, 1997). We were particularly influenced by the work of Falloon and colleagues (1984), who developed a structured, educational, skill-oriented approach to the family treatment of schizophrenia (*behavioral family management*; BFM). Falloon and colleagues tested the efficacy of BFM in relatively chronically ill schizophrenic patients who were randomly assigned to receive either this 9-month, home-based family therapy (in conjunction with a standard phenothiazine regimen) or a supportive, nondirective individual therapy (also in conjunction with phenothiazine). In 9-month and 2-year follow-ups (Falloon et al. 1982, 1985), patients receiving BFM and medication had fewer psychotic relapses; had better social, occupational, and familial relationships; and could be maintained on lower neuroleptic dosages than those receiving individual therapy and medication.

We reasoned that Falloon's psychoeducational approach could be adapted to the specific family problems associated with bipolar disorder, with the objective of modifying family risk factors (e.g., EE) that bode poorly for the disorder's outcome. Our approach—known as the *family-focused treatment* (FFT) of bipolar disorder—consists of four primary assessment and treatment modules (after Falloon et al. 1984; see Table 4–1): initial assessment phase, education about bipolar disorder, communication enhancement training, and training in problem-solving skills.

In our initial pilot study with bipolar patients (Miklowitz and Goldstein 1990), we conducted FFT with nine bipolar patients who had been discharged recently from the hospital after a manic episode and had returned to live with their parents or spouses. Treatment consisted of 21 hour-long sessions spread over 9 months and was generally conducted at the family's residence by two therapists. At the end of the 9-month pilot treatment, only one of the nine (11%) patients had relapsed, a rate that compares favorably with the 61% relapse rate among patients followed up naturalistically over 9 months with aggressively delivered medication (Miklowitz et al. 1988), or the 50% rate over 1 year observed among patients maintained in a carefully administered lithium carbonate protocol (Prien et al. 1984). From this pilot study, we (Miklowitz and Goldstein 1997) developed a manual for FFT, which is currently being used in two controlled experimental trials (see later in this chapter).

Initial Assessment Phase

FFT begins after the patient has begun to symptomatically remit from an acute manic or depressive episode. The first step is to assess thoroughly the functioning of the family or marital unit and the individuals within that unit. The therapist measures each relative's level of EE toward the index patient with the 1–1½ hour, semistructured

Table 4–1. Stages in the family-focused treatment of bipolar disorder

Initial assessment phase

Camberwell Family Interview for expressed emotion

Structured family interactional assessment

Education about bipolar disorder

Signs and symptoms of mania and depression

Variable courses of bipolar disorder

Theories of etiology and the vulnerability-stress model

Rationale for pharmacological and psychosocial treatments

How the family can help

Stigmatization and coping with the illness label

The episode as a trauma for the patient and family

Communication enhancement training

Listening actively

Offering positive feedback

Making positive requests for behavior change

Requesting changes in undesirable behaviors

Problem-solving skills

Defining the problem

"Brainstorming" possible solutions

Evaluating the pros and cons of each proposed solution

Choosing and implementing one or a combination of solutions

Crisis intervention (as needed)

Addressing specific life events

The "relapse drill"

Camberwell Family Interview (Vaughn and Leff 1976), which assesses the relative's emotional reactions to the patient's most recent psychiatric episode. Levels of criticism, hostility, or emotional overinvolvement inform the therapist of the patient's risk for recurrence and of key issues that need to be addressed in the family treatment (e.g., disruptive habits in family members, interpersonal boundaries within the family).

Equally and often more informative are structured 10-minute family interaction "samples" obtained a few weeks after the patient has been discharged from the hospital or has shown partial remission of an acute, nonhospitalized episode. In laboratory-based problem-solving discussions, the family or couple attempts to resolve two current conflicts identified in individual interviews. Through these assessments, the clinician learns a great deal about the family's styles of defining and generating solutions to conflict, the affective tone of their transactions, and the degree to which messages are communicated clearly or unclearly. Various coding systems exist for operationalizing these dimensions of family communication (e.g., the affective style coding system [Doane et al. 1981] or the Category System for Partner Interactions [Hahlweg et al. 1989]). The clinician uses these assessments to determine specific communication or problem-solving skills that need to be enhanced through the treatment. These assessments also often reveal what families do and do not understand about bipolar disorder, which directly informs the educational portion of the treatment.

Education About Bipolar Disorder

Ordinarily, the education module requires about seven sessions. The therapist uses a didactic format to acquaint the patient and his or her parents or spouse with the symptoms of mania and depression, the typical courses of bipolar disorder, and the factors that affect prognosis (e.g., medication nonadherence, severe family conflict, substance abuse). The therapist explains the roles that genetic vulnerability, biochemical imbalances, and stress play in precipitating illness episodes. Finally, the therapist continually emphasizes the importance of regular pharmacotherapy, with associated blood tests and medication-monitoring visits, and the potential benefits of combining psychosocial treatments with drug regimens. Family members are encouraged to maintain a low-stress home atmosphere and to moderate expectations for the patient's immediate adaptation to the workplace and social-familial environment.

Throughout this didactic portion, care is taken not to imply that family members or the patient is to blame for the onset of the disorder. This is done by normalizing family members' reactions to the patient's behavior and by making analogies between bipolar disorder and other biologically based illnesses requiring long-term medical maintenance (e.g., diabetes, hypertension).

An issue that often arises among bipolar patients and their family members is the stigma associated with the mental illness label. Patients with bipolar disorder are often quite high-functioning before the onset of the illness, and it is difficult for them and their significant others to accept that anything of consequence has happened. If they have been hospitalized, patients often recast hospitalization as the cause rather than the response to the episode (e.g., consider the patient who says, "All that happened is I couldn't sleep, so they locked me up"). In FFT, the therapist addresses denial gently but does not challenge it directly. He or she focuses on helping the patient to realize that many important life goals may still be attainable; that many highly intelligent, creative people have led successful lives while coping with this disorder; and that there may be ways to minimize the likelihood of recurrences.

The episode itself has often been a traumatic experience for the patient and family. The therapist encourages the patient to recount his or her hospital experiences and explore feelings about the treatment that was undertaken. The clinician also helps clarify that the family's support of (and, in some cases, initiation of) the hospitalization came out of concern for the patient's welfare rather than hostility, rejection, or abandonment. Finally, the clinician offers standard information about the nature and goals of inpatient care but also empathizes with the feelings of humiliation often experienced by patients and family members during the hospitalization period.

Communication Enhancement Training

The second FFT module, which requires seven or more sessions, involves teaching the family, or couple, skills that enhance communication. The earlier assessment tasks have usually identified qualities of the family's ongoing transaction patterns, but additional data are gleaned from the education portion (e.g., Do family members allow one another to complete sentences? Do discussions often escalate into arguments?). The therapist then acquaints the family with four basic communication skills: 1) listening actively, 2) offering positive feedback, 3) making positive requests for change in another family member's behavior, and 4) expressing negative feelings and requesting changes in undesirable behaviors.

The core therapeutic technique is structured role-playing. Two family members turn their chairs toward each other, and one is appointed the speaker and the other the listener. Family members are then given feedback and coached on effective communication strategies. For example, if one member of a dyad is appointed the listener, he or she is encouraged to keep eye contact, paraphrase the speaker's statements, and ask clarifying questions. Role-playing is usually repeated until a skill is mastered, and participants are then given between-session homework assignments to help them apply these skills outside of the sessions.

We have observed certain communication patterns that distinguish families coping with bipolar disorder from those coping with schizophrenia (Miklowitz et al. 1995). Bipolar patients, whom we found to be much more verbal in family transactions than were schizophrenic patients, often attempt to direct or control stressful family interactions through aggressiveness or assertiveness, frequently refusing to acknowledge the possible validity of family members' statements. These assertive or oppositional styles in bipolar patients are often accompanied by criticism or intrusiveness ("mind reading") from family members, which may engender further opposition from patients. In FFT, role-playing and between-session behavioral rehearsal are encouraged so that family members and patients learn to "call for time out," listen to and paraphrase each others' statements, and request specific changes in each others' behavior that are both feasible to implement and nonthreatening.

Problem-Solving Skills Training

The final module in FFT is the learning of conflict resolution (average of four to five sessions). Families of psychiatric patients often have long-standing, unresolved conflicts that escalate over time. In FFT, the family or couple is taught to identify specific family problems (e.g., housecleaning, cooking, coordinating use of the car) and to take a series of predetermined steps to define these problems and then generate, evaluate, choose, and implement solutions to them. A problem-solving recording sheet that family members complete during these exercises often facilitates and concretizes the process. The therapist again serves as a coach in the problem-solving process and avoids helping to generate or evaluate solutions. Eventually, the family is able to complete these exercises with little outside help.

Crisis Intervention

Throughout the 9 months of FFT, therapists often must depart from the skill-training modules to address specific life events that have occurred between sessions. For example, if a couple is contemplating divorce, the educational agenda is set aside so that issues within the marriage can be addressed. Training in communication and problem-solving skills can be adapted to help participants address these or related issues.

A specific form of crisis intervention is the *relapse drill* (Marlatt and Gordon 1985). When a patient has just been discharged from the hospital (which often coincides with the educational portion of FFT), he or she may show residual symptoms (e.g., hypomania) that, if untreated, could escalate into a full-blown episode. In the family education module, the patient and the family can be taught to identify the signs of an incipient relapse and to take steps to reduce the likelihood of its acceleration (e.g., arranging an emergency medication session with the patient's psychiatrist, having telephone numbers of important support sources available, or becoming acquainted with hospital resources). The format of this drill is very similar to (and is often that family's first exposure to) structured problem-solving.

Common Issues in the Family Treatment of Bipolar Disorder

Table 4–2 lists the core issues that arise in FFT with bipolar patients (see also Goldstein and Miklowitz 1994; Miklowitz and Goldstein 1997). Some of these issues have already been discussed: accepting the illness and the likelihood of future episodes, understanding the roles of medication in long-term maintenance, and restoring functional family relationships after the episode. What may be less obvious from the earlier discussion are two questions: "What role does stress play in the disorder?" and "How do we distinguish between what is the patient's illness and what is the patient's personality?"

Table 4–2.   Core themes in the psychoeducational family treatment of
bipolar disorder

Integration of the mood disorder episode

Acceptance of the vulnerability to future episodes

Dependence on medication for symptom control

Differentiation of personality traits from symptoms of the disorder

Significance of stress as a trigger for recurrences

Reestablishment of functional family relationships after the episode

The first question can be addressed by acquainting the family
with the vulnerability-stress/instability model. Specific examples are
obtained of stressors that appear to have elicited the patient's prior
episodes. Statements such as "You tend to develop symptoms when
work demands are at a maximum or when family conflict is highest"
are of practical use to patients and family members. Emphasis is
placed on the ways that communication and problem-solving skills
can be used in the future to minimize the impact of these stressors.

The second question, distinguishing personality from disorder,
is far more complex. In fact, it is often difficult for clinicians to make
this distinction. The prodromal, residual, or intermorbid subsyndromal periods of the disorder can be almost indistinguishable from
pathological personality traits (e.g., narcissism, impulsivity, dependence). Family members may view certain patient behaviors
(e.g., a downcast look, tearfulness) as signs of an incipient episode,
whereas the patient may angrily counter that these behaviors are his
or her typical ways of coping with life events.

There is no easy answer to this question, although it is helpful
to encourage within the family a discussion of how the patient's
personality appeared before the illness and to show distinctions
and draw similarities between his or her past and current behavior.
Most important, the patient must feel that he or she has a "self" separate from the disorder and that emotions he or she expresses from
here on will not invariably be interpreted by the family or the clinician as signs of a relapse. Appreciation of the patient's interpersonal strengths (e.g., his or her ability to make new friends) often
helps the patient to feel that he or she has not been reduced to a list
of symptoms.

Empirical Studies of the Family-Focused Treatment of Bipolar Disorder

Two randomized, controlled treatment studies are being conducted on the efficacy of FFT for bipolar disorder. One is at the University of California, Los Angeles (UCLA) (Goldstein and Miklowitz 1994), and the other at the University of Colorado, Boulder (Miklowitz et al. 1996). Both sites compare a group receiving 9 months of FFT and standard medication with a group receiving a comparison treatment and medication. In both studies, patients are recruited during an acute, often hospitalized, episode of illness and are followed up for 2 years as outpatients. FFT is delivered in 21 outpatient sessions administered over 9 months in titrated fashion (weekly for 3 months, biweekly for 3 months, monthly for 3 months), either in a clinic or at the family's home.

At the UCLA site, the comparison (no FFT) group receives two sessions of family education and 9 months of individually based patient management, with a patterning and frequency of sessions identical to that administered to the FFT group. Individual patient management consists of sessions with a counselor who offers crisis intervention, support regarding problems in living, and encouragement regarding pharmacological adherence. At the University of Colorado, the comparison treatment group also receives two sessions of family education but otherwise is followed up naturalistically for 9 months, with crisis intervention—delivered on an as-needed basis—and monthly telephone "checkups" but no regular patient management sessions. Other important design differences exist between the two studies, but these differences are beyond the scope of this discussion.

Both trials are in progress and therefore do not yet have data regarding the efficacy of FFT in the symptom management of bipolar disorder. However, we are observing in both studies high rates of "consumer acceptance" of the treatment. Families and patients have been highly compliant with sessions, early terminations have been few, and participants have consistently reported feeling that the work was beneficial (Miklowitz and Goldstein 1997; Miklowitz et al. 1996).

An Individual, Interpersonal Model

The family psychoeducational model has one important limitation: it assumes the availability of significant others. More traditional psychosocial approaches to bipolar disorder have involved individual psychotherapies (Jamison and Goodwin 1983). However, as is the case for family therapy, few studies exist on the efficacy of individual therapy as an adjunct to pharmacological maintenance in bipolar disorder.

Frank et al. (1994) have developed an individual, interpersonal psychotherapy for bipolar patients (*interpersonal and social rhythm therapy*; IP/SRT), which has its bases in two compatible models: the interpersonal psychotherapy of depression (Klerman et al. 1984) and the social rhythm stability hypothesis (Ehlers et al. 1988, 1993). This therapy, currently being evaluated in a controlled trial at the University of Pittsburgh (Frank et al. 1994), is a present-focused interpersonal treatment that views the core deficit in bipolar disorder as one of instability (Goodwin and Jamison 1990). That is, stable mood is hypothesized to be in part a function of the stability of social rhythms (patterns of daily activity and social stimulation) and the effects of this level of stability on biologically based circadian rhythms.

IP/SRT has three key objectives:

1. Patients learn to regulate social rhythms and sleep-wake cycles, as noted earlier in this chapter.
2. Patients learn to understand and renegotiate the interpersonal context associated with the onset of mood disorder symptoms. For example, the patient learns how interpersonal events exacerbate symptoms of mania or depression and how these symptoms affect their social relationships.
3. Patients learn to master conflicts associated with interpersonal loss experiences, disputes, deficits, and role transitions.

IP/SRT is carried out in four primary phases, as summarized in Table 4–3. Treatment duration varies, but after initial weekly sessions, treatment is titrated to biweekly and, then, if a clinical remission continues, to monthly sessions that continue for 2 years (or, outside of the context of a clinical trial, beyond 2 years).

Table 4–3.	Stages in the interpersonal and social rhythm therapy of bipolar disorder

Initial phase

Obtain history of the illness

Educate patient about recurrent affective disorder

Obtain an interpersonal inventory

Initiate the Social Rhythm Metric

Identify an interpersonal problem area

Intermediate and later phases

Develop a symptom management plan:

Search for triggers of social rhythm disruption

Regulate daily social and circadian rhythms

Find a healthy balance between rhythm regularity, activity, stimulation, and mood state

Explore and resolve interpersonal problem areas:

Grief over loss

Grief over the lost healthy self

Interpersonal disputes

Interpersonal deficits

Role transitions

Termination phase

Review treatment progress and areas needing improvement

Help patient cope with future stressors and prevent future episodes

Foster a sense of hope

Initial Phase of IP/SRT

The initial phase can begin while the patient is recovering from an acute episode or during a symptomatic remission. The patient and therapist first collaborate in gathering a thorough history of the illness, with a particular focus on the extent to which episodes may have been precipitated by changes in social and/or circadian rhythms (e.g., manic episodes preceded by transcontinental flights).

With the therapist's empathic guidance, the patient learns about recurrent affective disorder and the possible role of social and circadian rhythm disruption in precipitating his or her episodes. This phase also advances the goals of the patient's pharmacological treatments by identifying episodes that were precipitated by periods of drug nonadherence. Within a supportive therapeutic environment, the patient begins to see the toll the illness has taken on his or her life, which tends to decrease his or her denial about the reality of the disorder.

During this phase, patient takes an *interpersonal inventory*, a survey of the number and quality of relationships in the patient's familial and social network. This survey is central to identifying key interpersonal problem areas and planning the interpersonal interventions undertaken later.

The therapist introduces the patient to the Social Rhythm Metric assignment (Monk et al. 1990, 1991), a self-monitoring chart the patient completes at the end of each day, noting the timing of each of 17 daily activities (e.g., wake time, first contact with another person, meal times, bedtime), whether each occurred alone or with others present, and how stimulating (i.e., quiet versus interactive) these others were. The patient also rates his or her mood each day. As the patient gets more experience with completing the Social Rhythm Metric, he or she begins to see the dynamic interplay among instabilities in daily routines, patterns of social stimulation, sleep-wake times, and mood fluctuations. However, at this early stage of IP/SRT, no attempt is made to alter these daily rhythms.

The final goal of this phase is to identify an interpersonal problem area. The core problem areas—grief over loss, interpersonal disputes, interpersonal deficits, and role transitions—are similar to those described for unipolar-depressed patients (Klerman et al. 1984). However, special interpersonal problems accompany bipolar disorder, for example, "grieving the lost healthy self." This problem is a phenomenon that probably occurs in many debilitating, recurrent disorders but seems especially salient in bipolar disorder (Frank et al. 1994). Bipolar patients often speak of their lives as divided into two periods—before and after the illness began. They express grief reactions over the loss of their prior lifestyles, relationships, and abilities—reactions similar to those they might express about a close relative who had died. In other cases, patients may deny that any change has occurred and will discontinue their medications and attempt to return to their former jobs and relationships, often with disastrous results. As discussed in the next section, IP/SRT often involves allowing the patient to work through his or her grief about lost dreams and aspirations (Frank et al. 1994).

Intermediate and Later Phases of IP/SRT

As IP/SRT progresses, the work focuses on two goals: 1) development of a *symptom management plan*, in which the patient is encouraged to stabilize his or her daily routines, and 2) resolution of the interpersonal problem area(s) identified in the initial phase, with special emphasis on how these problems exacerbate symptoms and/or disrupt social rhythms. The patient continues to complete the Social Rhythm Metric. The therapist and patient search for environmental factors that trigger rhythm disruption (e.g., a waitressing job with constantly shifting work hours), and the patient is educated about the risks associated with rhythm irregularities. Gradually, the patient learns to standardize his or her daily routines and often sees the direct benefit of this regulation on his or her mood.

Some patients complain that stabilizing their daily routines makes their lives less exciting or spontaneous. Bipolar patients seem to crave variety and spontaneity, which may in part account for why they object to having their moods controlled by medication (Jamison et al. 1979). Thus, in IP/SRT, the therapist often helps the patient to find an appropriate balance between sleep and waking, activity and rest, social stimulation and solitude, with their associated mood consequences (Frank et al. 1994).

The intermediate and later phases of IP/SRT involve much work in the interpersonal domain. The patient learns to label problematic interpersonal patterns, to gain insight into how he or she is perceived by others, and to observe the bidirectional relationships between interpersonal distress and changes in mood. If the most recent episode involved grief over a loss, the therapist's task is to encourage a healthy mourning process that can involve exploring the real and symbolic meanings of this loss and the way this loss has changed the patient's life and his or her daily routines. For example, the death of a parent is usually accompanied by intense sadness but also may require changes in employment or residence, which may disrupt social rhythms.

As discussed above, bipolar patients frequently grieve about the person they once were. The therapist must encourage the patient to express painful feelings about lost hopes and aspirations and about the loss of important relationships that may have been central to the patient's preillness social network. However, the therapist expresses optimism about the patient's ability to develop new friendships, renew old ones, and achieve new, although perhaps less ambitious, goals. The patient is dissuaded from discontinuing medication as a way of testing whether the "former self" is still retrievable.

Bipolar patients are frequently involved in interpersonal disputes. Because bipolar patients seem prone to expect a great deal from others and often take somewhat egocentric views of their social relationships, they have frequent, often intense conflicts with others. These disputes can be exacerbated by mood disorder symptoms but also probably play their own role in precipitating or worsening symptomatic states. The IP/SRT therapist guides the patient toward identifying the typical patterns of dispute he or she has with parents, spouses, friends, or co-workers (e.g., often feeling let down, seeing others as withholding) and helps the patient become more tolerant and accepting of others. Sometimes, disputes within the therapeutic relationship can be examined as examples of the kinds of conflicts the patient has with significant others. The patient learns new ways to resolve interpersonal conflicts and to prevent these disputes from occurring in the future.

A minority of bipolar patients isolate themselves socially, sometimes because of interpersonal or social skill deficits but often because they fear the negative evaluations of others. This self-isolation can be particularly acute just after a major episode and appears similar to the *deficit syndrome* often seen in schizophrenia. These patients can be guided toward gradually developing new friendships, appraising relationships in more realistic ways, learning to take risks (e.g., facing possible rejection when attempting to renew a relationship with someone whom they treated badly during a manic episode), and setting goals for increasing the scope of their social and occupational activities. Certain forms of skill training, such as assertiveness techniques, are used sparingly but nevertheless supplement the more exploratory interventions.

Finally, many bipolar patients face role transitions just before or immediately after a major episode. Job loss frequently occurs as the patient begins to cycle into a new episode. These transitions often aggravate the patient's regrets about the perceived loss of his or her former self. Role transitions usually require that the patient develop new, more realistic life goals, adapt to a new lifestyle (e.g., get by on less money), and sometimes develop new friendships or relationships. The mistakes made during the episode (e.g., sexual indiscretions) can often force these transitions (e.g., if a previous lover terminates the relationship). The therapist helps the patient learn to accept the new terms and rules of his or her life, cope with the demands of the new role, and adjust his or her daily routines to adapt to new circumstances.

In exploring these interpersonal problem areas, the therapist continually helps the patient identify ways in which these problems could be avoided in the future. For example, if a patient works at a plant that is expecting layoffs, and he or she has a history of developing new episodes after job changes, the patient can begin to plan how to cope with a new financial situation should that be necessary, how existing friendships can be maintained, and how daily routines can be adapted to the expected change in job status. Likewise, if a patient has experienced problems when relatives visit for extended periods, the patient and the therapist can explore whether an anticipated visit can gracefully be shortened in planned duration and, if not, what strategies the patient can use to reduce or eliminate the disputes that typically arise with relatives during such visits.

Termination of Psychosocial Treatments

The goals of termination sessions in FFT and IP/SRT are quite similar and are discussed conjointly here. As in any therapy, the therapist reviews the progress the patient has made, explores areas with the patient that still need improvement, and helps him or her develop plans for coping with stressors in the future. The prodromal signs of the patient's major episodes are again reviewed, and plans are developed for averting or minimizing the impact of future episodes (e.g., acquainting family members with signs of recurrence or developing plans for obtaining emergency treatment). Most important, the therapist attempts to give the patient a sense of hope and optimism, highlighting the degree of personal control the patient can now muster in managing his or her affective disorder.

Although terminations are necessary in controlled trials of specified duration, a "thinning" of session frequency may be preferred in actual practice. Because bipolar patients are likely to continue pharmacological treatment indefinitely, the idea of continued but less frequent psychosocial treatment may make sense both to patients and to family members. Such ongoing contact enables the therapist to reinforce the continued use of skills and to intervene quickly when prodromal signs appear.

An Empirical Study of IP/SRT

As noted earlier, IP/SRT is being evaluated in a randomized, controlled maintenance trial at the University of Pittsburgh (Frank et al. 1994). This study compares initially manic or depressed bipolar patients receiving IP/SRT and medication with a group receiving drug therapy and a clinical status and symptom review treatment paradigm, the latter administered by the same treatment personnel who conduct IP/SRT. Patients are randomized to one of these two groups during an acute treatment phase and again at the beginning of a long-term maintenance phase.

The Pittsburgh Maintenance Therapies project has demonstrated good rates of subject retention in the IP/SRT group. So far, the program has also determined that patients in IP/SRT can be taught to maintain stability in their daily routines over the course of treatment (Frank 1995). The project will next be able to determine whether maintaining social rhythm stability leads to more sustained remissions of patients' affective disorder and fewer recurrences over the course of a long-term follow-up.

Other Controlled Trials of Psychosocial Treatment

In this chapter, we have focused on randomized experimental trials of only two forms of psychosocial therapy for bipolar disorder. Two other NIMH-funded, carefully designed trials of psychoeducational family or marital interventions are ongoing or have been completed, one at the Brown University School of Medicine (I. Miller and G. Keitner, principal investigators) and one at the Cornell University Medical College (J. Clarkin and I. Glick, principal investigators).

The Brown University trial compares three different groups: a standard medication group; a seven-session psychoeducation plus standard medication group; and a psychoeducation, family therapy, and standard medication group. This study will be able to examine the effects of family therapy over and above those of educating the patient and family about the symptoms and associated features of the disorder. The family therapy is based on the McMaster model, in which clinicians develop individualized treatment plans for families with respect to difficulties in problem solving, communication, affective involvement, affective responsiveness, roles within the family, and behavior control.

The recently completed Cornell University study examines an intervention for married couples in which one spouse has bipolar disorder. This psychoeducational and cogitive-behavioral intervention is used in conjunction with mood-stabilizing medications. Its specific goals are to encourage the spouse and the patient to develop more positive attitudes toward each other; to decrease negative, aversive marital interactions through improved problem solving and communication; and to engage the spouse as an ally in encouraging the patient's medication compliance. Clarkin et al. (1998) found that this psychoeducational intervention, when combined with medication, led to higher global functioning scores and better medication adherence in patients than did medication alone. However, the combined psychoeducational and pharmacological program did not lead to improved symptomatic functioning over medication alone during an 11-month treatment period.

Conclusions and Future Directions

It may strike the reader that the various psychosocial treatments currently being tested for bipolar disorder, although developed and conceptualized quite independently, represent similar conclusions regarding the necessary ingredients of a psychosocial treatment for this disorder. Each treatment is present focused and time limited; each typically begins during or shortly after an acute manic or depressive episode; each is delivered in the context of standard pharmacotherapy; each encourages adherence to drug regimens; each educates the patient (and often the family) about the disorder; and each offers practical techniques for coping with interpersonal, familial, and occupational stressors. Each treatment views episodes of bipolar disorder as traumatic for the patient and the family and gives participants a framework for understanding the disorder and integrating it into their daily living.

None of these treatment models argues that the benefits of psychosocial treatment derive directly from the patient's insight into early childhood events, as was the orientation of many early forms of psychotherapy for bipolar disorder (e.g., Cohen et al. 1954). Equally important, none of these approaches views coping with bipolar disorder as simply requiring the learning of rote skills, in the absence of exploring the meaning of the illness to the patient and his or her significant others.

Many questions still need to be addressed in this area. If psychosocial treatments are indeed found to be efficacious when delivered in combination with standard medications, then by what mechanisms do they operate? Can the effects of psychosocial intervention be attributed solely to their impact on the patient's pharmacological adherence? Do these interventions lead to reductions in levels of stress for the patient or the family? For what patient subpopulations, and under what conditions, is psychosocial treatment effective? At what stage of the disorder? Finally, in this era of managed health care, does the combination of psychotherapy and medication lower service utilization costs?

Bipolar disorder, even when treated carefully with the most modern approaches to pharmacotherapy, can be a quite debilitating illness. New forms of psychotherapy, if found to be effective, would be welcome additions to our standard pharmacological practices for this disorder. It is our hope that this discussion encourages readers to further acquaint themselves with these psychosocial approaches and to consider the applicability of these models to patients under their care.

References

Clarkin JF, Carpenter D, Hull J, et al: Effects of a psychoeducational intervention for married patients with bipolar disorder and their spouses. Psychiatr Serv 49:531–533, 1998

Cohen M, Baker G, Cohen RA, et al: An intensive study of 12 cases of manic-depressive psychosis. Psychiatry 17:103–137, 1954

Coryell W, Scheftner W, Keller M, et al: The enduring psychosocial consequences of mania and depression. Am J Psychiatry 150:720–727, 1993

Dion GL, Tohen M, Anthony WA, et al: Symptoms and functioning of patients with bipolar disorder six months after hospitalization. Hosp Community Psychiatry 39:652–657, 1988

Doane JA, West KL, Goldstein MJ, et al: Parental communication deviance and affective style. Arch Gen Psychiatry 38:679–685, 1981

Ehlers CL, Frank E, Kupfer DJ: Social zeitgebers and biological rhythms: a unified approach to understanding the etiology of depression. Arch Gen Psychiatry 45:948–952, 1988

Ehlers CL, Kupfer DJ, Frank E, et al: Biological rhythms and depression: the role of zeitgebers and zeitstorers. Depression 1:285–293, 1993

Falloon IRH, Boyd JL, McGill CW, et al: Family management in the prevention of exacerbations of schizophrenia: a controlled study. N Engl J Med 306:1437–1440, 1982

Falloon IRH, Boyd JL, McGill CW: Family Care of Schizophrenia. New York, Guilford, 1984

Falloon IRH, Boyd JL, McGill CW, et al: Family management in the prevention of morbidity of schizophrenia. Arch Gen Psychiatry 42:887–896, 1985

Fowles DC: Schizophrenia: diathesis-stress revisited. Annu Rev Psychol 43:303–336, 1992

Frank E: Regularizing social routines in patients with bipolar I disorder. Paper presented at the 34th annual meeting of the American College of Neuropsychopharmacology, San Juan, Puerto Rico, 1995

Frank E, Kupfer DJ, Ehlers CL, et al: Interpersonal and social rhythm therapy for bipolar disorder: integrating interpersonal and behavioral approaches. The Behavior Therapist 17:143–149, 1994

Gelenberg AJ, Kane JM, Keller MB, et al: Comparison of standard and low serum levels of lithium for maintenance treatment of bipolar disorder. N Engl J Med 321:1489–1493, 1989

Gershon ES: Genetics, in Manic-Depressive Illness. Edited by Goodwin FK, Jamison KR. New York, Oxford University Press, 1990, pp 373–401

Goldstein MJ, Miklowitz DJ: Family interventions for persons with bipolar disorder, in New Directions: Interventions With Families of the Mentally Ill. Edited by Hatfield A. San Francisco, CA, Jossey-Bass, 1994, pp 23–35

Goodwin FK, Jamison KR: Manic-Depressive Illness. New York, Oxford University Press, 1990

Goodwin FK, Zis AP: Lithium in the treatment of mania: comparisons with neuroleptics. Arch Gen Psychiatry 36:840–844, 1979

Hahlweg K, Goldstein MJ, Nuechterlein KH, et al: Expressed emotion and patient-relative interaction in families of recent-onset schizophrenics. J Consult Clin Psychol 57:11–18, 1989

Harrow M, Goldberg JF, Grossman LS, et al: Outcome in manic disorders: a naturalistic follow-up study. Arch Gen Psychiatry 47:665–671, 1990

Hirschfeld RMA, Clayton PJ, Cohen I, et al: Practice guideline for treatment of patients with bipolar disorder. Am J Psychiatry 151 (suppl):1–36, 1994

Hooley JM, Orley J, Teasdale JD: Levels of expressed emotion and relapse in depressed patients. Br J Psychiatry 148:642–647, 1986

Jamison KR, Akiskal HS: Medication compliance in patients with bipolar disorder. Psychiatr Clin North Am 6:175–192, 1983

Jamison KR, Goodwin FK: Psychotherapeutic issues in bipolar illness, in Psychiatry Update: The American Psychiatric Association Annual Review, Vol 2. Edited by Grinspoon L. Washington, DC, American Psychiatric Press, 1983, pp 319–345

Jamison KR, Gerner RH, Goodwin FK: Patient attitudes toward lithium. Arch Gen Psychiatry 36:866–869, 1979

Johnson SL, Roberts JE: Life events and bipolar disorder: implications from biological theories. Psychol Bull 117:434–449, 1995

Kavanagh D: Recent developments in expressed emotion in schizophrenia. Br J Psychiatry 160:601–620, 1992

Klerman GL, Weissman MM, Rounsaville BJ, et al: Interpersonal Psychotherapy of Depression. New York, Basic Books, 1984

Malkoff-Schwartz S, Frank E, Anderson E, et al: Stressful life events and social rhythm disruption in the onset of manic and depressive bipolar episodes: a preliminary investigation. Arch Gen Psychiatry 55:702–707, 1998

Markar HR, Mander AJ: Efficacy of lithium prophylaxis in clinical practice. Br J Psychiatry 155:496–500, 1989

Marlatt GA, Gordon JR (eds): Relapse Prevention. New York, Guilford, 1985

Miklowitz DJ: Family risk indicators in schizophrenia. Schizophr Bull 20: 137–149, 1994

Miklowitz DJ, Goldstein MJ: Behavioral family treatment for patients with bipolar affective disorder. Behav Modif 14:457–489, 1990

Miklowitz DJ, Goldstein MJ: Bipolar Disorder: A Family Focused Treatment Approach. New York, Guilford, 1997

Miklowitz DJ, Goldstein MJ, Nuechterlein KH, et al: Family factors and the course of bipolar affective disorder. Arch Gen Psychiatry 45:225–231, 1988

Miklowitz DJ, Goldstein MJ, Nuechterlein KH: Verbal interactions in the families of schizophrenic and bipolar affective patients. J Abnorm Psychol 104:268–276, 1995

Miklowitz DJ, Simoneau TL, Sachs-Ericsson N, et al: Family risk indicators in the course of bipolar affective disorder, in Interpersonal Factors in the Origin and Course of Affective Disorders. Edited by Mundt C, Goldstein MJ, Hahlweg K, et al. London, Gaskell Books, 1996, pp 204–217

Miklowitz DJ, Frank E, George EL: New psychosocial treatments for the outpatient management of bipolar disorder. Psychopharmacol Bull 32:613–621, 1996

Monk TH, Flaherty JF, Frank E, et al: The Social Rhythm Metric: an instrument to quantify daily rhythms of life. J Nerv Ment Dis 178:120–126, 1990

Monk TH, Kupfer DJ, Frank E, et al: The Social Rhythm Metric (SRM): measuring daily social rhythms over 12 weeks. Psychiatry Res 36:195–207, 1991

O'Connell RA, Mayo JA, Flatow L, et al: Outcome of bipolar disorder on long-term treatment with lithium. Br J Psychiatry 159:123–129, 1991

Post RM: Transduction of psychosocial stress into the neurobiology of recurrent affective disorder. Am J Psychiatry 149:999–1010, 1992

Post RM: Issues in the long-term management of bipolar affective illness. Psychiatric Annals 23:86–93, 1993

Potter WZ, Prien RF: Report from the NIMH Workshop on the Treatment of Bipolar Disorder. Rockville, MD, NIMH Division of Clinical Research, 1990

Priebe S, Wildgrube C, Muller-Oerlinghausen B: Lithium prophylaxis and expressed emotion. Br J Psychiatry 154:396–399, 1989

Prien RF, Kupfer DJ, Mansky PA, et al: Drug therapy in the prevention of recurrences in unipolar and bipolar affective disorders. Arch Gen Psychiatry 41:1096–1104, 1984

Shapiro DR, Quitkin FM, Fleiss JL: Response to maintenance therapy in bipolar illness. Arch Gen Psychiatry 46:401–405, 1989

Shaw E: Lithium noncompliance. Psychiatric Annals 16:583–587, 1986

Silverstone T, Romans-Clarkson A: Bipolar affective disorder: causes and prevention of relapse. Br J Psychiatry 154:321–335, 1989

Small JG, Klapper MH, Kellams JJ, et al: Electroconvulsive treatment compared with lithium in the management of manic states. Arch Gen Psychiatry 45:727–732, 1988

Strober AM, Morrell W, Lampbert C, et al: Relapse following discontinuation of lithium maintenance therapy in adolescents with bipolar I illness: a naturalistic study. Am J Psychiatry 147:457–461, 1990

Stromgren LS, Boller S: Carbamazepine in treatment and prophylaxis of manic-depressive disorder. Psychiatric Developments 4:349–367, 1985

Vaughn CE, Leff JP: The influence of family and social factors on the course of psychiatric illness. Br J Psychiatry 129:125–137, 1976

CHAPTER 5

Long-Term Outcome of Anticonvulsants in Affective Disorders

Robert M. Post, M.D.
Kirk D. Denicoff, M.D.
Mark A. Frye, M.D.
Gabriele S. Leverich, M.S.W.
Gabriela Cora-Locatelli, M.D.
Timothy A. Kimbrell, M.D.

*L*ithium therapy, even when used with adjunctive unimodal antimanic and antidepressant medication, is often inadequate in the long-term treatment of bipolar disorder. Naturalistic outcome studies (such as those described in Goldberg and Harrow, Chapter 1; Maj, Chapter 2; and Gitlin and Hammen, Chapter 3, of this volume) have led to an accelerated search for mood-stabilizing alternatives to lithium. Naturalistic follow-up studies of clinic populations have shown that bipolar disorder often recurs despite attempts to optimize lithium prophylaxis, and in a small percentage of patients, lithium loses its efficacy on long-term follow-up (Kukopulos et al. 1995; Maj et al. 1989; Post et al. 1993a). Patients who have bipolar disorder have a generally poorer prognosis than was previously thought, as preceding chapters of this volume indicate. Patients who were hospitalized for mania during adolescence and followed up until age 30 showed an extremely poor outcome; the effect of the illness was similar to that of schizophrenia and was substantially worse than for patients hospitalized with recurrent unipolar illness (Gillberg et al. 1993). These findings represent a prognosis significantly different than previously reported (Werry et al. 1991).

Although a variety of bipolar disorder subtypes and comorbidities are associated with a relatively poor response to lithium, either acutely or in initial prophylaxis (Post 1990a), we focus here on factors associated with loss of responsiveness to lithium during long-term maintenance treatment. The subtypes often associated with a relatively poor response to lithium prophylaxis include those patients with dysphoric mania, comorbid substance abuse, the episode pattern of depression-mania-well (intermorbid) interval (D-M-I) as opposed to the M-D-I sequence, or a negative family history for bipolar illness in first-degree relatives. However, even in patients initially responsive to lithium, two routes to nonresponsiveness exist: lithium efficacy loss via tolerance during long-term treatment and lithium discontinuation-induced refractoriness.

Lithium Efficacy Loss Via Tolerance During Long-Term Treatment

Maj et al. (1989) (see also Maj, Chapter 2, in this volume) reported breakthrough episodes in a substantial proportion of patients after 2 years of lithium treatment, even though these patients were initially completely responsive and in remission. Maj and colleagues observed isolated or periodic breakthrough episodes in these patients during 5 additional years of follow-up. These findings parallel our own retrospective life chart data in lithium nonresponders, indicating that 23 of 66 patients (34.8%) apparently became tolerant to the long-term effects of lithium during prophylaxis (Post et al. 1993b). Kukopulos et al. (1995) reported that 11 of 129 patients (8.5%) responded poorly to lithium, apparently as a result of tolerance. We stress these findings because parallel findings are beginning to emerge in studies of the anticonvulsants, as we note later in this chapter.

Lithium Discontinuation-Induced Refractoriness

In addition to this pattern of progressive efficacy loss during sustained and compliant lithium pharmacotherapy, another pattern has emerged called *lithium discontinuation-induced refractoriness*. We and others have observed a series of patients who showed sustained long-term prophylactic response to lithium, discontinued the drug, experienced a relapse, and then failed to re-respond to treatment reinstitution (Kukopulos et al. 1995; Post et al. 1992, 1993b). Baldessarini (1996) also found that patients responded significantly more poorly when lithium treatment was reinstituted after a period of discontinuation; the percentage of time spent ill while taking lithium increased from 18.9% ± 21.9% to 26.1 ± 24.1%. The reanalysis of these data no longer revealed a significant difference on this measure, but the need for neuroleptics was increased significantly.

These data may be interpreted from several perspectives. Most intriguing and disturbing is the possibility that additional episodes of affective illness propel the neurobiological mechanisms driving the illness to a new stage (Post 1992; Post and Weiss 1995) that is no longer responsive to lithium. This perspective converges with data indicating that the greater the number of episodes or the more illness morbidity that occurs before lithium prophylaxis begins, the greater the likelihood of lithium nonresponsiveness (Denicoff et al. 1997; Gelenberg et al. 1989; O'Connell et al. 1991; Sarantidis and Waters 1981; Swann et al. 1997). Thus, additional episodes during the lithium-discontinuation phase might provide greater illness burden and change the patient's long-term responsiveness to lithium. Recently, Coryell et al. (1998) reported that they observed no evidence of a lithium discontinuation–related refractoriness, although their study was confounded by the presence of unconfirmed lithium responders and a sample size not able to detect rare events or ones that might occur in only 5%–10% of the responsive population.

Anticonvulsant Mood Stabilizers

Carbamazepine and valproate are the best studied of the mood-stabilizing anticonvulsants. They are now widely accepted as adjuncts or alternatives to lithium in the treatment of bipolar disorder. The dihydropyridine L-type calcium channel blockers (CCBs) have an interesting potential anticonvulsant profile, and initial reports suggest they may also have some efficacy in the treatment and prevention of rapid fluctuations in manic and depressive moods and behavior. The high-potency anticonvulsant benzodiazepines clonazepam and lorazepam are widely used adjuncts in clinical practice. Lamotrigine and gabapentin, two anticonvulsants recently approved by the U.S. Food and Drug Administration (FDA) for adjunctive use in the treatment of epilepsy, have novel mechanisms of action and promising psychotropic profiles in preliminary studies.

Carbamazepine (Tegretol)

Considerable evidence supports carbamazepine's acute antimanic efficacy, including 19 double-blind studies of various designs (Post et al. 1996). These studies suggest that carbamazepine has approximately equal incidence, magnitude, and time course of clinical response compared with typical neuroleptics, and several studies suggest that carbamazepine is better tolerated. The acute antidepressant efficacy of carbamazepine is not as well established, although studies suggest that some patients who have treatment-refractory unipolar or bipolar affective disorders may show both acute and long-term prophylactic response (Coxhead et al. 1992; Dilsaver et al. 1996; Okuma et al. 1981; Post et al. 1986, 1997).

Most of the double-blind, placebo-controlled randomized comparison studies of carbamazepine in long-term prophylaxis have been criticized on methodological grounds (Prien and Gelenberg 1989), but taken together with a series of 14 studies (Post et al. 1996) and with the use of on-off-on trials and mirror-image designs, these comparison studies strongly support carbamazepine's prophylactic efficacy. Three large-scale randomized studies reported equal efficacy of lithium and carbamazepine (Greil et al. 1997a, 1997b; Wolf et al. 1997), although one found lithium better for those with euphoric mania and carbamazepine better for those with atypical presentations such as schizoaffective depression. Carbamazepine appears to be effective in the prevention of manic and depressive episodes in a subgroup of patients who took the drug alone and in another subgroup of patients with rapid-cycling bipolar disorder who took the drug in combination with lithium (Denicoff et al. 1997; Kishimoto 1992; Kramlinger and Post 1989; Okuma 1993).

However, another subgroup of patients showed a gradual loss of responsiveness to carbamazepine (Figure 5–1) and an increasing severity of episodes in a pattern similar to that observed in tolerance to lithium (Post 1990a, 1990b) and valproate (Post et al. 1993a) (Figure 5–2). We observed efficacy loss after an average of 2.8 years of prophylaxis in 45% of the responsive patients in a cohort of severely ill patients who were followed up for an average of 6.9 years (G. S. Leverich, R. M. Post, M. A. Frye, T. A. Kimbrell, K. Noe, unpublished data, 1998). Whether the same high incidence of efficacy loss via tolerance would be observed in patients who had less severe and refractory illness from the outset (i.e., those not referred to the National Institute of Mental Health, where we made these observations) remains to be determined. Indirect evidence, from a preclinical model of tolerance to the anticonvulsant effects of carbamazepine on amygdala-kindled seizures, suggests that loss of illness-driven compensatory adaptations might account in part for tolerance development and that switching to drugs with different mechanisms of action or retrying the same drug later may be worthwhile (Post and Weiss 1995; Weiss et al. 1995a).

The pharmacokinetics of carbamazepine are of considerable interest in relation to its multiple drug interactions. As in epilepsy, no distinct relation exists between carbamazepine blood levels and the degree of clinical response, although the blood level range of 4–12 µg/mL is most often associated with success and a minimum of side effects. However, individual titration of the dose to minimize side effects and maximize efficacy is the key to successful use of the drug, as wide individual differences exist in the doses and blood levels at which patients experience side effects (Tomson 1984). Because carbamazepine induces hepatic enzymes of the cytochrome P450 3A4 variety, agents that interfere with this process can be associated with marked increases in carbamazepine blood levels; and if a patient is near the side-effect threshold, side effects could emerge (Ketter and Post 1994; Ketter et al. 1995b, 1996). These agents include erythromycin and its antibiotic congeners, the CCBs verapamil and diltiazem (but not nimodipine, nifedipine, or isradipine),

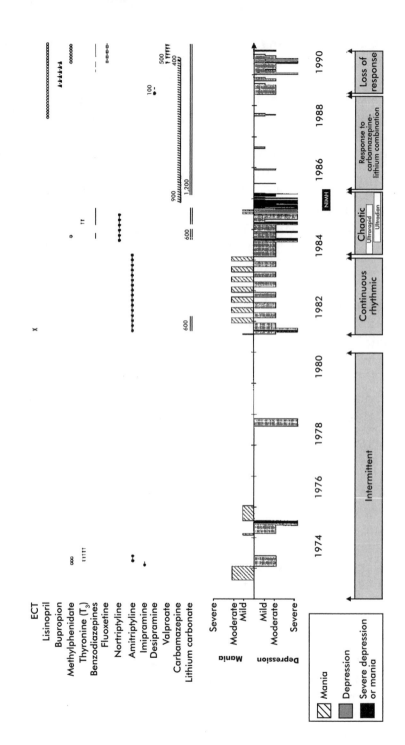

acetazolamide, propoxyphene (Darvon), the monoamine oxidase inhibitor isoniazid (but not phenelzine or tranylcypromine), fluvoxamine, and fluoxetine (see Ketter and Post 1994).

When carbamazepine is used in combination with valproate, the carbamazepine dosage often needs to be reduced because valproate displaces carbamazepine from binding sites, which increases free levels. It blocks the breakdown of the active 10,11-epoxide to an inactive diol metabolite, leading to a buildup of the active 10,11-epoxide that is not usually detectable in traditional plasma-level monitoring (Ketter and Post 1994).

Carbamazepine decreases the blood levels of a variety of compounds including haloperidol, bupropion, dicumarol, warfarin, and theophylline. Carbamazepine decreases the levels (and hence the efficacy) of birth control pills, a major concern necessitating the use of higher-dosage forms or alternative contraceptive techniques. Although carbamazepine markedly decreases the level of bupropion itself, it increases the levels of its hydroxy metabolite (Ketter et al. 1995a). Because bupropion is thought to have some antidepressant activity, monitoring levels of bupropion itself during carbamazepine treatment is not clinically worthwhile. Carbamazepine induces the metabolism of dexamethasone and increases free cortisol excretion. It thus invalidates the dexamethasone suppression test, because its use is associated with a high degree of false-positive escape

---

Figure 5–1 (see previous page). Phases in illness evolution and treatment response in a woman with bipolar II disorder. Life chart depicts clinical response to multiple treatment interventions with psychotropic agents, including anticonvulsants. Treatment with amitriptyline appears to have induced a clear pattern of rapid cycling, which progressed to ultrarapid (ultradian) cycling during subsequent treatment with nortriptyline. Lithium carbonate (600 mg/day) was of no apparent efficacy until augmentation was begun with carbamazepine (900 mg/day). Augmentation led to a complete resolution of hypomanic periods for more than 1 year, followed ultimately by a loss of response (increasing periods of breakthrough depression), presumably reflecting tolerance to carbamazepine. ECT = electroconvulsive therapy; NIMH = National Institute of Mental Health.

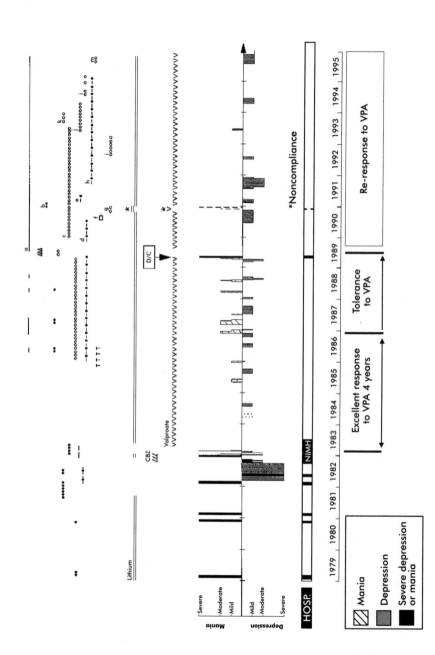

from dexamethasone suppression (Rubinow et al. 1984, 1986). However, Cora-Locatelli et al. (1996) suggested that the degree of escape from dexamethasone both before and during carbamazepine administration is correlated with severity of depression in women but not in men.

Valproate (Depakote)

Valproate and its enteric-coated divalproex sodium formulation (Depakote) are effective in the treatment of acute mania and have been approved by the FDA for this indication. This approval was based on a series of double-blind studies indicating significant antimanic effects of valproate over placebo at a magnitude approximately equal to lithium (Bowden et al. 1994; Emrich et al. 1980; Freeman et al. 1992; Pope et al. 1991; Post 1989). However, only 50% of the patients in Bowden et al.'s (1994) intend-to-treat analysis showed 50% improvement in their manic symptoms by the end of 3 weeks, again attesting to the relative inadequacy of either lithium or valproate in monotherapy for the treatment of acute mania.

Virtually no controlled studies have examined the use of valproate in the treatment of acute depression. However, several open-label trials have compared valproate with lithium in long-term prophylaxis, and the largest of these studies ($n = 121$ bipolar and 29 unipolar subjects) found approximately equivalent results (Lambert and Venaud 1992). A recent placebo-controlled study of val-

---

Figure 5–2 (see previous page). Tolerance and re-response to prophylactic effects of valproate (VPA) in a patient with bipolar I disorder. Lithium monotherapy was only partially effective in preventing recurrent episodes. After a brief and ineffectual trial of carbamazepine (CBZ), significant improvement was noted with valproate plus lithium for approximately 2 years. Breakthrough manic and depressive symptoms developed with increasing intensity, despite augmentation with fluoxetine and benzodiazepines. Valproate was discontinued temporarily and resumed after several months with an observed re-response of antimanic properties. Episodes of depression persisted, however, despite additional augmentation strategies.
NIMH = National Institute of Mental Health.

proate in long-term prophylaxis was associated with a relatively high attrition rate prior to study entry and an equivocal preventive effect of valproate in recurrent manic episodes (Bowden 1997). However, patients appeared to have fewer depressive recurrences, and remarkably, patients taking lithium experienced more episodes of depression compared with those patients taking the placebo (Bowden 1996).

Many patients with rapid-cycling bipolar disorder experience suppression or amelioration of manic and depressive recurrences during long-term treatment with valproate (Calabrese et al. 1992, 1993, 1994; Emrich et al. 1984; McElroy et al. 1988a, 1988b, 1992; Post 1990a; Post et al. 1996; Schaff et al. 1993). The drug is now widely used for prophylaxis, particularly in patients who do not respond adequately to lithium carbonate (Hirschfeld et al. 1994).

Bowden et al. (1996) proposed a relation between antimanic response and valproate blood levels within the range of 45–125 µg/mL. Jacobsen (1993) reported that patients with cyclothymic or mild bipolar II disorder might achieve therapeutic responses with lower valproate doses and blood levels, whereas patients with a more severe form of the illness required higher doses and blood levels. These observations are partially convergent with those of Bowden et al. (1996), indicating a better acute antimanic response in those patients having valproate blood levels greater than 45 µg/mL in the first week of treatment. Keck et al. (1993) suggested that loading doses of valproate (as divalproex sodium) can be achieved rapidly with minimal side effects in the treatment of acute mania. These investigators administered a 20 mg/kg dose of valproate on day 1. Whether this loading-dose strategy substantially decreases the time to remission remains to be determined, but preliminary analysis suggests that a considerable lag remains in the time course to full antimanic efficacy.

Unlike several other anticonvulsants, such as carbamazepine, phenytoin, and phenobarbital, valproate does not appear to yield clinically significant induction of hepatic metabolism of other drugs. In fact, valproate appears to be a weak enzyme inhibitor, but this weakness does not appear to cause many clinically significant drug interactions. An important exception is that valproate inhibition of epoxide hydrolase (Kerr et al. 1989) can yield increases in plasma carbamazepine-10,11-epoxide, which can cause increased therapeutic and toxic effects (Ramsay et al. 1990; Robbins et al. 1990). This effect, combined with increases in free carbamazepine and free carbamazepine-epoxide resulting from displacement from binding sites by valproate, can result in clinical neurotoxicity during carbamazepine plus valproate combination therapy, despite apparent therapeutic carbamazepine levels.

High-Potency Anticonvulsant Benzodiazepines as Adjunctive Treatments

In contrast to alprazolam, which has been associated with the induction of mania and cycling in several case studies (Arana et al. 1985), the anticonvulsant benzodiazepines clonazepam and lorazepam are now used widely as adjunctive treatments for insomnia and agitation associated with breakthrough manic or depressive episodes. The use of these agents as adjuncts is based on a database of controlled or partially controlled studies (Bradwejn et al. 1990; Busch et al. 1989; Chouinard et al. 1983, 1993; Edwards et al. 1991; Lenox et al. 1992), wide clinical experience, and the relative safety and better side-effects profiles of these agents compared with the neuroleptics. Many of the studies are confounded by the use of concomitant neuroleptics, but several studies indicate the utility of these agents. Kishimoto et al.'s (1988) open study reported an 84% moderate-to-marked improvement with clonazepam in 27 patients who had either unipolar major depression ($n = 18$) or bipolar depression ($n = 9$) but also reported a high incidence of efficacy loss via tolerance.

Unfortunately, no controlled studies have examined the use of clonazepam and lorazepam in long-term prophylaxis of bipolar disorder, although Sachs et al. (1990) and others suggested that these agents might be useful as adjunctive regimens in long-term treatment. Further controlled studies in this area are warranted.

Anticonvulsant Calcium Channel Blockers

A large clinical and preclinical database suggests that different types of CCBs can exert anticonvulsant effects in different seizure types and animal models. Increased serum calcium levels are detectable when a patient switches into mania (Carman et al. 1979). This observation has prompted the use of calcitonin to decrease serum calcium, leading to longer cycle intervals and less severe agitation (Carman et al. 1984). Although CCBs are not traditional anticonvulsants, they may exert their influence by mechanisms relevant to the action of some anticonvulsants.

The most widely used phenylalkylamine L-type CCB, verapamil, has a profile quite different from that of the dihydropyridine L-type CCBs, which in many instances appear to exert anticonvulsant and behavioral effects not shared by verapamil (Post et al., in press a). For example, the dihydropyridine CCBs can block cocaine-induced hyperactivity and the associated increase in dopamine overflow in the nucleus accumbens, whereas verapamil does not have this effect (Pani et al. 1990).

These data are interesting in light of the relatively poor efficacy of verapamil in the treatment of depression (Hoschl and Kozeny 1989) and its inadequacy in prophylaxis. In contrast, several double-blind, controlled studies suggest verapamil's efficacy in the treatment of acute mania (Dubovsky et al. 1986; Garza-Treviño et al. 1992), although findings have not been consistent across studies (Janicak et al. 1998).

The dihydropyridine L-type CCBs such as nimodipine appear to be more promising as mood stabilizers than are the phenylalkylamine L-type CCBs. Several controlled and open studies report mood stabilization with nimodipine in patients unresponsive to verapamil (Goodnick 1995; Manna 1991; McDermut et al. 1995; Pazzaglia et al. 1993). These data, taken with the preclinical studies we noted earlier in this chapter, suggest that differential efficacy may exist among the CCBs depending on whether they are used as antidepressants or as mood stabilizers.

A subgroup of patients with rapid and ultrarapid (ultradian)-cycling bipolar disorder did respond to nimodipine (Pazzaglia et al. 1993). This observation was reconfirmed in a double-blind study with a B-A-B-A (placebo-active-placebo-active) design (McDermut et al. 1995). Although approximately one-third of the first 30 patients who had refractory affective illness responded to nimodipine in monotherapy, many required another mood stabilizer such as carbamazepine in combination for a more complete response (Pazzaglia et al., in press).

These observations are interesting from the perspective that nimodipine blocks calcium influx through L-type calcium channels, whereas carbamazepine blocks calcium influx through N-methyl-D-aspartate (NMDA) receptors (Hough et al. 1996). As calcium entry via these channels could be additive and is discretely encoded at the level of gene transcription, it provides a basis for considering how putative increased intracellular calcium, noted in most studies of blood elements of patients with affective disorders, could be normalized by actions of two separate calcium entry points (Post et al., in press a).

Lamotrigine (Lamictal)

Initial add-on trials with lamotrigine, a newly approved anticonvulsant adjunct, reported that the drug had positive effects on mood and behavior and provided a sense of well-being in patients with refractory epilepsy. These observations led to several case reports (Fogelson and Sternbach 1997; Weisler et al. 1994) and a larger open study by Calabrese et al. (1996), which found evidence of a substantial degree of mood improvement in approximately 70% of patients when lamotrigine was used adjunctively or, in some cases, in monotherapy. Lamotrigine has also shown promise in open reports of depressed patients who have treatment-resistant bipolar disorder (Labbate and Rubey 1997; Sporn and Sachs 1997) and in at least one case series of rapid cycling (Fatemi et al. 1997).

Frye and associates (1998) have mirrored these findings in their preliminary analysis of the first 33 patients to enter a double-blind randomized trial comparing lamotrigine versus gabapentin versus placebo. Seventeen of these patients showed a good response to lamotrigine, having a moderate-to-marked degree of improvement on the revised version of the Clinical Global Impressions Scale for Bipolar Disorder (CGI-BP; Spearing et al. 1997). Most of these patients had failed multiple mood-stabilizer trials, in which drugs were used both in monotherapy and in combination before the clinical trial, suggesting that lamotrigine may have an added spectrum of action compared with some of the more widely used agents.

Interestingly, lamotrigine is reported to decrease the release of excitatory amino acids (Messenheimer 1995), although Waldmeier et al. (1995) have questioned whether this is the mechanism of action of lamotrigine. These investigators observed that although lamotrigine blocked sodium- and tetrodotoxin-induced release of excitatory amino acids at clinically relevant concentrations, it failed to do so in response to the more physiologically relevant electrically stimulated release of these amino acids. Moreover, carbamazepine and oxcarbazepine also exhibit these actions.

Thus, to the extent that lamotrigine appears to have differential and enhanced efficacy in treating some patients who have refractory epilepsy and, potentially, in treating patients who have refractory affective disorders (based on the highly preliminary data we noted earlier in this chapter), it might be more promising to look for novel mechanisms of action of this compound compared with traditional agents. Lamotrigine's reported effects on sodium influx might be pertinent to its actions in either epilepsy or affective disorders. Whether these actions are different from those of carbamazepine and phenytoin, which are potent in inducing a frequency- and use-dependent blockade of sodium channels (Schwarz and Grigat 1989; Willow et al. 1984), is unknown.

Gabapentin (Neurontin)

Gabapentin was recently approved by the FDA as an adjunct for the treatment of epilepsy. Gabapentin's mechanism of action is unknown, although it is a potent inhibitor of amino acid transport (Beydoun et al. 1995), and it appears to increase γ-aminobutyric acid (GABA) levels in the brain. However, even though gabapentin is a congener of GABA, it is not active at GABA receptors. Only preliminary reports support gabapentin's mood-stabilizing effect (Bennett et al. 1997; McElroy et al. 1997; Ryback et al. 1997; Schaffer and Schaffer 1997; Stanton et al. 1997; Young et al. 1997); however, a variety of gabapentin's properties make it of great potential interest for treatment of bipolar disorder. Dimond et al. (1996) reported positive effects on mood and well-being in patients who had epilepsy, and the drug appears to be effective against anxiety and insomnia in patients who have bipolar disorder, particularly when used as an adjunct to previously ineffective regimens.

The double-blind study of Frye et al. (1998) found that gabapentin monotherapy did not outperform placebo in a 6-week trial in refractory affective patients. Preliminary evidence indicates that gabapentin has no significant effect on lithium pharmacokinetics (Frye 1996). Gabapentin is not metabolized in the liver in humans and is excreted in the urine. This property, along with its lack of protein binding and effects on hepatic isoenzymes, makes it readily usable in combination with a variety of psychotropic and other anticonvulsant medications. Virtually no drug interactions are associated with gabapentin, in contrast to many of the other anticonvulsants. Also, gabapentin inhibits its own transport uptake into cells in high doses, so patients are relatively unlikely to overdose on it. However, because of this effect and its relatively short half-life, the drug appears to require three-times-daily administration rather than a single dose at bedtime.

Other Anticonvulsants

Mysoline. Mysoline has a useful adjunctive effect when given to patients who have treatment-refractory bipolar disorder (Hayes 1993). This finding is of considerable clinical interest and deserves follow-up in light of mysoline's effects on absence seizures and the potential involvement of novel mechanisms in this seizure type. Valproate, clonazepam, ethosuximide, and lamotrigine have been reported to have efficacy against absence seizures, whereas carbamazepine may exacerbate this seizure type in some individuals. Again, these data highlight the potential differential responsivity among patients who have different pathophysiologies and rhythmic subtypes in the seizure disorders and possibly in the affective disorders.

Phenytoin. Although claims of the efficacy of phenytoin in the treatment of depressive illness were widespread (Dreyfus 1981), few systematic studies supported these claims. However, one schizoaffective patient involved in a repeated on-off-on-off trial was responsive specifically to phenytoin (Freyhan 1995).

Felbamate. Felbamate has been approved by the FDA for use in the treatment of refractory epilepsy. This drug's unique profile of efficacy and side effects might be of considerable interest to patients who have affective disorders. However, the manufacturer of fel-bamate and the FDA have delimited the use of this agent to highly selective patient populations and instances of refractoriness, as a series of potentially lethal hematological and allergic side effects emerged during postmarketing surveillance.

Felbamate, as a glutamate antagonist–like compound, appears to have properties similar to the stimulants in terms of activation and side effects such as insomnia and weight loss. Felbamate is unlikely to receive wide clinical testing in the treatment of bipolar depression because of its potentially serious side effects. However, it might be considered a prototype drug so that other glutamate antagonists, perhaps with more favorable idiosyncratic side-effect profiles, might be tested in patients who have symptoms of atypical depression or bipolar disorder, including hypersomnia, carbohydrate craving, and decreased energy.

Endogenous Anticonvulsant Neuropeptides: Potential Implications for Pathophysiology and Treatment

A variety of neuropeptides, including thyrotropin-releasing hormone (TRH), cholecystokinin (CCK), and somatostatin, appear to have prominent anticonvulsant effects in animal model systems. TRH is the best studied of these neuropeptides. It showed promising initial results in a series of clinical trials attempting to enhance antidepressant effects (Kastin et al. 1972; Prange et al. 1972) but did not demonstrate benefits over placebo in subsequent studies (Benkert et al. 1974; Kiely et al. 1976; Mountjoy et al. 1974). However, this result may have been related to the administration paradigm (i.e., dose and patterning) or to tolerance development (Bassiri and Utiger 1973; Brooks et al. 1988).

Antidepressant Effect of Thyrotropin-Releasing Hormone

We reexplored the anticonvulsant effects of TRH by administering intrathecal TRH to eight patients who had treatment-refractory depression and then comparing the results with those associated with a sham infusion lumbar puncture procedure. We observed significant improvement in patients who received active TRH (500 μg) compared with placebo, in some cases resulting in dramatic but transient improvement in mood, anxiety, depression, and a subjective sense of cognitive clearing (Marangell et al. 1997). Two of the best intrathecal responders received intravenous or subcutaneous parenteral administration (500 μg) on a regular basis in an attempt to convert these acute challenge responses to more long-term therapeutic regimens (Callahan et al. 1997). These intractably ill patients improved for approximately 1 month before efficacy loss gradually emerged and tolerance appeared to develop. Whether a more long-term clinical response could be achieved with other dose regimens in less refractory patients is unknown.

The observation that parenteral and intrathecal TRH can exert acute and rapid-onset antidepressant effects suggests that TRH hypersecretion in some depressed patients (Banki et al. 1988; Kirkegaard et al. 1979) might be an endogenous compensatory adaptation rather than a part of the primary pathophysiology of depression (Post and Weiss 1992, 1996). These data raise the possibility that not only could therapeutic approaches to depression interfere with pathological processes, but some positive adaptive mechanisms such as the putative increases in TRH could be enhanced for therapeutics. Carbamazepine significantly increases TRH in the cerebrospinal fluid of patients who have affective disorders (Marangell et al. 1994). Whether this observation reflects events in the brain and/or is related to carbamazepine's mechanism of action in affective disorders or epilepsy is unknown. Together, these data suggest that TRH administration, either via the appropriate route of administration or indirectly via pharmacological manipulation, might eventually play a role in the acute treatment of affective disorders. Even if TRH is not useful in this way, this approach represents a potential paradigm for the manipulation of other putative adaptive neuropeptides for therapeutic purposes.

Tolerance Mechanisms

In the animal model of tolerance to the anticonvulsant effects of carbamazepine on amygdala-kindled seizures, the state of tolerance achieved was associated specifically with the failure of some putative positive seizure-induced adaptations to occur (Weiss et al. 1995a), including the normally seizure-induced increases in TRH and GABA$_A$ receptors. In the tolerant state, full-blown seizures broke through drug treatment, yet they selectively failed to induce some of the expected compensatory adaptations. Whether this result is related directly to the loss of carbamazepine efficacy is unknown, although this possibility is more probable considering the *time-off seizure effect* described in the next section.

Time-Off Seizure Effect: Evidence for Seizure-Induced Endogenous Anticonvulsant Mechanisms

The time-off seizure effect occurs in the animal model of tolerance when, after a sufficient period of time has passed since the induction of the last medication-free seizure, carbamazepine is no longer an effective anticonvulsant (Post and Weiss 1992; Weiss et al. 1995a). This effect suggests that some of the seizure-induced changes in kindling are necessary for carbamazepine's anticonvulsant effects, and after these changes have dissipated, carbamazepine is no longer effective. Similarly, the failure of some of these seizure-induced adaptations to occur in the tolerance phenomenon might be related to carbamazepine's gradual efficacy loss.

Implications for the Development of Efficacy Loss Via Tolerance

These considerations are perhaps worthy of further exploration for their potential clinical ramifications in instances of tolerance to carbamazepine in trigeminal neuralgia, epilepsy, and affective disorders (Frankenburg et al. 1988; Post et al. 1990). One could then ask whether the loss of illness-induced adaptations in these syndromes is related to the process of tolerance development.

In clinical settings, a pharmacodynamic tolerance effect has not been proved because lower blood levels or noncompliance could play a role in breakthrough episodes; however, in the preclinical seizure model, such an effect can be demonstrated readily. In the preclinical model, tolerance is contingent and fully dependent on the interaction of the drug with the episode being treated (Weiss et al.

1995a). If animals are exposed to similar amounts of the drug and a similar number of seizure episodes (i.e., the drug is given after the seizure has occurred), but in a temporally dissociated fashion, no tolerance develops. This observation indicates that the interaction of the presence of the drug with emerging illness episodes, and not mere exposure to the drug, is associated with the gradual efficacy loss.

The neurobiology of this type of tolerance requires specific exploration with the appropriate control groups (Weiss et al. 1995a). It is not enough to merely treat the animals with a drug regimen suitable for chronic illness and assess the resulting neurobiological adaptations. The drug and the episode being treated must be studied concomitantly in a tolerance paradigm and in a control group in which each occurs but not concurrently.

To the extent that this type of tolerance plays a role in the emergence of illness (highly likely when tolerance develops to the antinociceptive, anticonvulsant, and anti–affective disorder components of carbamazepine), one might need to explore this new field of associative pharmacology rather than the pharmacological and biochemical results of episodes and drug treatment in isolation. In the face of tolerance development, the preclinical model suggests the utility of switching to a new drug with a different mechanism of action that does not show cross-tolerance and then, after a time-off period, reexposing the patient to the initially effective agent. Theoretically, a time-off period should allow reemergence of the adaptive changes that may then be associated with efficacy renewal. Obviously, these highly preliminary formulations based on the preclinical models should be tested clinically in patients who have affective disorders.

Conclusion

We have examined a variety of anticonvulsant agents that appear to have either mood-stabilizing or unimodal antimanic or antidepressant properties. As a group, the mood-stabilizing anticonvulsants provide many options for treatment of bipolar disorder in lithium-nonresponsive patients. These agents may be helpful to patients who have treatment-refractory unipolar disorder, and lamotrigine appears to be particularly promising in this regard.

In addition to these pharmacological approaches, preliminary data suggest that repetitive transcranial magnetic stimulation (rTMS) of the brain may have an antidepressant effect (George et al. 1995, 1997). How well this approach may be adapted to the acute and long-term treatment of depression is unknown; however, initial case studies and sham-controlled randomized studies are positive. For example, one patient who failed to respond to more than 10 different antidepressant interventions over a 3-year period showed a complete response to rTMS. She experienced a renewed episode of depression 5 months later, despite attempts at pharmacoprophylaxis, and re-responded to rTMS on a second treatment. On a third occasion, a similar sequence was replicated when she experienced another breakthrough episode. If rTMS proves useful in treating refractory depression, rTMS might become an alternative to electroconvulsive therapy (ECT). This finding would be of considerable importance, as rTMS does not share many of the liabilities of ECT, including the need for anesthesia, the induction of a seizure, and the method's attendant effects on memory. Whether low frequencies, which are anticonvulsant against kindled seizures (Weiss et al. 1995b), are more or less effective than the 10–20 Hz frequencies so far utilized remains to be determined (Post et al., in press b).

Much work is needed to better evaluate long-term approaches to the treatment of refractory bipolar illness, especially its depressive components. Studies suggest that combinations of agents may be more effective than monotherapies. Examples of such combinations include the use of lithium and carbamazepine in patients who have rapid-cycling bipolar disorder (Denicoff et al. 1997; Okuma 1993) and the use of either carbamazepine (Pazzaglia et al. 1993, in press) or lithium (Manna 1991) with the CCB nimodipine. The development of appropriate treatment algorithms to optimally sequence these agents and to effectively use unimodal antidepressants is needed.

References

Arana GW, Pearlman C, Sahder RL: Alprazolam-induced mania: two clinical cases. Am J Psychiatry 142:368–369, 1985

Baldessarini RJ: Risks of discontinuing maintenance treatments (abstract). Paper presented at the 149th annual meeting of the American Psychiatric Association. New York, May 1996

Banki CM, Bissette G, Arato M, et al: Elevation of immunoreactive CSF TRH in depressed patients. Am J Psychiatry 145:1526–1531, 1988

Bassiri R, Utiger RD: Metabolism and excretion of exogenous thyrotropin-releasing hormone in humans. J Clin Invest 52:1616–1619, 1973

Benkert O, Martschke D, Gordon A: Comparison of T.R.H., L.H.-R.H., and placebo in depression. Lancet 2:1146, 1974

Bennett J, Goldman WT, Suppes T: Gabapentin for treatment of bipolar and schizoaffective disorders (letter). J Clin Psychopharmacol 17:141–142, 1997

Beydoun A, Uthman BM, Sackellares JC: Gabapentin: pharmacokinetics, efficacy, and safety. Clin Neuropharmacol 18:469–481, 1995

Bowden CL: Maintenance strategies for bipolar disorder (Abstract 17E). Paper presented at the 149th annual meeting of the American Psychiatric Association. New York, May 1996, p 301

Bowden CL: Long-term prophylactic treatment priorities in bipolar disorder (abstract). Abstracts of the 20th Collegium International Neuropsychopharmacologicum Congress, Vienna, Austria, September 1997. Eur Neuropsychopharmacol 7 (suppl 2):S123, 1997

Bowden CL, Brugger AM, Swann AC, et al: Efficacy of divalproex vs lithium and placebo in the treatment of mania. JAMA 271:918–924, 1994

Bowden CL, Janicak PG, Orsulak P, et al: Relation of serum valproate concentrations to response in mania. Am J Psychiatry 153:765–770, 1996

Bradwejn J, Shriqui C, Koszycki D, et al: Double-blind comparison of the effects of clonazepam and lorazepam in acute mania. J Clin Psychopharmacol 10:403–408, 1990

Brooks BR, Kalin N, Beaulieu DA, et al: Thyrotropin releasing hormone uptake into serum and cerebrospinal fluid following intravenous or subcutaneous administration. Neurol Res 10:236–238, 1988

Busch FN, Miller FT, Weiden PJ: A comparison of two adjunctive treatment strategies in acute mania. J Clin Psychiatry 50:453–455, 1989

Calabrese JR, Markovitz PJ, Kimmel SE, et al: Spectrum of efficacy of valproate in 78 rapid-cycling bipolar patients. J Clin Psychopharmacol 12 (suppl 1):53S–56S, 1992

Calabrese JR, Woyshville MJ, Kimmel SE, et al: Predictors of valproate response in bipolar rapid cycling. J Clin Psychopharmacol 13:280–283, 1993

Calabrese JR, Woyshville MJ, Rapport RT: Clinical efficacy of valproate, in Anticonvulsants in Mood Disorders. Edited by Joffe RT, Calabrese JR. New York, Marcel Dekker, 1994, pp 131–146

Calabrese JR, Bowden CL, Rhodes LJ, et al: Lamotrigine in treatment-refractory bipolar disorder (Abstract 36). Paper presented at the 149th annual meeting of the American Psychiatric Association. New York, May 1996, p 15

Callahan A, Frye MA, Marangell LB, et al: Comparative antidepressant effects of intravenous and intrathecal thyrotropin releasing hormone: confounding effects of tolerance and implications for therapeutics. Biol Psychiatry 41:264–272, 1997

Carman JS, Post RM, Runkle DC, et al: Increased serum calcium and phosphorous with the "switch" into manic or excited psychotic state. Br J Psychiatry 135:55–61, 1979

Carman JS, Wyatt ES, Smith W, et al: Calcium and calcitonin in bipolar affective disorder, in Neurobiology of Mood Disorders. Edited by Post RM, Ballenger JC. Baltimore, MD, Williams & Wilkins, 1984, pp 340–355

Chouinard G, Young SN, Annable L: Antimanic effect of clonazepam. Biol Psychiatry 18:451–466, 1983

Chouinard G, Annable L, Tumier L, et al: A double-blind randomized clinical trial of rapid tranquillization with I.M. clonazepam and I.M. haloperidol in agitated psychotic patients with manic symptoms. Can J Psychiatry 38:S114–S121, 1993

Cora-Locatelli G, Frye MA, Kimbrell TA, et al: Carbamazepine induces escape from dexamethasone suppression across mood disorder subtypes and panic disorder (Abstract NR444). Paper presented at the 149th annual meeting of the American Psychiatric Association. New York, May 1996, p 191

Coryell W, Solomon D, Leon AC, et al: Lithium discontinuation and subsequent effectiveness. Am J Psychiatry 155:895–898, 1998

Coxhead N, Silverstone T, Cookson J: Carbamazepine versus lithium in the prophylaxis of bipolar affective disorder. Acta Psychiatr Scand 85:114–118, 1992

Denicoff KD, Smith-Jackson EE, Disney ER, et al: Comparative prophylactic efficacy of lithium, carbamazepine, and the combination in bipolar disorder. J Clin Psychiatry 58:470–478, 1997

Dilsaver SC, Swann AC, Chen YW, et al: Treatment of bipolar depression with carbamazepine: results of an open study. Biol Psychiatry 40:935–937, 1996

Dimond KR, Pande AC, Lamoreaux L, et al: Effect of gabapentin (Neurontin) on mood and well-being in patients with epilepsy. Prog Neuropsychopharmacol Biol Psychiatry 20:407–417, 1996

Dreyfus J: A Remarkable Medicine Has Been Overlooked. New York, Simon and Schuster, 1981

Dubovsky SL, Franks RD, Allen S: Calcium antagonists in mania: a double-blind study of verapamil. Psychiatry Res 18:309–320, 1986

Edwards R, Stephenson U, Flewett T: Clonazepam in acute mania: a double blind trial. Aust N Z J Psychiatry 25:238–242, 1991

Emrich HM, Von Zerssen D, Kissling W, et al: Effect of sodium valproate in mania; the GABA hypothesis of affective disorders. Archives of Psychiatry and Neurological Sciences 229:1–16, 1980

Emrich HM, Dose M, Von Zerssen D: Action of sodium-valproate and of oxcarbazepine in patients with affective disorders, in Anticonvulsants in Affective Disorders. Edited by Emrich HM, Okuma T, Muller AA. Amsterdam, The Netherlands, Excerpta Medica, 1984, pp 45–55

Fatemi SH, Rapport DJ, Calabrese JR, et al: Lamotrigine in rapid-cycling bipolar disorder. J Clin Psychiatry 58:522–527, 1997

Fogelson DL, Sternbach H: Lamotrigine treatment of refractory bipolar disorder. J Clin Psychiatry 58:271–273, 1997

Frankenburg FR, Tohen M, Cohen BM, et al: Long-term response to carbamazepine: a retrospective study. J Clin Psychopharmacol 8:130–132, 1988

Freeman TW, Clothier JL, Pazzaglia P, et al: A double-blind comparison of valproate and lithium in the treatment of acute mania. Am J Psychiatry 149:108–111, 1992

Freyhan FA: Effectiveness of diphenylhydantoin in management of nonepileptic psychomotor excitement states. Arch Neurol Psychiatry 53:370–374, 1995

Frye MA: Gabapentin does not alter lithium pharmacokinetics. American Psychiatric Association 1996 Annual Meeting New Research Program and Abstracts (NR311). Washington, DC, American Psychiatric Association, 1996, p 151

Frye MA, Ketter TA, Osuch EA, et al: Gabapentin and lamotrigine monotherapy in mood disorder: an update, in CME Syllabus and Scientific Proceedings of the 151st Annual Meeting of the American Psychiatric Association. Washington, DC, American Psychiatric Association, 1998, p 150

Garza-Treviño ES, Overall JE, Hollister LE: Verapamil versus lithium in acute mania. Am J Psychiatry 149:121–122, 1992

Gelenberg AJ, Kane JM, Keller MB, et al: Comparison of standard and low serum levels of lithium for maintenance treatment of bipolar disorder. N Engl J Med 321:1489–1493, 1989

George MS, Wassermann EM, Williams WA, et al: Daily repetitive transcranial magnetic stimulation (rTMS) improves mood in depression. NeuroReport 6:1853–1856, 1995

George MS, Wassermann EM, Kimbrell TA, et al: Mood improvement following daily left prefrontal repetitive transcranial magnetic stimulation in patients with depression: a placebo-controlled crossover trial. Am J Psychiatry 154:1752–1756, 1997

Gillberg IC, Heligren L, Gillberg C: Psychotic disorders diagnosed in adolescence; outcome at age 30 years. J Child Psychol Psychiatry 34:1173–1185, 1993

Goodnick PJ: Nimodipine treatment of rapid cycling bipolar disorder (letter). J Clin Psychiatry 56:330, 1995

Greil W, Ludwig-Mayerhofer W, Erazo N, et al: Lithium vs. carbamazepine in the maintenance treatment of schizoaffective disorder: a randomized study. Eur Arch Psychiatry Clin Neurosci 247:42–50, 1997a

Greil W, Ludwig-Mayerhofer W, Erazo N, et al: Lithium versus carbamazepine in the maintenance treatment of bipolar disorders—a randomized study. J Affect Disord 43:151–161, 1997b

Hayes SG: Barbiturate anticonvulsants in refractory affective disorders. Ann Clin Psychiatry 5:35–44, 1993

Hirschfeld RMA, Clayton P, Cohen I, et al: Practice guideline for the treatment of patients with bipolar disorder. Am J Psychiatry 151 (suppl): 1–36, 1994

Hoschl C, Kozeny J: Verapamil in affective disorders: a controlled, double-blind study. Biol Psychiatry 25:128–140, 1989

Hough CJ, Irwin RP, Gao X-M, et al: Carbamazepine inhibition of N-methyl-D-aspartate-evoked calcium influx in rat cerebellar granule cells. J Pharmacol Exp Ther 276:143–149, 1996

Jacobsen FM: Low-dose valproate: a new treatment for cyclothymia, mild rapid cycling disorders, and premenstrual syndrome. J Clin Psychiatry 54:229–234, 1993

Janicak PG, Sharma RP, Pandey G, et al: Verapamil for the treatment of acute mania: a double-blind, placebo-controlled trial. Am J Psychiatry 155:972–973, 1998

Kastin AJ, Ehrensing RH, Schalch DS, et al: Improvement in mental depression with decreased thyrotropin response after administration of thyrotropin-releasing hormone. Lancet 2:740–742, 1972

Keck PE Jr, McElroy SL, Tugrul KC, et al: Valproate oral loading in the treatment of acute mania. J Clin Psychiatry 54:305–308, 1993

Kerr BM, Rettie AE, Eddy AC, et al: Inhibition of human liver microsomal epoxide hydrolase by valproate and valpromide: in vitro/in vivo correlation. Clin Pharmacol Ther 46:82–93, 1989

Ketter TA, Post RM: Clinical pharmacology and pharmacokinetics of carbamazepine, in Anticonvulsants in Mood Disorders. Edited by Joffe RT, Calabrese JR. New York, Marcel Dekker, 1994, pp 147–187

Ketter TA, Jenkins JB, Schroeder DH, et al: Carbamazepine but not valproate induces bupropion metabolism. J Clin Psychopharmacol 15: 327–333, 1995a

Ketter TA, Flockhart DA, Post RM, et al: The emerging role of cytochrome P450 3A in psychopharmacology. J Clin Psychopharmacol 15:387–398, 1995b

Ketter TA, Frye MA, Callahan AM, et al: Clinical pharmacokinetic update on anticonvulsants (abstract). Twentieth CINP Congress, 1996

Kiely WF, Adrian AD, Lee JH, et al: Therapeutic failure of oral thyrotropin-releasing hormone in depression. Psychosom Med 38:233–241, 1976

Kirkegaard C, Faber J, Hummer L, et al: Increased levels of TRH in cerebrospinal fluid from patients with endogenous depression. Psychoneuroendocrinology 4:227–235, 1979

Kishimoto A: The treatment of affective disorder with carbamazepine: prophylactic synergism of lithium and carbamazepine combination. Prog Neuropsychopharmacol Biol Psychiatry 16:483–493, 1992

Kishimoto A, Kamata K Sugihara T, et al: Treatment of depression with clonazepam. Acta Psychiatr Scand 77:81–86, 1988

Kramlinger KG, Post RM: The addition of lithium carbonate to carbamazepine: antidepressant efficacy in treatment-resistant depression. Arch Gen Psychiatry 46:794–800, 1989

Kukopulos A, Reginaldi D, Minnai G, et al: The long term prophylaxis of affective disorders. Adv Biochem Psychopharmacol 49:127–147, 1995

Labbate LA, Rubey RN: Lamotrigine for treatment-refractory bipolar disorder (letter). Am J Psychiatry 154:1317, 1997

Lambert PA, Venaud G: Comparative study of valpromide vs lithium in treatment of affective disorders. Nervure 5(2):57–65, 1992

Lenox RH, Newhouse PA, Creelman WL, et al: Adjunctive treatment of manic agitation with lorazepam versus haloperidol: a double-blind study. J Clin Psychiatry 53:47–52, 1992

Maj M, Pirozzi R, Kemali D: Long-term outcome of lithium prophylaxis in patients initially classified as complete responders. Psychopharmacology 98:535–538, 1989

Manna V: Bipolar affective disorders and role of intraneuronal calcium; therapeutic effects of the treatment with lithium salts and/or calcium antagonist in patients with rapid polar inversion. Minerva Medica 82: 757–763, 1991

Marangell LB, George MS, Bissette G, et al: Carbamazepine increases CSF thyrotropin-releasing hormone in affectively ill patients. Arch Gen Psychiatry 51:625–628, 1994

Marangell LB, George MS, Callahan AM, et al: Effects of intrathecal thyrotropin-releasing hormone (TRH) in refractory depressed patients. Arch Gen Psychiatry 54:214–222, 1997

McDermut W, Pazzaglia PJ, Huggins T, et al: Use of single case analyses in off-on-off-on trials in affective illness: a demonstration of the efficacy of nimodipine. Depression 2:259–271, 1995

McElroy SL, Keck PE Jr, Pope HG Jr, et al: Valproate in the treatment of rapid-cycling bipolar disorder. J Clin Psychopharmacol 8:275–279, 1988a

McElroy SL, Pope HG Jr, Keck PE Jr: Treatment of psychiatric disorders with valproate: a series of 73 cases. Psychiatrie Psychobiologie 3:81–85, 1988b

McElroy SL, Keck PE, Pope HG, et al: Valproate in the treatment of bipolar disorder; literature review and clinical guidelines. J Clin Psychopharmacol 12:42S–52S, 1992

McElroy SL, Soutullo CA, Keck PE Jr, et al: A pilot trial of adjunctive gabapentin in the treatment of bipolar disorder. Ann Clin Psychiatry 9:99–103, 1997

Messenheimer J: Lamotrigine. Epilepsia 36 (suppl 2):S87–S94, 1995

Mountjoy CG, Price JS, Weller M, et al: A double-blind crossover sequential trial of oral thyrotrophin-releasing hormone in depression. Lancet 1:958–960, 1974

O'Connell RA, Mayo JA, Flatow L, et al: Outcome of bipolar disorder on long-term treatment with lithium. Br J Psychiatry 159:123–129, 1991

Okuma T: Effects of carbamazepine and lithium on affective disorders. Neuropsychobiology 27:138–145, 1993

Okuma T, Inanaga K, Otsuki S, et al: A preliminary double-blind study of the efficacy of carbamazepine in prophylaxis of manic-depressive illness. Psychopharmacology 73:95–96, 1981

Pani L, Kuzmin A, Diana M, et al: Calcium receptor antagonists modify cocaine effects in the central nervous system differently. Eur J Pharmacol 190:217–221, 1990

Pazzaglia PJ, Post RM, Ketter TA, et al: Preliminary controlled trial of nimodipine in ultra-rapid cycling affective dysregulation. Psychiatry Res 49:257–272, 1993

Pazzaglia PJ, Post RM, Ketter TA, et al: Nimodipine monotherapy and carbamazepine augmentation in patients with refractory recurrent affective illness. J Clin Psychopharmacol (in press)

Pope HG, McElroy SL, Keck PE Jr, et al: Valproate in the treatment of acute mania. Arch Gen Psychiatry 48:62–68, 1991

Post RM: Use of anticonvulsants in the treatment of manic-depressive illness, in Clinical Use of Anticonvulsants in Psychiatric Disorders. Edited by Post RM, Trimble MR, Pippenger CE. New York, Demos, 1989, pp 113–152

Post RM: Alternatives to lithium for bipolar affective illness, in American Psychiatric Press Review of Psychiatry, Vol 9. Edited by Tasman A, Goldfinger SM, Kaufmann C. Washington, DC, American Psychiatric Press, 1990a, pp 170–202

Post RM: Prophylaxis of bipolar affective disorders. International Review of Psychiatry 2:277–320, 1990b

Post RM: Transduction of psychosocial stress into the neurobiology of recurrent affective disorder. Am J Psychiatry 149:999–1010, 1992

Post RM, Weiss SRB: Endogenous biochemical abnormalities in affective illness: therapeutic versus pathogenic. Biol Psychiatry 32:469–484, 1992

Post RM, Weiss SRB: The neurobiology of treatment-resistant mood disorders, in Psychopharmacology: The Fourth Generation of Progress. Edited by Bloom FE, Kupfer DJ. New York, Raven, 1995, pp 1155–1170

Post RM, Weiss SRB: A speculative model of affective illness cyclicity based on patterns of drug tolerance observed in amygdala-kindled seizures. Mol Neurobiology 13:33–60, 1996

Post RM, Uhde TW, Roy-Byrne PP, et al: Antidepressant effects of carbamazepine. Am J Psychiatry 143:29–34, 1986

Post RM, Leverich GS, Rosoff AS, et al: Carbamazepine prophylaxis in refractory affective disorders: a focus on long-term follow-up. J Clin Psychopharmacol 10:318–327, 1990

Post RM, Leverich GS, Altshuler L, et al: Lithium discontinuation-induced refractoriness: preliminary observations. Am J Psychiatry 149:1727–1729, 1992

Post RM, Ketter TA, Denicoff K, et al: Assessment of anticonvulsant drugs in patients with bipolar affective illness, in Human Psychopharmacology: Methods and Measures, Vol 4. Edited by Hindmarch I, Stonier PD. Chichester, England, Wiley, 1993a, pp 211–245

Post RM, Leverich GS, Pazzaglia PJ, et al: Lithium tolerance and discontinuation as pathways to refractoriness, in Lithium in Medicine and Biology. Edited by Birch NJ, Padgham C, Hughes MS. Lancashire, England, Marius Press, 1993b, pp 71–84

Post RM, Ketter TA, Pazzaglia PJ, et al: Rational polypharmacy in the bipolar affective disorders. Epilepsy Res 11 (suppl):153–180, 1996

Post RM, Frye MA, Denicoff KD, et al: Anticonvulsants in the long-term prophylaxis of depression, in Depression: Neurobiological, Psychopathological and Therapeutic Advances. Edited by Honig A, Van Praag HM. Sussex, England, Wiley, 1997, pp 483–498

Post RM, Pazzaglia PJ, Ketter TA, et al: Carbamazepine and nimodipine in refractory bipolar illness: efficacy and mechanisms, in Book IV: Pharmacotherapy of Mood and Cognition. Edited by Montgomery S, Halbreich U. Washington, DC, American Psychiatric Press (in press a)

Post RM, Kimbrell T, McCann U, et al: Repetitive transcranial magnetic stimulation as a neuropsychiatric tool: present status and future potential. J ECT (in press b)

Prange AJ Jr, Lara PP, Wilson IC, et al: Effects of thyrotropin-releasing hormone in depression. Lancet 2:999–1002, 1972

Prien RF, Gelenberg AJ: Alternatives to lithium for preventive treatment of bipolar disorder. Am J Psychiatry 146:840–848, 1989

Ramsay RE, McManus DQ, Guterman A: Carbamazepine metabolism in humans: effect of concurrent anticonvulsant therapy. Ther Drug Monit 12:235–241, 1990

Robbins DK, Wedlund PJ, Kuhn R: Inhibition of epoxide hydrolase by valproic acid in epileptic patients receiving carbamazepine. Br J Clin Pharmacol 29:759–762, 1990

Rubinow DR, Post RM, Gold PW: Neuroendocrine and peptide effects of carbamazepine: clinical and theoretical implications. Psychopharmacol Bull 20:590–594, 1984

Rubinow DR, Post RM, Gold PW, et al: Effect of carbamazepine on mean urinary free cortisol excretion in patients with major affective illness. Psychopharmacology 88:115–118, 1986

Ryback RS, Brodsky L, Munasifi F: Gabapentin in bipolar disorder (letter). J Neuropsychiatry Clin Neurosci 9:301, 1997

Sachs GS, Rosenbaum JF, Jones L: Adjunctive clonazepam for maintenance treatment of bipolar affective disorder. J Clin Psychopharmacol 10: 42–47, 1990

Sarantidis D, Waters B: Predictors of lithium prophylaxis effectiveness. Prog Neuropsychopharmacol 5:507–510, 1981

Schaff MR, Fawcett J, Zajecka JM: Divalproex sodium in the treatment of refractory affective disorders. J Clin Psychiatry 54:380–384, 1993

Schaffer CB, Schaffer LC: Gabapentin in the treatment of bipolar disorder (letter). Am J Psychiatry 154:291–292, 1997

Schwarz JR, Grigat G: Phenytoin and carbamazepine: potential- and frequency-dependent block of Na^+ currents in mammalian myelinated nerve fibers. Epilepsia 30:286–294, 1989

Spearing MK, Post RM, Leverich GS, et al: Modification of the Clinical Global Impressions (CGI) Scale for use in bipolar illness (BP): the CGI-BP. Psychiatry Res 73:159–171, 1997

Sporn J, Sachs G: The anticonvulsant lamotrigine in treatment-resistant manic-depressive illness. J Clin Psychopharmacol 17:185–189, 1997

Stanton SP, Keck PE Jr, McElroy SL: Treatment of acute mania with gabapentin (letter). Am J Psychiatry 154:287, 1997

Swann AC, Bowden CL, Petty F, et al: Mania: clinical and biological predictors of outcome. ACNP Scientific Abstracts, 1997, p 252

Tomson T: Interdosage fluctuations in plasma carbamazepine concentration determine intermittent side effects. Arch Neurol 41:830–834, 1984

Waldmeier PC, Baumann PA, Wicki P, et al: Similar potency of carbamazepine, oxcarbazepine, and lamotrigine in inhibiting the release of glutamate and other neurotransmitters. Neurology 45:1907–1913, 1995

Weisler RH, Risner ME, Ascher JA, et al: Use of lamotrigine in the treatment of bipolar disorder. American Psychiatric Association 1994 Annual Meeting New Research Program and Abstracts (NR611). Washington, DC, American Psychiatric Association, 1994, p 216

Weiss SRB, Clark M, Rosen JB, et al: Contingent tolerance to the anticonvulsant effects of carbamazepine: relationship to loss of endogenous adaptive mechanisms. Brain Res Rev 20:305–325, 1995a

Weiss SRB, Li XL, Rosen JB, et al: Quenching: inhibition of development and expression of amygdala kindled seizures with low frequency stimulation. NeuroReport 6:2171–2176, 1995b

Werry JS, McClellan JM, Chard L: Childhood and adolescent schizophrenic, bipolar, and schizoaffective disorders: a clinical and outcome study. J Am Acad Child Adolesc Psychiatry 30:457–465, 1991

Willow M, Kuenzel EA, Catterall WA: Inhibition of voltage-sensitive sodium channels in neuroblastoma cells and synaptosomes by the anticonvulsant drugs diphenylhydantoin and carbamazepine. Mol Pharmacol 25:228–234, 1984

Wolf C, Berky M, Kovacs G: Carbamazepine versus lithium in the prophylaxis of bipolar affective disorders: a randomised, double-blind 1-year study in 168 patients. Eur Neuropsychopharmacol 7 (suppl 2):S176, 1997

Young LT, Robb JC, Patelis-Siotis I, et al: Acute treatment of bipolar depression with gabapentin. Biol Psychiatry 42:851–853, 1997

Mixed-State Bipolar Disorders: Outcome Data From the NIMH Collaborative Program on the Psychobiology of Depression

Robert J. Boland, M.D.
Martin B. Keller, M.D.

*T*he possibility that patients could simultaneously exhibit both manic (or hypomanic) and depressive symptoms has long been recognized (Kraepelin 1921/1976); however, mania and depression are usually imagined as polar opposites. This thinking may explain why it is difficult even to agree on a definition of *mixed mania* (also called *dysphoric mania*) (McElroy et al. 1992). Most studies of mixed mania are limited by this lack of consistent criteria for the syndrome. For example, whether mixed mania is a distinct disorder, a subtype of mania, a particularly severe form of rapid cycling, or a transitional point between mania and depression is unclear. Because the course and treatment outcome of mixed mania have been the subject of increasing clinical and research interest, it may be useful to begin this chapter with a brief overview of the concept and definition of mixed states.

In DSM-IV (American Psychiatric Association 1994), mixed

states are defined by the simultaneous presence of a full manic and a full major depressive syndrome. Several studies have examined the dimensional, rather than categorical, aspects of depression when it arises concomitantly with a manic syndrome (Bauer et al. 1994; McElroy et al. 1992). Notably, Cassidy and colleagues (1997) found that only certain depressive symptoms had predictive value in diagnosing the mixed state. Anhedonia, fatigue, feelings of worthlessness or guilt, and recurrent thoughts of death or suicide all were useful in diagnosing mixed-state bipolar disorders. However, changes in weight, sleep, psychomotor performance, and concentration/cognition were less robustly associated with a mixed-state diagnosis. These investigators identified a "depressive mood factor" in mania, involving a bimodal distribution among bipolar patients, which suggests that mixed mania is a unique bipolar subtype (Cassidy et al. 1998). Although DSM-IV does not classify subsyndromal depression during mania (or subsyndromal mania during a major depressive episode) as a mixed state, evidence from empirical studies has not yet identified the most useful operational definition for mixed mania.

Given the existing ambiguities about the defining characteristics of mixed states, the difficulty involved in reaching a consensus on the disorder's features is not surprising. Prevalence rates vary widely. Goodwin and Jamison (1990) determined that at least 40% of the subjects in studies on mania published between 1969 and 1989 had mixed mania. McElroy and colleagues (1992) reported an overall mean prevalence of 31% for mixed mania among acutely manic patients. Similarly, statements about the demographics of this disorder are inconsistent and often contradictory.

Reports of the disorder's course are somewhat more consistent. Kraepelin (1921/1976) believed that mixed mania was a more virulent form of *manic-depressive insanity,* and most subsequent authors have agreed. Most studies on mixed mania suggest that patients with this disorder take longer to recover from an acute episode (Keller 1985, 1988). Patients with mixed mania also seem to relapse sooner, and more often, than do patients with other forms of bipolar disorder (Tohen et al. 1990). Similarly, patients with mixed mania may respond more poorly to both the acute and the prophylactic phases of treatment (McElroy et al. 1992). Dilsaver and colleagues

(1993) reported a rate of treatment response for mixed mania that was about one-half that of patients with pure mania. Unfortunately, many of these conclusions are based on case reports, and few controlled studies exist to help resolve these issues. However, one recent study examined 179 bipolar subjects who were randomized to receive divalproex sodium, lithium carbonate, or placebo; patients who had depressive symptoms responded preferentially to divalproex sodium (Swann et al. 1997).

Clinicians need more information about this disorder, particularly because mixed mania appears to be more common than originally thought. Furthermore, mixed-affective symptoms may be relevant to the course and expected treatment response of bipolar disorder.

In this chapter, we review recent data regarding mixed mania. These data are from the National Institute of Mental Health (NIMH) Collaborative Program on the Psychobiology of Depression, an ongoing large-scale study in which standardized information about a large population of subjects helps us to better understand this disorder. After reviewing the design and pertinent results from this research program, we present a case to illustrate the clinical significance of the major findings.

The NIMH—Clinical Research Branch Collaborative Program on the Psychobiology of Depression—Clinical Studies (Collaborative Depression Study)

Overview

The Collaborative Depression Study (CDS) was designed to study the natural course of unipolar and bipolar mood disorders. It is a prospective, long-term follow-up study of the psychopathology and treatment of the disorders and the psychosocial functioning of people who have them (Katz and Klerman 1979). The 955 subjects who entered the study were recruited from those seeking psychiatric treatment through inpatient and outpatient treatment facilities at five medical centers.[1] The research program is ongoing, with plans to continue for at least 17 years of follow-up on all subjects.

Diagnoses

Diagnoses were based on the Research Diagnostic Criteria (RDC; Spitzer et al. 1985). The *mixed/cycling group* of bipolar patients comprised three subtypes: those with mixed-affective symptoms, those with single-cycling episodes, and those with multiple-cycling episodes. The mixed subgroup had manic (or hypomanic) and depressive symptoms intermingled throughout the day. Patients in either of the cycling subgroups experienced periods of mania alternating with depression that were not separated by an intervening well period of at least 8 weeks (the criteria for recovery). The single-cycling group had multiple periods of mania and one period of depression, whereas the multiple-cycling group also had multiple periods of depression.

Assessment Tools

Several standardized assessment tools were administered at the time of intake, including the Schedule for Affective Disorders and Schizophrenia (SADS; Spitzer and Endicott 1979). At each 6-month follow-up, the subjects were given the Longitudinal Interval Follow-up Evaluation (LIFE) (Keller et al. 1987; Shapiro and Keller 1979). The investigators determined changes in psychopathology, measured to the week, with the Psychiatric Status Rating (PSR), which quantifies the severity of symptoms on a six-point scale (Keller et al. 1992).

Definitions of Course Change Points

Recovery was defined as at least 8 consecutive weeks with no more than two mild symptoms (as rated on the LIFE scale). *Relapse* was defined as fulfillment of RDC criteria for an episode of major depressive

---

[1] Research centers participating in the CDS include Columbia University (New York City), Harvard University (Boston, Mass.), the University of Iowa (Iowa City), Rush-Presbyterian-St. Luke's Medical Center (Chicago, Ill.), and Washington University (St. Louis, Mo.).

disorder, minor depression, mania, hypomania, or schizoaffective disorder after an 8-week period of recovery from an affective disorder. (Thus, the time to relapse could not be less than 9 weeks.)

Assessment of Treatment

Although the investigators did not participate in decisions about treatment, they did collect information on the intensity and appropriateness of somatotherapy. They rated treatment for depressive symptoms as follows: *High-intensity treatment* was defined as at least 200 mg of imipramine hydrochloride (IMI) or its equivalent, 45 mg of phenelzine sulfate, or 900 mg of lithium carbonate for 4 consecutive weeks; or a course of electroconvulsive therapy. *Moderate-intensity treatment* was defined as the equivalent of at least 100 mg of IMI, 30 mg of phenelzine, or 600 mg of lithium for 4 consecutive weeks. The investigators rated treatment for manic symptoms as *high* (at least 900 mg of lithium, a course of electroconvulsive therapy, or at least 500 mg of chlorpromazine or its equivalent) or *moderate* (600 mg or more of lithium or at least 300 mg of chlorpromazine or its equivalent).

Analyses

We review here analyses made at two points in the study: after the first 155 patients with bipolar disorder had been followed up for 6 months to 2 years (*Time I*) (Keller et al. 1986) and after the entire sample of patients with bipolar disorder had been followed up for 5 years (*Time II*) (Keller et al. 1993).

Sample characteristics. For these analyses, study subjects were chosen who had a history of mania but no history of schizoaffective disorder; subjects with bipolar II disorder were excluded. These subjects tended to be in their mid- to late 30s, with a mean age of 37 years. They were of varied social class and of roughly equal gender mix (45% were men and 55% women).

Among the first 155 subjects to enter the study (Time I), 63 were manic at the time of entry and 25 were depressed. Of the remaining 67 subjects, 7 met criteria for a mixed episode and 60 for a rapid-cycling episode. Half of the subjects in the cycling group had only one period of mania or hypomania and one period of depression (i.e., single cycling). The other half had multiple periods of mania or hypomania and depression (i.e., multiple cycling). The median follow-up period for these subjects was 18 months.

Among the 172 subjects studied at the 5-year follow-up (Time II), 69 had pure mania, 27 had pure depression, and 76 had mixed/cycling symptoms. Only 1% of the patients in the index manic group were lost to follow-up while still in the index episode, compared with 4% of the index depressed subjects and 8% of the mixed/cycling subjects.

Time to recovery. Subjects entering the study with an index episode of mania recovered faster than did the other subjects. At Time I, the pure manic group had a median time to recovery of 5 weeks, compared with a median of 9 weeks for the depressed group and 14 weeks for the mixed/cycling group. The difference between the manic and the mixed/cycling groups was significant.

At Time II, patients with pure manic symptoms continued to recover faster than the other groups, with a median time to recovery of 6 weeks, compared with 11 weeks for the depressed group and 17 weeks for the mixed/cycling group. These differences in rate of recovery were most marked in the period just after entry into the study.

Predictors of recovery. For those patients who were manic on entry into the study, several variables predicted the time to recovery. A longer duration of major depressive disorder before entry predicted a longer time to recovery: a tenfold increase in prior duration predicted a doubling of the time from entry to recovery. A greater number of previous major affective episodes was associated with more subsequent affective relapses; however, this variable also predicted a shorter time to recovery from an individual episode. Thus, 55% of the patients in their first episode of illness recovered in less than 6 months, whereas 73% of patients with one or two prior episodes and 90% of patients with three or more prior episodes recovered in the same amount of time.

For patients who were depressed at the time of entry into the study, a longer prior duration of illness also predicted a longer time to recovery. In this group, a diagnosis of *secondary major depressive bipolar disorder*, in which the first affective episode was preceded by another RDC disorder (such as alcoholism or other substance abuse), also predicted a longer time to recovery.

In the mixed/cycling group, a psychotic subtype of major depressive disorder and *endogenous features* (defined as an SADS score of at least 5) were most strongly associated with a longer time to recovery. Psychotic patients had a 37% probability of recovery by 6 months, compared with 65% for the nonpsychotic patients. The time to recovery was similar for both mixed and cycling patients.

Probability of chronicity. The probability of chronicity also differed across groups. After 2 years, only 4% of those entering the study with a manic episode had not yet recovered, compared with 15% of those in the depressed group, and 28% of those in the mixed/cycling group. By 5 years, 100% of the patients with pure mania had recovered from their index episode, compared with 89% of the patients with pure depression and 83% of the patients with mixed/cycling symptoms. For subjects entering with mania and not recovering by the first year, the probability of recovering by the second year was 60%. This recovery rate was significantly higher than in the other groups: Only 32% of depressed patients and 24% of mixed/cycling patients who had not recovered by the first year did so by the second year.

Changes in polarity. Of the patients who were manic at the time of entry into the study, 30% developed depression after entry but before recovery. Half of the patients still manic 12 weeks after entry cycled to depression before recovery. The median time to recovery for this group was 18 weeks, and the probability of remaining ill 1 year after cycling was 26%. Similarly, for those depressed at entry, 20% developed mania before recovery, and 80% of these patients did not recover after cycling.

Treatment received. When we analyzed the treatment received, we found that approximately 75% of the subjects in each group received both high intensity and sustained levels of somatotherapy. Most of the remaining subjects received moderate levels of treatment. Thus, although the naturalistic design did not allow for analyses of the effects of treatment on outcome, inadequate treatment was not likely to be responsible for a lack of recovery.

Time to relapse. As explained above, the time to relapse, by definition, could not be less than 9 weeks. For the relapse analysis, we reclassified subjects who changed polarity before a recovery based on their new symptoms. For example, of the patients with an index manic episode, 29% developed a depressive episode before recovery; this group was reclassified into the depressive group for relapse analysis.

Relapse was slowest for the manic group and similar for the depressed and mixed/cycling groups. In the first 3 months, the cumulative probability of relapse was similar for all three groups. However, by 6 months, the manic group had a 20% cumulative probability of relapse, compared with 33% for the depressed group and 36% for the mixed/cycling group. By the end of the first year, the manic group had a 48% probability of relapse, and the mixed/cycling group had a 57% chance of relapse. The depressed group's time to relapse was similar to that of the mixed/cycling group. By 5 years, the manic group had an 81% chance of relapse, compared with 91% for the mixed/cycling group. Relapse was also more severe in the mixed/cycling group: 59% of the mixed/cycling subjects relapsed into a major affective episode, compared with 38% of the pure manic subjects. The groups did not differ in the treatment they received before relapse.

First prospective episode. As subjects were already in their index episode on entry into this study, some information about this episode (such as initial onset) was necessarily retrospective. The 5-year follow-up allowed us to examine the course of the next episode— thus allowing for a prospective analysis. Observations of this first prospective episode were consistent with observations of the index episode. Subjects who entered the study with a mixed/cycling episode had the lowest cumulative probability of recovery from a subsequent episode. During the first prospective episode, rates of recovery in all groups were similar for the first 6 months and then began to diverge, with 78% of the manic group (grouped by index episode) recovering, compared with 58% of the index mixed/cycling group. By 3 years, the recovery rate was 100% for the index manic group, compared with 87% for the index mixed/cycling group. The depressed group had a small sample size, which limited comparability with the other groups; however, this group's rate of recovery seemed comparable to that of the index manic group.

Summary

The CDS found that the course and outcome of bipolar disorder in subjects entering the study differed significantly, depending on the subjects' initial symptoms. Most striking was the difference between subjects entering the study with a manic episode and those entering with a mixed/cycling episode. Differences between these groups in recovery rate, rate of chronicity, relapse rate, and rate of recovery from the next episode of disease were statistically significant and were large enough to be of clinical relevance.

The following case illustrates some of the principles and the practical significance of the CDS findings:

Ms. A, a 51-year-old married woman, presented to a psychiatrist with complaints of "depression." She did so quite reluctantly, saying that her daughter had insisted she find help. Ms. A felt she had been depressed since she had a hysterectomy a year ago. She reported being anergic and unable to get out of bed for as long as a month after the operation. Her gynecologist, presuming menopause as the cause of her complaints, prescribed estrogen replacement therapy (Premarin), which provided some relief, but she continued to complain of dysphoria. In this context, her internist prescribed amitriptyline (50 mg/day). Soon after, while still depressed, Ms. A began gambling compulsively at a nearby casino, despite never having any previous interest in gambling. She denied symptoms of euphoria during this time.

At the time of her initial presentation, Ms. A complained of initial and middle insomnia, little initiative, guilty ruminations (mainly about her considerable gambling losses), poor energy, and poor concentration. She reported that she felt hopeless about her life, but she denied suicidality.

Ms. A worked as an insurance examiner and had three adult

children. She reported numerous interpersonal problems with her family and felt they resented and blamed her for the family discord. She had a family history of alcohol abuse (father and mother) and depression (mother).

On initial examination, Ms. A was alert and well dressed. She was anxious, almost tearful at times. Her speech was clear and coherent, but the examiner noted it to be "pressured." Ms. A denied having delusions, hallucinations, or suicidal intent.

The psychiatrist considered a diagnosis of bipolar disorder at the time. However, because Ms. A denied experiencing isolated manic symptoms without concomitant depressive ideation (e.g., she reported feeling depressed even while gambling), the psychiatrist gave her a diagnosis of major depression and initiated treatment for this disorder.

Ms. A was started on nortriptyline (amitriptyline was discontinued), which was increased gradually over 6 weeks to a therapeutic dose (with blood-level monitoring). During this period, Ms. A continued to complain of depressive symptoms, although she did sleep better. However, her gambling increased over this period, and she lost most of her family's savings. In this context, she developed increasing suicidal ideation, overdosed on her nortriptyline, and then drove her car into a tree. Although she was not seriously injured, she was medically hospitalized for several days and then transferred—against her will—to an inpatient psychiatric facility. She was hospitalized there for 1 week, during which time her nortriptyline was discontinued and paroxetine (20 mg/day) was started.

Shortly after her hospitalization, Ms. A returned to her psychiatrist, tearful and angry. She resented having been hospitalized. She seemed to suspect a sinister purpose in "locking her away." When the psychiatrist explored these fears, Ms. A revealed a robust delusional scheme. She explained that in her job she gradually began to understand the presence and influence of the Mafia at all levels of society. She believed the Mob had been responsible for her hospitalization and was also responsible for the large amounts of money she lost at the casino. She felt that only she had the power and knowledge to defeat the Mafia and was "biding [her] time" until she "exposed" it. Though Ms. A was at first hesitant and suspicious while describing these details, her delusions became increasingly grandiose, and she appeared almost elated with her own power and influence.

The psychiatrist, alarmed at what appeared to be a new-onset psychosis, insisted on contacting a family member—something Ms. A had previously forbidden. She was reluctant but agreed.

Ms. A's daughter gave a different perspective. She reported that her mother had had frequent episodes of depression as long as the daughter could remember, often accompanied by the current "anxious" symptoms. The daughter also reported that her mother had had previous episodes of paranoia, often to the point of delusional ideation. She felt her mother had periods of "normalcy" between the "mood swings" but that these episodes were becoming more rare and shorter lived.

The psychiatrist revised the diagnosis to bipolar disorder, mixed type. Ms. A was started on lithium but complained of sedation, weight gain, tremors, and polyuria, even at subtherapeutic doses. The psychiatrist then prescribed divalproex sodium, slowly increasing the dose to 1,500 mg/day over the next 2 months. At 6-month follow-up, Ms. A had remained relatively stable on this dose with fewer mood swings and little desire to gamble. She continued, however, to have residual suspiciousness and to complain of occasional dysphoria.

Discussion

Ms. A's case demonstrates both the difficulty and the importance of recognizing and treating mixed mania. As in this case, the disorder is frequently misinterpreted. Ms. A's bias toward reporting the symptoms that most disturbed her (dysphoria and other depressive symptoms), and the clinician's misconception of mania and depression as mutually exclusive, likely led the clinician to rely too heavily on certain symptoms and behaviors in making the initial diagnosis. A more careful examination and greater consideration of the atypical aspects of Ms. A's case (e.g., her pressured speech on examination or her sudden interest in gambling) would have better clarified these issues. Earlier contact with the family would also have aided the diagnosis. Frequently, only longitudinal examination of a patient clearly identifies this syndrome.

This case also demonstrates the chronic nature of this disorder. As shown in the CDS, patients with mixed-state bipolar illness recover slowly. Indeed, throughout Ms. A's treatment (over 9 months), she never showed a period of full remission. The poor outcome in this disorder is even more dramatic when one considers the risk of suicide in this population. In examining patients with mania, Dilsaver and colleagues (1994) found that although only 2% of patients with pure mania were judged to be suicidal, 55% of patients with "depressive mania" were suicidal. Similarly, suicidality was more prevalent in mixed-state than in pure manic patients and appeared to be related to the severity of concurrent depressive symptoms (Strakowski et al. 1996).[2] Ms. A's sudden and serious suicide attempt underscores these risk factors.

That Ms. A worsened when taking an antidepressant emphasizes the importance of proper treatment. Little information exists on the proper pharmacotherapy of mixed mania; however, at least one study confirmed the higher risk of recurrence when patients take antidepressant medications alone (Prien et al. 1988). Indeed, Ms. A became paranoid and suicidal during this period.

Even with the use of appropriate mood stabilizers, Ms. A did not show a full remission; however, she improved greatly. Her active psychotic symptoms and impulsive behaviors decreased. Her gambling decreased, and she made no subsequent suicide attempts. As noted earlier in this chapter, few controlled studies exist to guide treatment of this disorder, although lithium may be useful in the treatment of acute mixed mania (McElroy et al. 1992). Preliminary reports also support the use of valproate and possibly other anticonvulsants in this population (McElroy et al. 1992; Swann et al. 1997), and Ms. A seemed to show at least a partial response to this treatment. Several preliminary studies have reported more dramatic acute symptom improvement in mixed mania with anticonvulsant mood stabilizers instead of lithium (Freeman et al. 1992; Frye et al. 1996; Keck et al. 1996). Further controlled studies, naturalistic trials, and long-term maintenance phase studies are needed in order to corroborate the potential differences in treatment outcome for mixed mania with anticonvulsant mood stabilizers versus lithium.

In summary, the findings of the CDS demonstrate convincingly

---

[2] See also Goldberg and Kocsis, Chapter 7, in this volume for a more detailed discussion of suicidality and depression in bipolar disorder.

that mixed mania is a particularly severe subtype of bipolar disorder. All aspects of bipolar disorder, including course and outcome, time to recovery, and risk of relapse and recurrence, appear to be worse in this form of the disorder. The patient's response to treatment may also be poor for this subtype of mania, although more information is needed in this area. Given the risk of chronicity and recurrence of mixed mania, efforts are needed to better understand and treat this virulent form of bipolar disorder.

References

American Psychiatric Association: Diagnostic and Statistical Manual of Mental Disorders, 4th Edition. Washington, DC, American Psychiatric Association, 1994

Buer MS, Whybrow PC, Gyulai J, et al: Testing definitions of dysphoric mania and hypomania. J Affect Disord 32:201–211, 1994

Cassidy F, Murray E, Forest K, et al: The performance of DSM-III-R major depression criteria in the diagnosis of bipolar mixed states. J Affect Disord 46:79–81, 1997

Cassidy F, Forest K, Murray E, et al: A factor analysis of the signs and symptoms of mania. Arch Gen Psychiatry 55:27–32, 1998

Dilsaver SC, Swann AC, Shoaib AM, et al: Depressive mania associated with nonresponse to antimanic agents. Am J Psychiatry 150:1548–1551, 1993

Dilsaver SC, Chen Y-W, Swann AC, et al: Suicidality in patients with pure and depressive mania. Am J Psychiatry 151:1312–1315, 1994

Freeman TW, Clothier JL, Pazzaglia P, et al: A double-blind comparison of valproate and lithium in the treatment of acute mania. Am J Psychiatry 149:108–111, 1992

Frye MA, Altshuler LL, Szuba MP, et al: The relationship between antimanic agent for treatment of classical or dysphoric mania and length of hospital stay. J Clin Psychiatry 57:17–21, 1996

Goodwin FK, Jamison KR: Manic-Depressive Illness. New York, Oxford University Press, 1990, p 48

Katz M, Klerman GL: Introduction: overview of the clinical studies program. Am J Psychiatry 136:49–51, 1979

Keck PE Jr, Nabulsi AA, Taylor JL, et al: A pharmacoeconomic model of divalproex vs. lithium in the acute and prophylactic treatment of bipolar I disorder. J Clin Psychiatry 57:213–222, 1996

Keller MB: Chronic and recurrent affective disorders: incidence, course and influencing factors, in Chronic Treatments in Neuropsychiatry. Edited by Kemali D, Racagni G. New York, Raven, 1985, pp 111–120

Keller MB: The course of manic-depressive illness. J Clin Psychiatry 49:4–6, 1988

Keller MB, Lavori PW, Coryell W, et al: Differential outcome of pure manic, mixed/cycling, and pure depressive episodes in patients with bipolar illness. JAMA 255:3138–3142, 1986

Keller MB, Lavori PW, Friedman B, et al: Longitudinal interval follow-up evaluation: a comprehensive method of assessing outcomes in prospective longitudinal studies. Arch Gen Psychiatry 44:540–548, 1987

Keller MB, Lavori PW, Mueller TI, et al: Time to recovery, chronicity, and levels of psychopathology in major depression: a five-year prospective follow-up of 431 subjects. Arch Gen Psychiatry 49:809–816, 1992

Keller MB, Lavori PW, Coryell W, et al: Bipolar I: a five-year prospective follow-up. J Nerv Ment Dis 181:238–245, 1993

Kraepelin E: Manic-Depressive Insanity (1921). Translated by Barclay RM. Edinburgh, Scotland, Livingstone. Reprint, New York, Arno Press, 1976

McElroy SL, Keck PE, Pope HG, et al: Clinical and research implications of the diagnosis of dysphoric or mixed mania or hypomania. Am J Psychiatry 149:1633–1644, 1992

Prien RF, Himmelhoch JM, Kupfer DJ: Treatment of mixed mania. J Affect Disord 15:9–15, 1988

Shapiro RW, Keller MB: Longitudinal Interval Follow-up Evaluation (LIFE). Boston, Massachusetts General Hospital, 1979

Spitzer RL, Endicott J: Schedule for Affective Disorders and Schizophrenia (SADS), 3rd Edition. New York, Biometrics Research Division, New York State Psychiatric Institute, 1979

Spitzer RL, Endicott J, Robins E: Research Diagnostic Criteria for a Selected Subgroup of Functional Disorders, 2nd Edition. New York, Biometrics Research Division, New York State Psychiatric Institute, 1985

Strakowski SM, McElroy SL, Keck PE Jr, et al: Suicidality among patients with mixed and manic bipolar disorder. Am J Psychiatry 153:674–676, 1996

Swann AC, Bowden CL, Morris D, et al: Depression during mania. Arch Gen Psychiatry 54:37–42, 1997

Tohen M, Waternaux CM, Tsuang MT: Outcome in mania: a 4-year prospective follow-up of 75 patients utilizing survival analysis. Arch Gen Psychiatry 47:1106–1111, 1990

CHAPTER 7

Depression in the Course of Bipolar Disorder

Joseph F. Goldberg, M.D.
James H. Kocsis, M.D.

*D*epression is common in the longitudinal course of bipolar disorder, although debate has arisen about its optimal treatment and
management. Uncertainties exist about whether depressive episodes differ phenomenologically in unipolar and bipolar patients,
whether mood stabilizers alone afford suitable treatment for both
manic and depressive phases of illness, how antidepressant medications may affect the short- and long-term courses of illness, and what
prognostic significance depressive episodes may hold in terms of
functioning and outcome for bipolar patients. In this chapter, we review these principal issues regarding the nature of depression in patients who have bipolar disorder, as well as current knowledge
about treatment and outcome for episodes of bipolar depression.

Phenomenology of Depression in Mania

Modern diagnostic systems such as DSM-IV (American Psychiatric
Association 1994) equate mania with bipolarity; depressive episodes
are typically viewed as an inevitable occurrence for most patients
who have acute mania. Nonetheless, some manic patients may never
develop depression. So-called *unipolar mania* has been suggested to

occur in one-quarter or more of some manic inpatients and may predominate among men (Abrams et al. 1979). Several investigators have questioned the validity of the concept of unipolar mania and have maintained that a careful history often identifies untreated depressive episodes (Nurnberger et al. 1979; Pfohl 1982).

Depressive episodes may occur at any time during the long-term natural history of bipolar disorder, and they tend to be of longer duration than are manic episodes (Angst 1981; Roy-Byrne et al. 1985). In the classic literature, Kraepelin (1921/1976) noted that depression typically preceded or followed mania in at least half of the cases he observed. Thus, the careful assessment of cycling in an affective episode may often reveal biphasic or triphasic patterns with depressive features that might otherwise elude detection. Contemporary investigators have observed that among men, manic and depressive episodes occur with similar frequency, whereas in women depressive episodes are typically more common than are manias or hypomanias (Goodwin and Jamison 1990). Bipolar patients also have significantly more episodes of depression than do unipolar-depressed patients (Roy-Byrne et al. 1985).

Longitudinal studies have found that patients who initially exhibit mania are likely to have predominantly manic relapses, whereas those who initially exhibit depression tend to have more depressive than manic recurrences (Perris and d'Elia 1966; Quitkin et al. 1986). Life chart data for a tertiary-care sample of bipolar patients treated at the National Institute of Mental Health (NIMH) suggest that a majority had both manic and depressive recurrences (Roy-Byrne et al. 1985). Similarly, within community-based clinical samples, naturalistic follow-up data such as that from the Chicago Follow-up Study indicate that a majority of bipolar patients (approximately 60%) had both manic and depressive recurrences at 2 years or 4–5 years after index hospitalization (Goldberg et al. 1995).

Depression as the
Initial Symptom of Bipolar Illness

How often do patients who have major depression eventually cycle into mania? Among children and adolescents with an affective disorder, follow-up studies suggest that a very early age at onset for depression confers a high risk (20%–30%) for subsequent bipolarity (Kovacs 1996). The likelihood for future mania also appears greater when depressed children or adolescents have a rapid onset of symptoms, psychomotor retardation, or psychotic features (Akiskal et al. 1983; Strober et al. 1982).

In adults, conversion rates from unipolar depression to bipolar disorder appear lower than in depressed children and adolescents. Dunner et al. (1976) reviewed records of bipolar I and bipolar II patients at the lithium clinic of the New York State Psychiatric Institute and found that 21% had been hospitalized initially for a "unipolar" major depression, whereas the remainder initially exhibited mania or hypomania. The authors used these data to estimate the degree of heterogeneity in broad samples of bipolar patients who initially exhibit unipolar depression and calculated that a patient with recurrent depression has approximately a 5% chance of becoming bipolar. No differences were reported between the bipolar I and bipolar II cohorts in their frequencies of depression predating the onset of mania or hypomania; however, bipolar patients drawn from specialized, tertiary-care academic centers may not be representative of typical bipolar patients. Other investigators have found that rates of conversion from unipolar depression to bipolar I disorder may be as high as 20%–40% (Akiskal et al. 1983; Rao and Nammalvar 1977).

Akiskal and colleagues (1983) noted that bipolar disorder was more likely to emerge among depressed patients when the onset of the depression occurred prior to age 25 years, atypical (hypersomnic-retarded) depressive features were evident, family histories of bipolar illness were present, or affective episodes occurred in the postpartum period or after induction by psychotropic medications.

Akiskal and colleagues (1995) examined the psychological and temperamental characteristics associated with depression in patients with bipolar disorder and, using a factor analysis, found that mood lability, high levels of energy-activity, daydreaming, and social anxiety significantly differentiated the unipolar-depressed patients who eventually had clear hypomania from the unipolar patients who did not.

Distinguishing Bipolar
From Unipolar Depression

Many investigators have compared the quality and severity of depressive symptoms among bipolar and unipolar patients. Delusions or hallucinations are common for most bipolar I manic patients, and current data tend to support the impression that psychosis is also more common among bipolar-depressed than unipolar-depressed patients (Goodwin and Jamison 1990). Detailed efforts to distinguish bipolar from unipolar depression have focused on clinical signs, premorbid characteristics, genetic–family history data, and treatment outcome.

Beigel and Murphy (1971) were among the first to compare the clinical features of depression in unipolar and bipolar patients. These authors observed that bipolar-depressed patients had less agitation, anxiety, and somatization than did unipolar-depressed patients. Katz et al. (1982) reported similar findings as part of the NIMH Clinical Research Branch Collaborative Study on the Psychobiology of Depression. Other investigators have noted that when bipolar patients become depressed, their episodes are typically of relatively short duration and are often characterized by diurnal variation, morning worsening, mood lability, and periods of derealization; in contrast, unipolar depression is often associated with episodes of longer duration, suicidality, initial insomnia, and weight loss (Mitchell et al. 1992). Psychomotor retardation is more common among bipolar-depressed than unipolar-depressed patients (Goodwin and Jamison 1990). Several genetic studies have found a higher frequency of first-degree relatives with affective illness among bipolar-depressed than unipolar-depressed patients (Goodwin and Jamison 1990).

From a clinical perspective, making an accurate cross-sectional diagnosis of bipolar depression may not always be straightforward. For example, in a patient with a major depressive episode but who reports a remote, prior diagnosis of mania or hypomania, the clinician may find it difficult to confirm accurately a previous bipolar episode based on accounts from the patient, corroborative historians, or past clinicians. At the same time, some clinicians or depressed patients may fail to identify previously undiagnosed episodes of mania or hypomania, especially if the episodes were never treated. Reliable diagnoses of bipolar II disorder are often difficult to make with reasonable certainty (see Coryell, Chapter 12, in this volume).

Some forms of depression that appear to be treatment-resistant and do not respond to adequate, sequential antidepressant trials may prompt the clinician to consider or reconsider the primary diagnosis, including the possibility of an underlying bipolar disorder. Nonprototypical forms of mania have been described that may further confound the diagnosis of severe, complex, or treatment-resistant forms of affective illness. Akiskal (1996) emphasized the heterogeneous nature of bipolar illness along the lines of a broad clinical spectrum. For example, the concepts of *soft bipolar signs, cyclothymia,* or *pseudounipolar disorder* have been used to describe some patients with recurrent depression who may show a hyperthymic temperament or low-grade mood instability yet never have mania or hypomania (Akiskal et al. 1985; Goodwin and Jamison 1990). Still other patients may have a major depressive episode initially but not reveal an underlying predisposition to bipolar disorder until later in the course of their illness.

Distinguishing agitated depression from mixed or dysphoric mania also can pose a challenge for even the most experienced clinician. Some clinical investigators have suggested that goal-directedness may be an essential feature by which to distinguish manic from depressive agitation. Similarly, diminished sleep is typically associated with fatigue in depression but undiminished energy in mania. In the absence of longitudinal data, it may at times be more difficult to differentiate depression from dysphoric mania in a bipolar patient than it is to identify depression in a patient with schizophrenia or schizoaffective disorder (Goodwin and Jamison 1990).

The differential diagnosis of bipolar depression is further complicated at times when attempting to delineate borderline character pathology or other Cluster B personality traits from dysphoric presentations of mania (Bolton et al. 1996). Longitudinal data and ancillary information such as a family history of bipolar disorder or past response to empiric trials of a mood stabilizer can sometimes support or clarify a predisposition to bipolar disorder in patients with depression.

Suicide in Bipolar Disorder

Approximately 19% of bipolar patients commit suicide (Goodwin and Jamison 1990), and the risk for suicidality appears higher during mixed or depressive phases of mania than during pure manic phases of illness (Dilsaver et al. 1994; Goldberg et al., in press b; Strakowski et al. 1996). Studies have suggested that suicide may be more likely to occur during the first few years after illness onset, with rates of completed suicide diminishing over time (Goodwin and Jamison 1990). Suicide attempts also appear to occur significantly more often among alcoholic than nonalcoholic bipolar patients (Feinman and Dunner 1996; Morrison 1974). Data from our studies at the Payne Whitney Clinic suggest that mixed-state bipolar patients may have a specific vulnerability for recurrent suicidality over time, which may be associated with lower remission rates from acute affective episodes (Goldberg et al., in press b). Other authors have noted that bipolar patients attempt suicide more often than do unipolar-depressed patients (Lester 1993). In addition, stressful life events are a common antecedent (>60%) of completed suicide in both bipolar and unipolar patients, although the nature of the stressful life events relate to self-damaging behaviors more often in bipolar than in unipolar patients (Isometsa et al. 1995).

Lithium use has been associated with a sixfold reduction in the rate of suicide attempts among bipolar patients (Tondo et al. 1997, 1998) and may also be superior to carbamazepine in preventing suicidal behaviors. In a 2.5-year prospective follow-up study of 378 bipolar patients, Thies-Flechtner and colleagues (1996) observed that none of nine suicide completions or five suicide attempts occurred during lithium treatment.

Comorbidity in Bipolar Depression

Affective disorders that co-occur with other psychiatric or medical disorders often appear more difficult to treat than are those occurring alone, and they may lead to greater functional disability over time. Sharma et al. (1995) compared frequencies of comorbidity in 24 unipolar-depressed and 25 bipolar-depressed patients. Although overall rates of any current comorbid diagnosis were significantly higher among unipolar (96%) than bipolar (56%) patients, both current and lifetime abuse of alcohol or other substances was significantly more common among bipolar-depressed than unipolar-depressed patients. Comorbid anxiety or agitation are particularly common in bipolar patients (see Himmelhoch, Chapter 13, in this volume).

Substance abuse is highly prevalent in bipolar disorder, although some debate exists as to whether it is more likely to occur during a manic or a depressive phase of illness. In contrast to unipolar depression, substance abuse among bipolar patients may arise more often as a symptom related to the recklessness and psychomotor acceleration of a manic episode, rather than as part of a depressive phase of illness. For example, some authors have observed that, often, bipolar patients who use cocaine do so during manic phases of illness, potentially in an effort to intensify high periods, rather than using the drug to self-medicate depression (Brady and Sonne 1995). Similarly, many bipolar patients use alcohol in the context of manic impulsivity, rather than in depressive phases of illness (Brady and Sonne 1995).

Other forms of comorbidity, such as panic or other anxiety disorders, are common in bipolar illness (Chen and Dilsaver 1995) and may add to the overall risk for suicidality, although empirical studies have not determined whether comorbid anxiety is more frequent during manic or depressed episodes.

Treatments for Bipolar Depression

Two of the central controversies surrounding the treatment of bipolar depression involve 1) the limited efficacy of current therapies and 2) questions about the safety of antidepressant therapies in bipolar disorder, because such therapies have been reported to trigger or evoke manic episodes. These two issues are related in that mood stabilizers, widely considered to be the mainstay of treatment for bipolar disorder in all its phases, may not always lead to remission of depressive symptoms when used without antidepressant agents.

Antidepressant medications, electroconvulsive therapy (ECT), and possibly other somatic antidepressant treatments have been linked to the induction of mania in some bipolar patients (see

Coryell, Chapter 12, in this volume). Wehr and Goodwin (1987) described the phenomenon of mania induced by the use of tricyclic antidepressants (TCAs) in bipolar patients. These investigators used a controlled study design, although reports from the 1950s found that mania or hypomania developed after the use of imipramine (Goodwin and Jamison 1990). Uncertainty exists about which antidepressants other than TCAs may hasten a manic phase of illness. Some investigators have suggested that selective serotonin reuptake inhibitors (SSRIs) may be less likely to precipitate mania than are TCAs (Peet 1994), although reports of SSRI-induced manias also exist (Howland 1996; Vesely et al. 1997). Which bipolar patients are most vulnerable to pharmacologically induced mania also remains poorly understood, although estimates of the overall risk for mania or hypomania induced by TCAs or other antidepressants are in the range of 30%–70% (Goodwin and Jamison 1990; Zornberg and Pope 1993). Hence, many clinicians and investigators urge the use of extreme caution when prescribing any antidepressant for a bipolar patient.

Treatment algorithms such as the Expert Consensus Guidelines (Frances et al. 1996) advocate the use of bupropion or an SSRI as first-line treatment choices for bipolar depression; second-line agents include monoamine oxidase inhibitors (MAOIs), venlafaxine, and nefazodone; TCAs are described as *low-rated second-line agents* that should be avoided in bipolar-depressed patients who have histories of antidepressant-induced mania or rapid cycling.

Many clinicians anecdotally recommend the use of smaller-than-usual doses of antidepressants for shorter-than-usual periods of time during depressive phases of illness. Some clinicians advocate ensuring the presence of a "therapeutic" blood level of a primary mood stabilizer before adding any antidepressant medication as a form of protection against precipitating mania, although this clinical practice has not been investigated rigorously.

Mood Stabilizers

Early investigations compared the antidepressant effects of lithium on depressed patients who had histories of mania or hypomania with the effects of lithium on those who had no such histories

(Goodwin et al. 1969, 1972). More than one-half of the bipolar-depressed patients showed at least partial improvement, whereas nearly one-third had complete remission from depression when taking lithium alone. Among the unipolar-depressed patients in these samples, those with recurrent episodes also were more likely to show at least a partial response to lithium than were patients with single episodes. These authors suggest that the frequency, or *cyclicity,* of affective episodes (regardless of polarity) may affect the likelihood of treatment response to lithium.

The extent to which lithium is effective for bipolar depression, either acutely or prophylactically, remains an empirical question with limited research data available. In two multicenter studies, lithium monotherapy was comparable to imipramine monotherapy in preventing depressive recurrences among bipolar patients (Prien et al. 1973, 1984). However, the addition of a TCA (imipramine) to lithium did not enhance the efficacy of lithium alone in preventing depressive relapses among bipolar patients (Kane et al. 1981; Prien et al. 1984). By contrast, another study found that lithium was superior to imipramine after 3 weeks of treatment for the depressive phase of bipolar disorder (Worrall et al. 1979). In a noncontrolled study, half of all bipolar II or cyclothymic patients had a depressive relapse during lithium prophylaxis (Peselow et al. 1982).

Anticonvulsant mood stabilizers have gained popularity among patients who have treatment-resistant forms of bipolar disorder (see Post et al., Chapter 5, in this volume). Their use specifically in dysphoric mania (see also Boland and Keller, Chapter 6, in this volume) or in pure depressive phases of illness has received particular attention. According to initial reports, divalproex sodium may have some advantage over lithium in the treatment of mixed mania (Bowden et al. 1994), although it has not shown efficacy as monotherapy for depression without concurrent manic features in bipolar patients.

Lamotrigine and gabapentin are among the newest anticonvulsants being used "off label" with increasing frequency in the treatment of bipolar disorder. Lamotrigine may have antidepressant effects among rapid-cycling bipolar patients (Calabrese et al. 1996). In a preliminary open trial of lamotrigine add-on or monotherapy in 39 bipolar patients who had treatment-refractory depression, overall depression ratings improved moderately or markedly in 69% of the sample, and remissions were sustained for at least 6 months (Calabrese et al. 1997). In another open-label study, five of nine bipolar patients with treatment-resistant depression showed no significant symptoms after an average of 5 weeks of treatment with lamotrigine (Sporn and Sachs 1997). Frye et al. (1998) reported preliminary results of a 6-week double-blind trial involving lamotrigine, gabapentin, or placebo, in which significant improvement was observed in patients with treatment-refractory bipolar depression who received lamotrigine. Further large-scale controlled clinical trials are needed for these and other new anticonvulsants (e.g., topiramate, tiagabine) that could have potential antidepressant properties in bipolar disorder.

Lithium combined with an anticonvulsant mood stabilizer may provide greater protection from affective relapse during maintenance treatment than when lithium alone is used to stabilize mood (Solomon et al. 1997). Further studies are needed to determine whether combinations of mood stabilizers offer superior prophylaxis against depressive and manic recurrences.

Antidepressants

Antidepressant agents given without a mood stabilizer are rarely advocated in the treatment of bipolar disorders. Yet, because lithium or anticonvulsant mood stabilizers may not always be effective in severe bipolar-depressed states, antidepressant medications are usually considered at some point for many bipolar patients. Many clinicians initiate treatment for bipolar depression by optimizing one or more mood stabilizers and then adding an antidepressant medication if the response is suboptimal. Treatment guidelines also distinguish severe from mild major depressive episodes in bipolar disorder. In severe nonpsychotic depression, a mood stabilizer combined with an antidepressant is recommended, whereas in milder major depressions, a sequential approach, starting with a mood stabilizer alone, is recommended (Frances et al. 1996).

Antidepressants are generally not recommended for long-term treatment of depression in bipolar patients. The potential danger of antidepressant-induced mania or hypomania has inspired a search for agents less likely to induce cycling. At the same time, depressive phases of illness may be especially resistant to treatment with first-line antidepressant medications (Sachs 1996), prompting a need for safe and effective antidepressant agents for the treatment of bipolar depression.

Case reports and clinical trials have suggested that two classes of antidepressant medications—MAOIs and the atypical antidepressant bupropion—may have better efficacy for bipolar depression and may be less likely to precipitate mania than are other antidepressants. Data regarding the use of MAOIs are derived mainly from a controlled study that found tranylcypromine to be superior to imipramine in treating anergic depression among 56 bipolar outpatients (Himmelhoch et al. 1991). Bupropion in the treatment of bipolar depression has been associated with antidepressant efficacy combined with a lower-than-expected risk of inducing manic episodes (Sachs et al. 1994). Several case reports have suggested that bupropion may exert a prophylactic effect in bipolar illness (Shopsin 1983), whereas others have found that it may also precipitate mania (Fogelson et al. 1992; Zubieta and Demitrack 1991).

Few systematic data exist on the safety and efficacy of SSRIs in the treatment of bipolar depression. A small, naturalistic chart review found that paroxetine was associated with remission from depression in 65% of patients whose bipolar disorder was formerly resistant to treatment, whereas only 10% cycled into mania (Baldassano et al. 1995). Similarly, fluoxetine was associated with an 86% rate of improvement after 6 weeks of treatment in 89 bipolar-depressed patients (Benfield et al. 1986), and the drug is efficacious among bipolar II patients who had depression (Simpson and De Paulo 1987). However, one double-blind study found a 19% rate of switching into mania or hypomania during fluoxetine treatment for bipolar depression (Cohn et al. 1989).

Data have become available from the first randomized placebo-controlled trial of paroxetine compared with imipramine for bipolar depression (Pitts et al. 1997). These authors observed comparable efficacy between the two antidepressants but a higher switch rate into mania with imipramine (8.3%) than with paroxetine (0%). They also found significantly more anticholinergic side effects with imipramine than with paroxetine. Further clinical trials are needed to assess the efficacy and rates of treatment-emergent mania with other SSRIs, such as sertraline or fluvoxamine, and other agents such as venlafaxine, nefazodone, or mirtazapine.

Electroconvulsive Therapy

Interest in the use of ECT has been renewed recently. Today, it is often considered the treatment of choice for psychotic depression and for use in pregnant, treatment-resistant, or psychotically depressed bipolar patients (Frances et al. 1996; Sachs 1996; Small et al. 1988). The overall response to ECT in bipolar and unipolar depression appears to be comparable, although few studies exist in this area (Goodwin and Jamison 1990). Some investigators have reported that the risk for treatment-induced mania may be higher when using unilateral-nondominant rather than bilateral ECT, suggesting that bilateral treatment may be preferable for most depressed patients (Sachs 1996). The risk of treatment-induced mania may be lower with ECT in general than with pharmacotherapies for mania. Thus, ECT may offer some advantage over other antidepressant treatments with regard to its effect on subsequent cycling and the long-term course of illness.

Alternative Treatments

Other somatic therapies for bipolar depression, particularly in treatment-resistant cases, have been described in noncontrolled studies or case reports, although data from rigorous clinical trials are scarce. Novel strategies include neuroleptics, calcium channel blockers, hypermetabolic thyroid hormone, biogenic amine precursors, phototherapy, sleep deprivation, ascorbic acid, methylene blue, ethylenediaminetetraacetic (EDTA) acid, and in women, hormone therapy (estrogen/progesterone) (see Dubovsky and Buzan 1997; Sachs 1996). Such alternative treatment approaches have a smaller database of evidence in support of their efficacy and safety and await further systematic study.

Certain dopamine agonists used to treat Parkinson's disease also may have antidepressant properties, including pergolide (Bouckoms and Mangini 1993) and pramipexole (Corrigan and Evans 1997; DeBattista and Schatzberg 1998). Pramipexole has been found in preliminary case reports to improve depression among bipolar patients without inducing mania (Goldberg et al., in press a). Controlled trials with these agents are needed to further assess their safety and efficacy for bipolar depression.

Psychotherapy

Specific psychotherapies targeted at affective symptoms have been developed. Advances in this area, notably in cognitive psychotherapy, interpersonal psychotherapy for bipolar disorder, and social rhythm therapy, are discussed in greater detail in Miklowitz and Frank, Chapter 4, in this volume.

In the treatment of bipolar depression, psychotherapies are advocated as helpful second-line measures that enhance psychosocial support, improve medication compliance, and monitor key features of the illness such as sleep hygiene and cyclicity and potential complications such as substance abuse or suicidality. Psychosocial factors such as the loss of an important relationship or changes in work, school, home life, or other interpersonal areas profoundly influence functioning in bipolar patients. Whether life stresses in bipolar patients may predispose a given individual to depressive versus manic recurrences is not well described. The kindling model of bipolar illness (see Post et al., Chapter 5, in this volume) also postulates that psychosocial stresses may be especially important in the first few episodes of bipolar illness; if so, psychotherapy and other psychosocial interventions could play an especially important role if initiated early in the course of illness.

In summary, treatment approaches to depression in the course of bipolar disorder are often varied and based at times on limited empirical data. The following case describes the development of depressive episodes in a rapid-cycling bipolar patient who underwent a number of successive pharmacotherapeutic trials before achieving mood stabilization with lamotrigine.

Ms. A, a 40-year-old woman, reported a lifelong history of mood swings, beginning with a hypomanic episode at age 15 and a major depression at age 18. Recently, she had developed rapid cycling, which lithium partially but incompletely suppressed. Ms. A was unable to tolerate carbamazepine or valproate because of a variety of side effects. She developed a predominant pattern of frequent episodes of depression, which responded to antidepressants but led quickly to hypomanias. Supraphysiological thyroid dosing achieved further partial relief. Cycling continued in a less frequent and malignant fashion, which allowed Ms. A to work and socialize more productively. Finally, lamotrigine was introduced with a gradual taper of thyroid supplement and lithium. She has sustained a marked improvement for more than 9 months. The lack of episodes of depression or hypomania during this interval on lamotrigine constitutes her longest euthymic period in many years.

Summary

Depressive episodes may signal the onset of bipolar illness in 5%–40% of patients with affective disorders, especially when accompanied by psychosis, early age at and rapidity of onset, and psychomotor retardation or other atypical depressive features. Depression and dysphoric-manic states markedly impair psychosocial functioning for many bipolar patients and have been associated with an increased risk for comorbid psychiatric disorders, treatment resistance, and suicide.

Standard pharmacotherapies for depression often increase the danger of antidepressant-induced cycling into mania, which may worsen both short- and long-term courses of illness. Lithium and the anticonvulsant mood stabilizers are often the mainstay of treatment, at times augmented with brief courses of antidepressants. When used on a short-term basis, bupropion, tranylcypromine, and some SSRIs may be less likely to induce cycling than are TCAs and other antidepressants. Other important treatment approaches include ECT and psychotherapy. Judicious pharmacology and early clinical interventions—before patterns of kindled episodes or treatment resistance develop—appear critical in minimizing the effects of depression on the long-term course of bipolar disorder.

References

Abrams R, Taylor MA, Hayman MA, et al: Unipolar mania revisited. J Affect Disord 1:59–68, 1979

Akiskal HS: The prevalent clinical spectrum of bipolar disorders: beyond DSM-IV. J Clin Psychopharmacol 16(1):4S–14S, 1996

Akiskal HS, Walker P, Puzantian VR, et al: Bipolar outcome in the course of depressive illness: phenomenologic, familial, and pharmacologic predictors. J Affect Disord 5:115–128, 1983

Akiskal HS, Downs J, Jordan P, et al: Affective disorders in referred children and younger siblings of manic-depressives: mode of onset and prospective course. Arch Gen Psychiatry 42:996–1003, 1985

Akiskal HS, Maser JD, Zeller PJ, et al: Switching from "unipolar" to bipolar II: an 11-year prospective study of clinical and temperamental predictors in 559 patients. Arch Gen Psychiatry 52:114–123, 1995

American Psychiatric Association: Diagnostic and Statistical Manual of Mental Disorders, 4th Edition. Washington, DC, American Psychiatric Association, 1994

Angst J: Course of affective disorders, in Handbook of Biological Psychiatry. Edited by Van Praag HM, Lader MH, Rafaelson OJ, et al. New York, Marcel Dekker, 1981, pp 225–242

Baldassano CF, Sachs GS, Stoll AL, et al: Paroxetine for bipolar depression: outcome in patients failing prior antidepressant trials. Depression 3:182–186, 1995

Beigel A, Murphy DL: Differences in clinical characteristics accompanying depression in unipolar and bipolar affective illness. Arch Gen Psychiatry 24:215–220, 1971

Benfield P, Heel RC, Lewis SP: Fluoxetine: a review of its pharmacodynamic and pharmacokinetic properties, and therapeutic efficacy in depressive illness. Drugs 32:481–508, 1986

Bolton S, Gunderson JG: Distinguishing borderline personality disorder from bipolar disorder: differential diagnosis and implications. Am J Psychiatry 153:1202–1207, 1996

Bouckoms A, Mangini L: Pergolide: an antidepressant adjuvant for mood disorders? Psychopharmacol Bull 29:207–211, 1993

Bowden CL, Brugger AM, Swann AC, et al: Efficacy of divalproex vs. lithium and placebo in the treatment of mania. JAMA 271:918–924, 1994

Brady KT, Sonne SC: The relationship between substance abuse and bipolar disorder. J Clin Psychiatry 56 (suppl 3):19–24, 1995

Calabrese JR, Fatemi SH, Woyshville MJ: Antidepressant effects of lamotrigine in rapid cycling bipolar disorder (letter). Am J Psychiatry 153:1236, 1996

Calabrese JR, Bowden CL, McElroy SL, et al: Lamotrigine in bipolar disorder: preliminary data. CME Syllabus and Scientific Proceedings of the 150th Annual Meeting of the American Psychiatric Association. Washington, DC, American Psychiatric Association, 1997, p 85

Chen Y-W, Dilsaver SC: Comorbidity of panic disorder in bipolar illness: evidence from the Epidemiologic Catchment Area Survey. Am J Psychiatry 152:280–282, 1995

Cohn JB, Collins G, Ashbrook E, et al: A comparison of fluoxetine, imipramine and placebo in patients with bipolar depressive disorder. Int Clin Psychopharmacol 4:313–322, 1989

Corrigan M, Evans D: Pramipexole, a dopamine agonist, in the treatment of major depression. Paper presented at the 36th annual meeting of the American College of Neuropsychopharmacology, Waikoloa, HI, December 8–12, 1997

Coryell W, Andreason NC, Endicott J, et al: The significance of past mania or hypomania in the course and outcome of major depression. Am J Psychiatry 144:309–315, 1987

DeBattista C, Schatzberg AF: Pramipexole augmentation of SSRIs in treatment-resistant major depression. Poster 189 presented at the 38th annual meeting of the New Clinical Drug Evaluation Unit (NCDEU) Program, Boca Raton, FL, June 10–13, 1998

Dilsaver SC, Chen Y-W, Swann AC, et al: Suicidality in patients with pure and depressive mania. Am J Psychiatry 151:1312–1315, 1994

Dubovsky SL, Buzan RD: Novel alternatives and supplements to lithium and anticonvulsants for bipolar affective disorder. J Clin Psychiatry 58: 224–242, 1997

Dunner DL, Fleiss JL, Fieve RR: The course of development of mania in patients with recurrent depression. Am J Psychiatry 133:905–908, 1976

Feinman JA, Dunner DL: The effect of alcohol and substance abuse on the course of bipolar affective disorder. J Affect Disord 37:43–49, 1996

Fogelson DL, Bystritsky A, Pasnau R: Bupropion in the treatment of bipolar disorders: the same old story? J Clin Psychiatry 53:443–446, 1992

Frances A, Docherty JP, Kahn DA: The Expert Consensus Guideline Series: treatment of bipolar disorder. J Clin Psychiatry 57 (suppl 12A):1–88, 1996

Frye MA, Ketter TA, Osuch EA, et al: Gabapentin and lamotrigine monotherapy in mood disorder: an update, in CME Syllabus and Scientific Proceedings of the 151st Annual Meeting of the American Psychiatric Association. Washington, DC, American Psychiatric Association, 1998, p 150

Goldberg JF, Harrow M, Grossman LS: Recurrent affective syndromes in bipolar and unipolar mood disorders at follow-up. Br J Psychiatry 166: 382–385, 1995

Goldberg JF, Frye MA, Dunn RT, et al: Pramipexole in refractory bipolar depression (letter). Am J Psychiatry (in press a)

Goldberg JF, Garno JL, Leon AC, et al: Recurrent suicidal ideation is associated with non-remission from acute mixed mania. Am J Psychiatry (in press b)

Goodwin FK, Jamison KR: Manic-Depressive Illness. New York, Oxford University Press, 1990

Goodwin FK, Murphy DL, Bunney WE Jr: Lithium carbonate treatment in depression and mania. Arch Gen Psychiatry 21:486–496, 1969

Goodwin FK, Murphy DL, Dunner DL, et al: Lithium response in unipolar versus bipolar depression. Am J Psychiatry 129:44–47, 1972

Himmelhoch JM, Thase ME, Mallinger AG, et al: Tranylcypromine versus imipramine in anergic bipolar depression. Am J Psychiatry 148:910–916, 1991

Howland RH: Induction of mania with serotonin reuptake inhibitors. J Clin Psychopharmacol 16:425–427, 1996

Isometsa E, Heikkinen M, Henriksson M, et al: Recent life events and completed suicide in bipolar affective disorder; a comparison with major depressive suicides. J Affect Disord 33:99–106, 1995

Kane JM, Quitkin FM, Rifkin A, et al: Prophylactic lithium with and without imipramine for bipolar I patients: a double-blind study. Psychopharmacol Bull 17:144–145, 1981

Katz MM, Croughan J, Secunda S, et al: Behavioural measurement and drug response characteristics of unipolar and bipolar depression. Psychol Med 12:25–36, 1982

Kovacs M: Presentation and course of major depressive disorder during childhood and later years of the life span. J Am Acad Child Adolesc Psychiatry 35:705–715, 1996

Kraepelin E: Manic-Depressive Insanity and Paranoia (1921). Translated by Barclay RM. Edited by Robertson GM. Edinburgh, Scotland, Livingstone. Reprint, New York, Arno Press, 1976

Lester D: Suicidal behavior in bipolar and unipolar affective disorders: a meta-analysis. J Affect Disord 27:117–121, 1993

Mitchell P, Parker G, Jamieson K, et al: Are there any differences between bipolar and unipolar melancholia? J Affect Disord 25:97–106, 1992

Morrison JR: Bipolar affective disorder and alcoholism. Am J Psychiatry 131:1130–1133, 1974

Nurnberger J, Roose SP, Dunner DL, et al: Unipolar mania: a distinct clinical entity? Am J Psychiatry 136:1420–1423, 1979

Peet M: Induction of mania with selective serotonin re-uptake inhibitors and tricyclic antidepressants. Br J Psychiatry 164:549–550, 1994

Perris C, d'Elia G: A study of bipolar (manic-depressive) and unipolar recurrent major depressive psychoses; X: mortality, suicide, and life cycles. Acta Psychiatr Scand 42 (suppl 194):172–183, 1966

Peselow ED, Dunner DL, Fieve RR, et al: Lithium prophylaxis of depression in unipolar, bipolar II, and cyclothymic patients. Am J Psychiatry 39: 747–775, 1982

Pfohl B, Vasquez N, Nasrallah H: Unipolar vs. bipolar mania: a review of 247 patients. Br J Psychiatry 141:453–458, 1982

Pitts CD, Young ML, Oakes R: Comparative safety of paroxetine versus imipramine in the treatment of bipolar depression. Poster 13 presented at the annual meeting of the New Clinical Drug Evaluation Unit (NCDEU), May 1997

Prien RF, Caffey EM, Klett CJ: Prophylactic efficacy of lithium carbonate in manic-depressive illness: report of the Veterans Administration and National Institute of Mental Health Collaborative Study Group. Arch Gen Psychiatry 28:337–341, 1973

Prien RF, Kupfer DJ, Mansky PA, et al: Drug therapy in the prevention of recurrences in unipolar and bipolar affective disorders: report of the NIMH Collaborative Study Group comparing lithium carbonate, imipramine, and a lithium carbonate–imipramine combination. Arch Gen Psychiatry 41:1096–1104, 1984

Quitkin FM, Rabkin JG, Prien RF: Bipolar disorder: Are there manic-prone and depressive-prone forms? J Clin Psychopharmacol 6:167–172, 1986

Rao AV, Nammalvar N: The course and outcome in depressive illness: a follow-up study of 122 cases in Madurai, India. Br J Psychiatry 130:392–396, 1977

Roy-Byrne PR, Post RM, Uhde TW, et al: The longitudinal course of recurrent affective illness: life chart data from research patients at the NIMH. Acta Psychiatr Scand 71 (suppl 317):1–32, 1985

Sachs GS: Treatment-resistant bipolar depression. Psychiatric Clin North Am 19:215–236, 1996

Sachs GS, Lafer B, Stoll AL, et al: A double-blind trial of bupropion versus desipramine for bipolar depression. J Clin Psychiatry 55:391–393, 1994

Sharma V, Mazmanian D, Persad E, et al: A comparison of comorbid patterns in treatment-resistant unipolar and bipolar depression. Can J Psychiatry 40:270–274, 1995

Shopsin B: Bupropion's prophylactic efficacy in bipolar affective illness. J Clin Psychiatry 44(5, sec 2):163–169, 1983

Simpson SG, DePaulo JR: Fluoxetine treatment of bipolar II depression. J Clin Psychopharmacol 11:52–54, 1987

Small JG, Klapper MH, Kellams JJ, et al: Electroconvulsive treatment compared with lithium in the management of manic states. Arch Gen Psychiatry 45:727–732, 1988

Solomon DA, Ryan CE, Keitner GI, et al: A pilot study of lithium carbonate plus divalproex sodium for the continuation and maintenance treatment of patients with bipolar I disorder. J Clin Psychiatry 58:95–99, 1997

Sporn J, Sachs G: The anticonvulsant lamotrigine in treatment-resistant manic-depressive illness. J Clin Psychopharmacol 17:185–189, 1997

Strakowski SM, McElroy SL, Keck PE Jr, et al: Suicidality among patients with mixed and manic bipolar disorder. Am J Psychiatry 153:674–676, 1996

Strober M, Carlson G: Bipolar illness in adolescents with major depression: clinical, genetic, and psychopharmacologic predictors in a three- to four-year prospective follow-up investigation. Arch Gen Psychiatry 39:549–555, 1982

Thies-Flechtner K, Müller-Oerlinghausen B, Seibert W, et al: Effect of prophylactic treatment on suicide risk in patients with major affective disorders: data from a randomized prospective trial. Pharmacopsychiatry 29(3):103–107, 1996

Tondo L, Jamison KR, Baldessarini RJ: Effect of lithium maintenance on suicidal behavior in major mood disorders, in The Neurobiology of Suicide: From the Bench to the Clinic. Edited by Stoff DM, Mann JJ. New York, Annals of the New York Academy of Sciences, Vol 836, 1997

Tondo L, Baldessarini RJ, Hennen J, et al: Lithium treatment and risk of suicidal behavior in bipolar disorder patients. J Clin Psychiatry 59:405–414, 1998

Vesely C, Fischer P, Goessler R, et al: Mania associated with serotonin reuptake inhibitors (letter). J Clin Psychiatry 58:88, 1997

Wehr TA, Goodwin FK: Can antidepressants cause mania and worsen the course of affective illness? Am J Psychiatry 144:1403–1411, 1987

Worrall EP, Moody JP, et al: Controlled studies of the acute antidepressant effects of lithium. Br J Psychiatry 135:255–262, 1979

Zornberg GL, Pope HG Jr: Treatment of depression in bipolar disorder: new directions for research. J Clin Psychopharmacol 13:397–408, 1993

Zubieta JK, Demitrack MA: Possible bupropion precipitation of mania and a mixed affective state. J Clin Psychopharmacol 11:327–328, 1991

CHAPTER 8

Comparison of Open Versus Blinded Studies in Bipolar Disorder

Charles L. Bowden, M.D.

*I*n this chapter, I discuss the clinical course of treatments for bipolar disorder and how investigators and practicing clinical psychiatrists are able to work in the difficult arena of bipolar disorder and achieve some reliability in their observations.

Illness Course Variables
Aiding the Study of Bipolar Disorder

The results I describe here are quite encouraging. For all the complexities of bipolar disorder, clinicians have one real advantage not present in most psychiatric disorders: the *sine qua non* of the diagnosis of bipolar disorder, at least bipolar I, is the presence of manic episodes. This characteristic has contributed to the development of the three mood stabilizers: lithium, valproate, and carbamazepine. In particular, the effectiveness of divalproex sodium and carbamazepine emerged largely from clinician-driven observations of the benefits of these medications in bipolar disorders. These two drugs did not emerge through impetus initiated by research psychopharmacological firms but out of psychiatrists' clinical practices.

The presence of mania makes assessment of treatment efficacy relatively easy. The criteria for mania are met principally through observable signs, as opposed to inferences or subjective experiences that patients relate but that clinicians can access only indirectly. Thus, most of what occurs during a bipolar I manic episode is observable even to the casual observer. Episodes not only are observable but also recur, and they do so with substantial frequency. As a result, clinicians can observe mania as well as use the recurrence of these episodes as an index of whether treatments are accomplishing their intended goal—to reduce the frequency of episodes.

Several other indices of outcome are also relatively reliable. These indices include the higher frequencies at which people with bipolar disorder commit suicide, divorce, remarry, declare bankruptcy, and change jobs. For example, one might ask whether cognitive therapy interventions in bipolar disorder reduce the frequency of suicide. The question is relatively easy to answer, because bipolar disorder entails countable phenomena. If a person attempts or commits suicide, terrible though it is, clinicians can assess the occurrence of this event reliably.

Table 8–1 presents data from a study in Denmark that showed the mortality rate in bipolar disorder to be four times higher than expected, not because these patients had adverse effects to lithium therapy, and not only because they had higher frequencies of suicide, but also because of increased mortality from cardiovascular disease and a number of accidental causes of death (Aagaard and Vestergaard 1990). These high rates may be related indirectly to risk-taking behaviors characteristic of the illness. These observations allow clinicians to use outcomes, other than symptomatic outcomes,

Table 8–1.   Five-year mortality in bipolar patients treated with lithium

Medical cause	Rate[a]
Uncertain cause	30.7
Cardiovascular	3.3
Pneumonia	10.7
Other causes	1.05
Total	4.35

[a]Rate is presented as the multiple of the rate expected from age- and sex-matched population norms.

that are linked closely to bipolar disorder. These outcomes can then be quantified in ways that offer an advantage over studies of other psychiatric disorders such as panic disorder and generalized anxiety disorder.

Few placebo-controlled studies have examined bipolar disorder. Table 8–2 lists the placebo-controlled studies that contributed to the regulatory approval of lithium for treatment of acute mania and the one placebo-controlled, parallel-group study. The early studies were inadequate by today's standards in several ways: they did not operationalize diagnostic criteria, they were crossover studies that would not be adequate in today's regulatory climate, and the early investigators did not have the use of the reliable rating procedures used in our study (Bowden et al. 1994) or in Pope et al.'s study (1991) of divalproex sodium. Nevertheless, by determining the patient's lithium response categorically—assessing these patients as complete, partial, or nonresponders, thereby taking advantage of the specificity of manic symptoms—these investigators were able to assess response reliably and sensitively (Goodwin et al. 1969). Indeed, the magnitude of the drug-placebo difference was about as great in the one parallel-group study as in the earlier crossover trials. Phrased differently, it is almost impossible to enroll a patient in a study of bipolar disorder, especially of acute manic episodes, unless

Table 8–2.　Lithium response in acute mania, placebo-controlled trials

Study	Type	Number of patients	% Response[a]
Schou et al. 1954	CO	38	[b]
Maggs 1963	CO	28	[c]
Goodwin et al. 1969	CO	12	75
Stokes et al. 1971	CO	38	75
Bowden et al. 1994	PG	36	49
Overall		152	64

Note.　CO = crossover; PG = parallel group.
[a]Response = 40% or greater improvement over baseline, or equivalent thereof.
[b]Crossover number not determinable.
[c]% responding not determinable, but response to lithium was greater than response to placebo.

the patient has the disease, or to call a person a clear-cut responder unless he or she is indeed responding. Some false-negative results may occur, in that some people who have manic or hypomanic episodes may not have been recognized as such because of exclusion criteria. Also, the course of bipolar disorder can contribute to underdiagnosis, especially early in the illness, because of patients who have one or more depressive episodes before the first episode of mania. Nevertheless, for those patients whom we diagnose as having bipolar disorder, we can have great confidence in the accuracy of the diagnosis and the clarity of the patients' response to treatments.

Study Limitations

Although the above-mentioned characteristics of bipolar disorder lend credibility to many open studies or comparison studies that have methodological limitations, it may be difficult to meaningfully or confidently interpret studies of bipolar disorder. This difficulty usually arises because critical information was not included, a small number of patients were studied, or data came from only one or two studies, without confirmation across studies. The following studies illustrate these problems.

One study of lithium in acute mania included placebo-treated patients in a crossover design (Schou et al. 1954). However, the report did not indicate the number of patients who were randomly crossed-over or the way they were assessed. A few studies of other medications used a placebo comparison. The positive reports on the calcium channel blocker verapamil are illustrative of problems with small-size studies with inconsistent methodologies. The first placebo-controlled trial of verapamil involved only seven subjects, one of whom received no placebo in the crossover design (Dubovsky et al. 1986). Another study with 12 patients did not specify diagnostic criteria nor whether patients were in an illness episode (Giannini et al. 1984).

The largest study to compare verapamil and lithium reported equivalent response rates, but neuroleptic use was much higher in verapamil-treated patients (Garza-Treviño et al. 1992). Randomized assignment, in which the patient has an equal likelihood of receiving the treatments under study at the starting point, provides a much more powerful test of hypotheses (see next section). For example, in a study of clonidine, which some open trials found to be effective in the treatment of mania, a random assignment design indicated that the drug was equal to placebo (Janicak et al. 1989). Janicak et al.'s randomized comparison of verapamil with placebo showed no difference in response between verapamil and placebo (Janicak et al. 1998). A randomized comparison of verapamil and lithium reported that lithium was significantly better than verapamil in alleviating acute manic symptoms (Walton et al. 1995); however, investigators knew which drug the patients were receiving, weakening the conclusions to be drawn.

This summary of studies on verapamil illustrates the importance of randomization, blinding, and placebo control in key clinical studies to establish efficacy for a medication. Blinding is needed to ensure that bias favoring one treatment over another is not a factor in outcome assessment. Placebo control ensures that reported success is not simply a consequence of noncritical interpretation of response or response that is essentially the natural course of the disorder when nonspecific interventions are used. Evidence indicates that specific drug benefits occur largely among patients who have moderate or marked illness severity, whereas placebo responsiveness is observed largely among patients who have mild illness severity (Uhlenhuth et al. 1997).

Placebo-controlled trials need to be implemented judiciously because potentially beneficial treatments are being withheld for a period of time from patients who receive some form of placebo therapy. For a more extensive discussion of the ethical and scientific aspects of placebo-controlled studies, see Rothman and Michels (1994). These authors address the importance of factors such as limiting placebo trials to situations in which efficacy has not been established. They do not acknowledge the nonspecific benefits of educational, psychosocial, and environmental structuring associated with randomization to placebo drug in psychiatric studies. Only when a drug can be shown to provide improvement, beyond the often substantial improvement provided by necessary caring support, can one conclude that the drug per se is efficacious.

Although randomized and blinded placebo-controlled studies

are important in all areas of medicine, their role in psychiatry is particularly important because of the partial benefits of these supportive psychotherapeutic measures. These benefits are generally more apparent in mildly ill rather than severely ill patients (Uhlenhuth et al. 1997). This has two important implications. Open reports of patients with mild symptoms may be misleadingly positive. Fortunately, this is unlikely to be the case in a manic episode because of its inherent severity. Second, it is now clear that studies that use placebo assignment need to enroll and treat patients with at least moderate illness severity to increase the likelihood of an effective treatment yielding statistical superiority over placebo. For bipolar disorder, this is more an issue for studies of prophylactic efficacy (Bowden et al. 1997).

The importance of conducting a study that includes a placebo needs to be determined in relation to the disease under consideration. Certainly, the ravages of untreated bipolar disorder warrant use of scientifically sound designs to improve the efficacy and safety of treatments. Placebo treatments should be continued only as long as necessary to answer the medically important question being addressed. Generally, acute treatment studies, measured in weeks, are more appropriate for placebo designs than are studies requiring months to address maintenance questions. The number of patients studied on placebo needs to be sufficient to answer the question but not larger than needed to meet the study's statistical projections. Fortunately, the availability of one or two well-designed controlled trials in a disease and treatment area aids greatly in interpreting the larger number of open and non-placebo-controlled studies.

Comparison of Open and Controlled Studies of Valproate in Acute Mania

Randomized assignment, in which patients have an equal likelihood of receiving the treatments under study, provides a much more powerful test of hypotheses. The completion of two well-designed and executed randomized, parallel-group, placebo-controlled studies of divalproex sodium allows for a comparison of the results achieved in these rigorous studies with those reported in open or comparator trials. Response to valproate has been studied in open or nonplacebo comparison trials involving more than 300 patients with varyingly well-defined manic states. The first study of valproate's effectiveness in bipolar disorder was published in 1966 (Lambert et al. 1966). Several open trials and a smaller number of comparator studies followed. In general, these open studies from Europe and the United States indicated an aggregate response rate, for moderate or better response, of about two-thirds of patients receiving valproate (see Table 8–3).

The outcomes are quite similar in the open and active comparator studies to those in the two placebo-controlled trials. These results indicate that one can generally have confidence in open trials of valproate in bipolar disorder. In general, the smaller number of patients in a study, the less reliable the results. For example, in a report based on only eight patients, a shift in two patients changes the response rate by 25%. Nevertheless, both small and larger studies were generally encouraging, with an aggregate response rate of greater than 60%, and led to placebo-controlled studies (Bowden et

Table 8–3.   Valproate response in acute mania

Study	Type	Number of patients	% Response
Placebo-controlled studies			
Pope et al. 1991	P	36	65
Bowden et al. 1994	P	179	54
Overall placebo-controlled		215	56
Open or comparator studies			
Emrich and Wolf 1992	C	12	75
Brennan et al. 1984	C	8	75
Prasad 1984	O	7	71
McElroy et al. 1988	O	56	59
Brown et al. 1989	O	233	64
Post et al. 1989	C	13	54
Calabrese and Delucchi 1990	O	31	61
Lambert 1984	O	20	50
Overall open or comparator		380	63

Note.   P = placebo-controlled study; C = comparator study; O = open study.

al. 1994; Pope et al. 1991). In these two studies with better methodological designs, response rates were similar to those reported in open and non-placebo-controlled comparisons. A major reason for these relatively similar response rates is the specificity conferred by the requirements for the diagnosis of mania and for a clinical response in mania.

In our study (Bowden et al. 1994), patients were assigned randomly to divalproex sodium, lithium, or placebo. The results showed that the placebo-treated group had much less improvement over the 3 weeks of this study of hospitalized acutely manic bipolar I patients than did either the divalproex sodium–treated or the lithium-treated patients. In the aggregate, we observed no difference in response between the two active medications. The response to the two active treatments represented a very large response. We analyzed this response using effect-size determination and standard tests of statistical significance. *Effect size* indicates the magnitude of difference between two treatments. In general, a practicing psychiatrist could recognize an effect size of around 0.5 or so in a patient, and an effect size of around 0.8 or greater would be quite large: the difference between illness at the point of entry into treatment and that at the time of recovery or when the patient is ready for discharge from the hospital. The effect size for divalproex sodium was large at 1.01, that for lithium was 0.79, and that for placebo was small at only 0.30. These effect sizes for divalproex sodium and lithium in the treatment of acute mania are larger than one generally sees in studies of approved antidepressant or antianxiety agents. The Pope et al. (1991) study randomized 17 patients to divalproex sodium and 19 to placebo. Yet this relatively small study showed a highly significant difference in overall improvement (54% versus 5%; $P = .001$) because the investigators were able to show the clear response to divalproex sodium and to document the low response to placebo. Thus, even with relatively small sample sizes, clinically meaningful differences are likely to be observed between an effective drug and placebo in acute mania, in contrast to those differences often observed in studies of major depression. However, the relatively small difference in effectiveness between two effective compounds such as divalproex sodium and lithium precludes any reasonable likelihood of establishing a significant difference between the two with attainable size samples. By contrast, studies of panic disorder often have placebo response rates higher than 30%, with the consequence that it becomes difficult to establish a real difference between the placebo and the medication.

Currently available rating scales contribute to our ability to recognize treatment-related changes in mania. We chose the Mania Rating Scale (Secunda et al. 1985) as the primary rating scale for our study (Bowden et al. 1994). This scale puts items on mania in two different groups: the so-called *Manic Syndrome* subscale and the *Behavior and Ideation* subscale from the Schedule for Affective Disorders and Schizophrenia (SADS; Endicott and Spitzer 1978). These two scales have high interrater reliability and test-retest reliability (Endicott and Spitzer 1978), the ability to distinguish manic patients from nonmanic subjects and healthy control subjects (Secunda et al. 1985), and sensitivity to change with pharmacotherapy (Swann et al. 1986).

Our study found that the Manic Syndrome subscale, composed of five items quite specific to mania (elevated mood, less need for sleep, excessive energy, excessive activity, and grandiosity) showed the greatest change with treatment with both divalproex sodium and lithium. The Behavior and Ideation subscale showed less change with treatment, indicating that signs and symptoms characteristic of, but not specific for, mania (irritability, motor hyperactivity, accelerated speech, racing thoughts, and poor judgment) are less sensitive to the effects of antimanic drugs. The sensitivity of the Manic Syndrome subscale allowed us to test more conclusively the question of the responsivity of mixed mania to lithium and divalproex sodium. Earlier studies of lithium in mixed manic patients had left unanswered the question of whether the poor response of mixed patients reflected treatment refractoriness per se or indicated that lithium is relatively ineffective in the treatment of mixed mania. A large open study (Calabrese and Delucchi 1990) and a small comparative study (Freeman et al. 1992) indicated good effectiveness of divalproex sodium in mixed mania. We found a clinically significant response to lithium in 81% of patients with pure mania, compared with a response rate of 37% among the mixed manic patients. By contrast, the response to divalproex sodium was equivalent among those patients with pure and mixed mania (67% and 70%, respectively) (Bowden 1998). These results are quite similar to those from open and controlled studies. Table 8–4 shows results in acute mania with lithium treatment in two randomized studies (Himmelhoch et al. 1982; Prien et al. 1988) and one open (Secunda et al. 1985) study. In each instance, the patients with pure or classical manic episodes responded much better than did those with mixed manic episodes. One open, naturalistic maintenance-phase study had analogous results (Keller et al. 1986). The probability of remaining ill for a 1-year period after initiation of treatment for an illness episode was 7% for patients who entered the study in a purely manic episode, 20% for those who entered in a depressed episode, and 32% for those who entered in a mixed manic episode (Keller et al. 1986). An open study by Calabrese and Delucchi (1990) assessed the effectiveness of divalproex sodium in rapid-cycling patients and showed high rates of response in mixed manic patients; these rates did not differ from those observed in patients who had pure mania.

Table 8–5 summarizes baseline demographic and clinical characteristics of patients enrolled in open versus blinded, placebo-controlled studies. Age at study entry, number of years from onset of the bipolar disorder, sex, and initial severity of illness are quite similar across studies. Design features generally account for any apparent differences. For example, Pope et al. (1991) enrolled only women not potentially capable of becoming pregnant; thus, their study included a smaller percentage of women. Particularly interesting is the Global Assessment Scale (GAS) score, an index of overall functional impairment. Each of the studies showed essentially the same high level of impairment in patients, with GAS scores in the 30s. Four of the studies obtained information on prior response to lithium treatment during an acute manic episode. The studies reported a narrow

Table 8–4.   Response to lithium among manic patients

Study	Mixed manic patients	Pure manic patients
Himmelhoch et al. 1976	42	81
Secunda et al. 1985	29	91
Prien et al. 1988	36	59

Table 8–5. Demographic characteristics of patients in clinical trials in mania

Study	N	Average age at study entry (years)	Age range (years)	Sex (male/ female)	Age at onset of illness (years)	GAS	Prior lithium effective (%)
Bowden et al. 1994	179	39±11	18–65	52/48	22	36	48
Freeman et al. 1992	27	—	—	22/78	—	29	41
Pope et al. 1991	36	37	18–65	72/28	25	31	[a]
Small et al. 1991	48	38	22–73	44/56	24	37	—
Calabrese and Delucchi 1990	55	41±13	—	42/58	25	—	46
Lerer et al. 1987	34	40	23–65	46/54	—	—	54
Secunda et al. 1985	19	44	23–74	63/37	—	36	—

Note. GAS = Global Assessment Scale score. The index of severity has a range of 0–100.
[a]Failure of response to lithium or intolerance to lithium was a requirement for inclusion in this study.

range of 41%–54% of patients with prior good response to lithium. The Pope et al. (1991) study had a condition for eligibility that the patients had not responded to lithium treatment; thus, the item was not meaningfully answerable for that study.

In the aggregate, open studies in mania have similar results, include the same types of patients, and provide relatively reliable data when compared with similar parameters from placebo-controlled studies. This characteristic of such studies is linked to clinicians' ability to reliably diagnose and rate change in signs and symptoms and otherwise reduce confounding factors in studies of mania. With both lithium and divalproex sodium, serum drug levels can be measured to ensure that patients are receiving doses of these medications adequate to provide a benefit if a benefit can be obtained. This measurement prevents patients who failed to receive a clinically effective dose from being included in the analysis, thereby ensuring that the drug's effectiveness is not underestimated.

Investigators should be able to use open study data to complement randomized placebo-controlled study data because the latter type of study is so methodologically difficult. A study assessing the maintenance-phase effectiveness of divalproex sodium, lithium, and placebo allowed us to assess from a different perspective the characteristics of patients who enter such rigorously designed trials (Bowden 1995). Patients had to be acutely manic at study entrance and then be successfully treated in an open fashion with any medication except depot neuroleptics. After response and stabilization were achieved, patients were randomized to treatment with divalproex sodium, lithium, or placebo in a 2:1:1 ratio. Because of the study's duration, caution by both investigators and patients may have led to some of the more severely ill patients being screened out. At an interim point in the study, we had screened 466 patients to enroll 67 subjects. Table 8–6 indicates the reasons that patients were not eligible for enrollment. The largest single factor was that the patients did not meet the criteria for a bipolar disorder, generally because they did not have a full manic episode (Bowden 1995).

Discussion of these studies raises a related issue. Given the difficulties in studies of bipolar disorder, a detailed description of illness characteristics of a particular sample becomes important. Not only does it aid in making sense of the results obtained, but it allows for

Table 8–6. Reasons for screening failure in study of mania prevention ($N = 577$)

Reason	Percent failing for this reason
Not bipolar	32
Refusal of consent	17
Illness episode longer than allowed	13
No second episode in past 3 years	11
Intolerant to valproate or lithium	4
History of drug abuse	5
Other illness present	4
Concurrent medication	3
Other reason	11

more meaningful comparison of results across studies. The remarkably similar GAS scores in the studies that provided such information attests both to the severity of illness in the patients and to the comparability of patients across the studies.

Reasons for Differences in Clinical Practice Results Compared With Controlled Trials

Numerous design features important for research purposes can reduce response rates compared with those obtained in clinical practice. Use of adjunctive medications, which may aid in nonspecific but important symptom control (e.g., insomnia, delusions, hostility), are likely to be disallowed or strictly controlled in clinical trials. Indeed, failure to do so tends to confound interpretation of studies. Because patients doing well on a regimen are unlikely to enter a study requiring an episode of illness, those enrolled in clinical trials may be more chronically ill or may have more treatment-refractory illness than are those seen in clinical practice. Adjunctive psychotherapy may also be curtailed so as to test the effectiveness of the drug of interest. Ethical and cost considerations often necessitate somewhat short trial periods, thus cutting off some patients who might respond at a slower rate. These features generally result in 10%–20% lower response or improvement rates in published studies than are likely to be attained in clinical practice.

Not all variables reduce response rates. If patients receive large amounts of other medications, for example, as occurred in most carbamazepine trials, or if only patients who complete the trial are analyzed, rather than all who entered the study, response rates may be inflated. For example, Lerer et al. (1987) did not include four patients who dropped out of a study because of worsening of symptoms or intolerance to lithium, thereby reporting a higher response rate than the correct rate of 61%. Especially for longer, maintenance-phase studies, biases may prevent particularly severely ill patients from being enrolled, out of concern that ineffective treatment protocols would increase the patients' risk of relapse. Maintenance trials are likely to require more frequent visits, give increased attention to adherence to medications, and provide more nonspecific support than the patient would receive in standard care, further reducing relapse rates. Although such concern is clearly justified for both the investigator and the patient, continuation rates in the study might appear more favorable than would occur in actual clinical practice.

Illness Course From the Perspective of Complex Cases

In this chapter, I emphasize the utility and degree of confidence that experimental clinical trials in bipolar disorder can provide. Each of these issues is important in the treatment and clinical course of bipolar disorder, but each cannot be studied easily or solely in an experimental paradigm. Experimental studies are difficult at best, and misleading at worst, when they involve patients with bipolar disorders that are so unusual as to be unique for many purposes. For example, one could select a sample of patients who have secondary bipolar disorders, but the variety of primary medical disorders would make it difficult to justify group analysis. Narrowing the focus to a single disorder, such as the first case reported here with bipolar disorder secondary to multiple sclerosis, would make it impossible to collect a large sample. Also, ethical concerns and medical necessity usually warrant individualization of treatment regimens in such patients; thus, the benefits of a standardized protocol may be minimally obtainable. Most experimental data come from acute trials, whereas bipolar disorder is usually lifelong. With these caveats in mind, I present three case studies intended to link some of the results from experimental studies to individual patient experience over time. These cases address secondary mania, changing tolerability to mood stabilizers over time, and combined mood stabilizer treatment. Each case has implications for treatment adherence.

Case Involving Secondary Mania

At age 38, Ms. A, a college-educated, part-time pianist, developed multiple sclerosis. Visual, motor, speech, and gait abnormalities were present at the outset, with fluctuating severity of impairment. Ten years later, while taking no medications, she had a full manic episode that lasted 10 weeks, followed by an episode of depression that lasted 3 months. Lithium was started, and a serum level of 0.75 mEq/L was needed for good control of manic episodes. Despite her psychiatrist's efforts to establish rapport and improve Ms. A's understanding of the illness, Ms. A avoided appointments and reduced her lithium intake because of the cognitive impairment side effects she experienced with therapeutic doses. She referred to the lithium as "taking her mind away." The reduced dosage produced significant impairment, including rambling speech, rapid shifts in attention, reduced sleep, volatile anger, and lack of recognition that she was clinically ill, even when she was reminded gently. She was functionally impaired, accomplishing little in household, intellectual, social, or cultural pursuits. She required a high level of attention from her husband.

After reassessment, lithium was tapered over a 3-week period and divalproex sodium was started at a dose of 1,000 mg, yielding a valproate level around 70 μg/mL. Her manic symptoms began to recede within 3 days and had stopped within 2 weeks. She had no adverse effects nor depressive symptoms. Her pleasure with her markedly improved cognitive status was immense. She resumed household, cultural, and avocational interests. Her relationship with her husband improved, and she assumed more independence of function. Once stabilized, Ms. A's useful insight into her illness and effective dealing with the limitations imposed by multiple sclerosis improved markedly. She also realistically recollected her prior manic behavior, which she had been unable to do before. Her family history was negative for any history of mood disorder. She has had full remission of bipolar symptomatology for 2 years and has faithfully taken prescribed divalproex sodium. Since her mood disorder began, her motor impairments from multiple sclerosis did not change.

Pertinent in Ms. A's case is that secondary mania may not develop coincident with the onset of a primary neurological condition, and it may develop even when the primary condition is otherwise clinically stable. Ms. A had good symptomatic control from lithium, but only at serum levels that caused severe, functionally impairing cognitive side effects. Divalproex sodium was effective at levels nominally needed in nonneurologically impaired adults and had no adverse cognitive or neuromuscular effects. Indeed, the cognitive deficits often associated with lithium were shown to diminish remarkably when divalproex sodium was substituted for lithium in an open case series (Stoll et al. 1996). Symptomatic control for Ms. A led to substantial functional improvement, despite the persisting multiple sclerosis. Case reports of patients with multiple sclerosis responsive to lithium and to carbamazepine have also been published.

Case Involving Changing Tolerability to Mood Stabilizers

At age 28 years, Ms. B, a married teacher, became profoundly depressed and experienced nihilistic delusions, social withdrawal, hypersomnia and daytime napping, tearfulness, a strong sense of guilt, and a loss of usual volume of speech. Her insight and judgment were severely limited. A pattern of onset of depression from late August to mid October with gradual resolution from late December to February, largely unrelated to several heterocyclic antidepressants prescribed at adequate doses, recurred for 8 years. Reevaluation indicated that Ms. B had several-day periods of exuberant mood, elevated energy, uncharacteristic assertiveness, a rush of ideas and plans, both after the end of depressive episodes and randomly throughout the year. Her family history was positive for recurrent depression and problems associated with impulse control. A presumptive diagnosis of bipolar II disorder was made, and she started taking lithium.

Ms. B improved within 3 weeks. Over the next 4 years, she had mild depressive episodes in the fall, which responded to increased doses of antidepressants. Adverse effects were mild, limited to constipation and weight gain of 20 pounds. Ms. B decided that she was well and discontinued all medications without consultation. A psychotic depression ensued 4 months later, and reinstitution of medications brought the symptoms under control.

At age 52, Ms. B began to complain of frequent short-term memory lapses that interfered with her teaching and caused embarrassment. Reduction of either lithium or desipramine resulted in return of mild depressive symptoms. Divalproex sodium was gradually substituted for lithium. Despite adequate serum levels, depression returned and lithium was restarted. Over a 10-week period, the depression gradually abated, but cognitive impairment returned. Ms. B was retired from her job on medical disability. Because of her adverse reaction to lithium, Ms. B was given a trial with carbamazepine and, subsequent to its failure to provide benefit, with divalproex sodium. Ms. B, who had opposed the first trial change in mood stabilizers, was amenable to the second trial. Her cognitive function returned to normal, and she maintained euthymia. The medical retirement was rescinded, and she resumed her job.

Ms. B's case illustrates several features about forms of bipolar disorder. Bipolar disorder presents with purely depressive symptoms for many years and in episodes in many patients. Even when hypomania occurs, it may be mild, functionally enabling rather than disabling, and evanescent. These characteristics can make recognition difficult. Seasonally affected bipolar disorders present both opportunities and difficulties in treatment. Anticipation of seasonal onset can yield early control. Effectiveness of treatments can be confounded by the intrinsic seasonal abatement of an episode. Lithium and antidepressants were generally but not fully effective for many years, and Ms. B tolerated them satisfactorily. As Ms. B aged, her susceptibility to the cognitive impairing effects of lithium increased, although she continued to require such levels for illness prophylaxis. A medication tried unsuccessfully, in this instance divalproex sodium, may warrant retrial if reasonable doubts exist as to the adequacy of the trial. Finally, the importance of close follow-up and psychological support, even after many years of treatment by the same psychiatrist, is underscored by Ms. B's decision to discontinue treatment while ostensibly doing well.

Case Involving Combined Mood Stabilizer Treatment

Mr. C, a 42-year-old divorced man, had experienced mixed manic and depressive episodes one to three times per year since adolescence. He also had ultradian cycles of subthreshold mood disturbance, both depressive and hypomanic, between major episodes. The episodes contributed to two divorces, other social problems, vocational difficulties, and overspending. Treatment had been episodic, in part because of characteristic adverse effects to many antidepressants, lithium, and carbamazepine. Despite being symptomatic more than half of the time annually, Mr. C had successfully launched a small business.

Two doses of fluoxetine (Prozac) appeared to dramatically improve his depressed mood and energy, but continued dosing invariably caused hypomanic symptoms. Mr. C became severely depressed, despondent, guilt filled, hopeless, and mildly suicidal. He was socially withdrawn and unable to carry out his substantial work responsibility. He lost confidence and was painfully indecisive. Treatment with lamotrigine, an antiepileptic agent thought to have mood-improving properties was started (Calabrese et al. 1996; Walden et al. 1996). Mr. C's mood improved within 2 days. He soon resumed good social and vocational function, his confidence improved, and he made difficult decisions well. His sleep continued to be light, and he woke several times during the night. A short-acting benzodiazepine aided sleep.

Mr. C experienced periods of speeded thoughts, excessive anger, impulsivity, and anxiety with paniclike onset. Although distressing to Mr. C, these episodes were not evident on repeated examination, except for moderate anxiety and rapid speech. Because of cognitive adverse effects from lithium and carbamazepine, divalproex sodium was added at a dose of 750 mg, which provided a serum level of 64 µg/mL. Mr. C's hypomanic symptoms abated, but his appetite increased and he gained 10 pounds within 2 weeks. The dose was reduced, yielding a serum level of around 30 µg/mL. Mr. C continued to do well with the combined regimen of lamotrigine and divalproex sodium.

As is often the case, this person's symptoms were often minimally observable in office visits. We must rely on subjectively reported symptoms or observations in such cases. Mr. C also had an early response to treatment that was not adequately sustained. It is therefore necessary to reconsider therapy that was initially satisfactory and make in-course additions of new medications to achieve a fully adequate response or to reduce the dose of or discontinue medications with adverse effects that interfere with function or efficacy. Mr. C's case also exemplifies the need in bipolar disorder for close follow-up and an open, effective doctor-patient relationship.

Conclusion

Psychiatrists and other professionals caring for patients with bipolar disorder face a complex and challenging, but gratifying, task. Although treatment efficacy, especially for mania and mood stabilization, is quite high, efficacy is not always achieved, because of fluctuating manifestations of the illness, poor toleration of medications, or failure to modify treatment regimens promptly when conditions deteriorate. Attention to the large amount of practical new information and treatment techniques emerging from both scientifically rigorous studies and empirical observations can positively affect treatment outcomes.

References

Aagaard J, Vestergaard P: Predictors of outcome in prophylactic lithium treatment: a 2-year prospective study. J Affect Disord 18:259–266, 1990

Bowden CL: Treatment of bipolar disorder, in Textbook of Psychopharmacology, 2nd Edition. Edited by Schatzberg AF, Nemeroff CB. Washington, DC, American Psychiatric Press, 1998, pp 733–745

Bowden CL, Brugger AM, Swann AC, et al: Efficacy of divalproex vs lithium and placebo in the treatment of mania. JAMA 271:918–924, 1994

Bowden CL, Swann AC, Calabrese JR, et al: Maintenance clinical trials in bipolar disorder: design implications of the divalproex-lithium-placebo study. Psychopharmacol Bull 33:693–699, 1997

Brennan MJW, Sandyk R, Borseek D: Use of sodium-valproate in the management of affective disorders: basic and clinical aspects, in Anticonvulsants in Affective Disorders. Edited by Emrich HM, Okuma T, Muller AA. Amsterdam, The Netherlands, Excerpta Medica, 1984, pp 56–65

Brown D, Silverstone T, Cookson J: Carbamazepine compared to haloperidol in acute mania. Int Clin Psychopharmacol 4:229–238, 1989

Calabrese JR, Delucchi GA: Spectrum of efficacy of valproate in 55 patients with rapid-cycling bipolar disorder. Am J Psychiatry 147:431–434, 1990

Calabrese JR, Fatemi SH, Woyshville MJ: Antidepressant effects of lamotrigine in bipolar rapid cycling (letter). Am J Psychiatry 153:1236, 1996

Dubovsky SI, Franks RD, Allen S, et al: Calcium antagonists in mania: a double blind study of verapamil. Psychiatry Res 18:309–320, 1986

Emrich HM, Wolf R: Valproate treatment of mania. Prog Neuropsychopharmacol Biol Psychiatry 16:691–701, 1992

Endicott J, Spitzer R: A diagnostic interview: the Schedule of Affective Disorders and Schizophrenia. Arch Gen Psychiatry 35:837–844, 1978

Freeman TW, Clothier JL, Pazzaglia P, et al: A double-blind comparison of valproate and lithium in the treatment of acute mania. Am J Psychiatry 149:108–111, 1992

Garza-Treviño ES, Overall JE, Hollister LE: Verapamil versus lithium in acute mania. Am J Psychiatry 149:121–122, 1992

Giannini AJ, House WL, Loiselle RH: Antimanic effects of verapamil. Am J Psychiatry 141:1602–1603, 1984

Goodwin FK, Murphy DL, Bunney WE Jr: Lithium carbonate treatment in depression and mania: a longitudinal double-blind study. Arch Gen Psychiatry 21:486–496, 1969

Himmelhoch JM, Mulla D, Neil JF, et al: Incidence and significance of mixed affective states in a bipolar population. Arch Gen Psychiatry 33:1062–1066, 1976

Himmelhoch JM, Fuchs CZ, Symons BJ: A double-blind study of tranylcypromine treatment of major anergic depression. J Nerv Ment Dis 170:628–634, 1982

Janicak PG, Sharma RP, Easton M, et al: A double-blind, placebo-controlled trial of clonidine in the treatment of acute mania. Psychopharmacol Bull 25:243–245, 1989

Janicak PG, Sharma RP, Pandey G, et al: Verapamil for the treatment of acute mania: a double-blind, placebo-controlled trial. Am J Psychiatry 155:972–973, 1998

Keller MB, Lavori PW, Coryell W, et al: Differential outcome of pure manic, mixed/cycling, and pure depressive episodes in patients with bipolar illness. JAMA 255:3138–3142, 1986

Lambert PA: Acute and prophylactic therapies of patients with affective disorders using valpromide (dipropylacetamide), in Anticonvulsants in Affective Disorders. Edited by Emrich HM, Okuma T, Muller AA. Amsterdam, The Netherlands, Excerpta Medica, 1984, pp 33–44

Lambert PA, Cavaz G, Borselli S, et al: Action neuropsychotrope d'un nouvel anti-epileplique: le depamide. Annals of Medical Psychology 1:707–710, 1966

Lerer B, Moore N, Meyendorff E, et al: Carbamazepine versus lithium in mania: a double-blind study. J Clin Psychiatry 48:89–93, 1987

Maggs R: Treatment of manic illness with lithium carbonate. Br J Psychiatry 109:56–65, 1963

McElroy SL, Keck PE Jr, Pope HG Jr, et al: Valproate in the treatment of rapid-cycling bipolar disorder. J Clin Psychopharmacol 8:275–279, 1988

Pope HG Jr, McElroy SL, Keck PE Jr, et al: Valproate in the treatment of acute mania: a placebo-controlled study. Arch Gen Psychiatry 48:62–68, 1991

Post RM, Rubinow DR, Uhde TW, et al: Dysphoric mania: clinical and biological correlates. Arch Gen Psychiatry 46:353–358, 1989

Prasad AJ: The role of sodium valproate as an antimanic agent. Pharmatherapeutica 4:6–8, 1984

Prien RF, Himmelhoch JM, Kupfer DJ: Treatment of mixed mania. J Affect Disord 15:9–15, 1988

Rothman KJ, Michels KB: The continuing unethical use of placebo controls. N Engl J Med 331:394–398,1994

Schou M, Juel-Nielson N, Stromgren E, et al: The treatment of manic psychoses by administration of lithium salts. J Neurol Neurosurg Psychiatry 17:250–260, 1954

Secunda S, Katz MM, Swann A, et al: Mania: diagnosis, state measurement and prediction of treatment response. J Affect Disord 8:113–121, 1985

Small JG, Klapper MH, Milstein V, et al: Carbamazepine compared with lithium in the treatment of mania. Arch Gen Psychiatry 48:915–921, 1991

Stokes PE, Shamoian CA, Stoll PM, et al: Efficacy of lithium as acute treatment of manic-depressive illness. Lancet 1:1319–1325, 1971

Stoll AL, Locke CA, Vuckovic A, et al: Lithium-associated cognitive and functional deficits reduced by a switch to divalproex sodium: a case series. J Clin Psychiatry 57:356–359, 1996

Swann AC, Secunda SK, Katz MM, et al: Lithium treatment of mania: clinical characteristics, specificity of symptom change, and outcome. Psychiatry Res 18:127–141, 1986

Uhlenhuth EH, Matuzas W, Warner TD, et al: Methodological issues in psychopharmacological research. Growing placebo response rate: the problem in recent therapeutic trials? Psychopharmacol Bull 33:31–39, 1997

Walden J, Hesslinger B, van Calker D, et al: Addition of lamotrigine to valproate may enhance efficacy in the treatment of bipolar affective disorder. Pharmacopsychiatry 29:193–195, 1996

Walton SA, Berk M, Brook S: Superiority of lithium over verapamil in mania: a randomized, controlled, single-blind trial. J Clin Psychiatry 57: 543–546, 1995

CHAPTER 9

Bipolar Disorder and Comorbid Substance Use Disorder

Mauricio Tohen, M.D., Dr.P.H.
Carlos A. Zarate Jr., M.D.

*O*utcome studies of mania have been conducted for as long as the diagnosis has been recognized. Kraepelin (1921/1976) acknowledged the importance of outcome data by differentiating the major psychoses into three types: dementia praecox, manic-depressive illness, and paranoia. *Dementia praecox* was defined as an illness with a deteriorating course, in contrast to *manic-depressive illness,* which was episodic with full recovery between episodes and a good prognosis (Kraepelin 1921/1976). Many outcome studies have been conducted over the years; however, the findings have been inconsistent. Inconsistencies may be the result of a number of factors, including nonsystematic sampling, loss of patients to follow-up, differences in diagnostic criteria, varying degrees of comorbidity in bipolar samples, and differences in methods used for outcome measurement collection and analysis (Bratfos and Haug 1968; Fleiss et al. 1976; Hastings 1958; Keller et al. 1987; Kraepelin 1921/1976; Shobe and Brion 1971). In addition, such discrepancies may be partly the result of the heterogeneity of studies that include a combination of multiple-episode and first-episode subjects. Several studies suggest that previous episodes of major affective disorders are a strong predictor of relapse (Keller et al. 1986; Tohen et al. 1990a, 1990b; Zis and Goodwin 1979). One study suggests that the outcome after a first episode of mania differs from that after multiple episodes. Keck and colleagues (1995) reported that patients with multiple manic episodes required significantly longer hospitalizations and longer lengths of stay than did manic patients experiencing their first episodes.

In this chapter, we address one of the major variables that contributes to the heterogeneity seen in outcome findings in mania: substance use disorder (SUD). We also address issues regarding outcome patterns seen after initial episodes of bipolar disorder, drawing on data from the McLean-Harvard First-Episode Mania Project. We also present an approach to studying the specific problem of comorbidity of bipolar disorder and substance abuse.

Bipolar disorder is a major public health problem. According to the Epidemiologic Catchment Area (ECA) study of the National Institute of Mental Health (NIMH) (Robins et al. 1984), the lifetime prevalence of a manic episode is 0.8%, and the point prevalence is 0.4%, meaning that at any given time, bipolar disorder affects 1 million people in the United States. Another epidemiological survey suggests that mania may even be more prevalent than originally estimated. The National Comorbidity Survey (NCS) reported a lifetime prevalence of 1.6% for a manic episode (Kessler et al. 1994), compared with 0.8% according to the ECA study (Robins et al. 1984). These data must be compared with the prevalence for nonaffective psychoses (including schizophrenia, schizophreniform disorder, schizoaffective disorder, delusional disorder, and atypical psychosis) of 0.6% in the NCS. Despite the apparently higher prevalence of bipolar disorder, the number of federal grants funded to study schizophrenia exceeds those to study bipolar disorder. Furthermore, the amount of money that the pharmaceutical industry spends in the development of drugs for schizophrenia also exceeds the amount spent on drugs for bipolar disorder. From a public health perspective, bipolar disorder demands further attention.

Psychiatric Comorbidity in Bipolar Disorder

Psychiatric comorbidity has been defined as "the presence of an antecedent or concurrent psychiatric syndrome in addition to the principal diagnosis" (Strakowski et al. 1995). Comorbidity in mania (*complicated mania*) has been defined as the presence of nonaffective DSM-III-R Axis I psychiatric diagnoses or serious or potentially life-threatening medical illness, but not well-controlled conditions (Black et al. 1988; Strakowski et al. 1992; Tohen et al. 1998; see also Winokur, Chapter 10, in this volume). The prevalence of comorbidity in population-based studies is high. Data from the NCS indicate that 19.3% of the United States population have a psychiatric disorder at some time in their lives and 26.6% have an SUD (Kessler et al. 1994). In the ECA study, 54% of subjects who were mentally ill had two or more conditions (Regier et al. 1990). The prevalence of comorbidity in the NCS also was high, at 56% (Kessler et al. 1994). In the McLean-Harvard First-Episode Mania Project, the comorbidity in 41 manic and mixed-state bipolar patients was 51.2%, of which 39.0% had at least one other psychiatric diagnosis and 22.0% had a comorbid medical disorder (Strakowski et al. 1992; Tohen et al. 1996). More than one comorbid diagnosis was found in 22% of the sample. The University of Cincinnati Mania First-Episode Project reported a higher rate of psychiatric comorbidity among bipolar patients (66%, or 47 out of 71 patients) (Keck et al. 1995). Keck et al. (1995) found no differences in rates of psychiatric comorbidity between first- and multiple-episode manic patients: first-episode manic patients had a psychiatric comorbidity rate of 71% ($n = 24$), and multiple-episode manic patients had a psychiatric comorbidity rate of 62% ($n = 23$). The same authors reported a higher rate (45%) for multiple comorbidity (defined as more than one Axis I diagnosis other than bipolar disorder) than did the McLean-Harvard First-Episode Mania Project (39%).

Bipolar Disorder and Comorbid Substance Use Disorder

The rate of comorbidity between bipolar disorder and substance-related disorders is high. Substance abuse and its associated behaviors may lead psychiatrists and family members to fail to recognize bipolar disorder (Hirschfeld et al. 1994). Conversely, the diagnosis of SUD may be overlooked in patients who have bipolar disorder. Furthermore, substance abuse may affect the course of illness, perhaps by decreasing compliance with treatment (Jamison and Akiskal 1983; Weiss et al. 1998) or by affecting response to lithium (Albanese et al. 1994). In a recent report, Weiss and colleagues (1998) found that compliance with mood stabilizer treatment was significantly higher among bipolar patients with SUD when valproate, rather than lithium, was the primary pharmacotherapy.

Among all Axis I conditions, bipolar disorder has the highest prevalence of comorbid substance use. An early age at onset of bipolar illness appears more often among those who develop substance abuse comorbidity than among those who do not (Feinman and Dunner 1996). Prevalence rates of alcohol or drug abuse in patients with bipolar disorder have been estimated to range from 21% to 58% (Brady and Lydiard 1992).

A large epidemiological study reported that the prevalence of comorbid SUD in patients with bipolar disorder is 60.7%, three times higher than in patients with depression (Regier et al. 1990). In this study, 46.2% received an alcohol abuse or dependence diagnosis, and 40.7% received a drug abuse or dependence diagnosis. The odds of a bipolar patient having a comorbid SUD compared with the general population are 8 to 1. Only antisocial personality disorder has a higher prevalence of comorbid SUD.

In the McLean-Harvard First-Episode Mania Project, women were 6.4 times more likely than men to have a history of comorbid substance abuse or dependence (36% among women versus 6.3% among men) (Strakowski et al. 1992; Tohen et al. 1996). The prevalence of drug abuse or dependence was 17.1% (24% among women versus 6.3% among men). Subjects who had a history of drug abuse or dependence were 3.2 times more likely to have another comorbid psychiatric diagnosis. Even more striking, Keck and colleagues (1995) reported that the prevalence rates for alcohol abuse or dependence and psychoactive substance abuse or dependence were 39% and 32%, respectively. In addition, the authors found no differences in the prevalence of alcohol and psychoactive substance abuse and dependence between first- and multiple-episode mania.

The foregoing epidemiological surveys indicate that SUD and affective disorders commonly co-occur. However, it is not clear why this association is so high. Several constructs may be useful in explaining this association:

- The two conditions are caused by the same biochemical abnormality (Hastings 1958).
- Certain psychiatric disorders may be risk factors for addictive disorders or modifiers of their course (Bratfos and Haug 1968).
- Mood disorders are secondary to the SUD (i.e., the result of intoxication or withdrawal symptoms) (Shobe and Brion 1971).
- A self-medication effect may exist (Khantzian 1985; Sonne et al. 1994).

The last explanation listed above remains controversial. Contrary to the expectation that bipolar patients would use an "upper" such as cocaine when depressed and would use a "downer" such as alcohol when euphoric, findings indicate that bipolar patients more frequently used cocaine during mania (Weiss and Mirin 1987). Therefore, the so-called *self-medication hypothesis* is not clearly validated. However, patients may seek heightened excitement during manic phases, which might lead them to use cocaine.

Mixed Bipolar Disorder and Substance Use Disorder

Mixed manic episodes (see Boland and Keller, Chapter 6, in this volume) have been associated with a higher prevalence of comorbid SUD than have euphoric manic states (Himmelhoch and Garfinkel 1986; Himmelhoch et al. 1976; Keller et al. 1986; Sonne et al. 1994; Tohen et al. 1996). Keller and colleagues (1986) found that patients with mixed or cycling forms of bipolar disorder had a 13% rate of concurrent alcoholism. Sonne and colleagues (1994) reported that bipolar patients with SUD were more likely to have dysphoric and irritable mood states and were twice as likely to experience more rapid mood swings than were bipolar patients without SUD. However, one study did not find a difference in the prevalence of comorbid alcohol and psychoactive abuse or dependence between patients with pure mania and patients with mixed mania (40% and 38%, respectively) (McElroy et al. 1995). Differences in the reported rates of substance abuse or dependence may be the result of differences in the populations under study or may depend on the definition of mixed mania used (McElroy et al. 1992, 1995).

It is not clear why mixed mania and SUD appear to be associated. Investigators have postulated that bipolar disorder is a "kindled" phenomenon because the course of the illness is often characterized by acceleration with successively shortened periods of remission between episodes (Post 1992; Post and Weiss 1989; Post et al. 1981). Cocaine and alcohol intoxication or withdrawal may produce this neuronal kindling and, as a result, may worsen the course of bipolar disorder by causing rapid cycling or mixed symptoms. The potential exists for behavioral sensitization to occur as a result of repeated cocaine use in bipolar patients, which may bear on underlying mechanisms of bipolar disorder.

Sonne and colleagues (1994) suggest that bipolar patients with SUD were more likely to have an earlier onset of mood disorder and to have more psychiatric hospitalizations than were bipolar patients without SUD. In contrast, some authors suggest that patients with bipolar disorder and alcoholism do better in treatment than do subjects with other affective syndromes. O'Sullivan et al. (1988) found that alcoholic patients with bipolar disorder functioned better during a 2-year follow-up period than did primary alcoholic patients or alcoholic patients with unipolar affective disorder. Similarly, Hasin and colleagues (1989) found that patients with bipolar II disorder were more likely to have early remission of alcoholism than were patients with schizoaffective disorder or bipolar I disorder. However, in these two studies, the treatment outcome measured was remission of alcoholism rather than affective stability or remission of affective symptoms.

Chronology of Bipolar Disorder and Comorbid Substance Use Disorder

Although substance abuse is common in bipolar disorder, it is unclear whether substance abuse is 1) a sequela of the mood instability inherent in the illness, 2) a risk factor for precipitating or perpetuating affective episodes (Weiss and Mirin 1987), 3) an attempt at self-medication of symptoms, or 4) an intoxication or withdrawal state that mimics primary affective symptoms (Hesselbrock et al. 1985). Winokur (Chapter 10, in this volume) discusses the complexities of this issue more fully in the specific case of alcoholism and bipolar disorder.

A first step in examining this problem would be to clarify the chronology of onset of principal and comorbid diagnoses (Strakowski et al. 1995). To study the sequence of two conditions, a cross-sectional assessment in multiple-episode patients carries the risk of producing biased results. To untangle the confounding factors behind this problem, it is preferable to study patients at the onset of the illness and then follow-up with them longitudinally. This approach led to the initiation of the McLean-Harvard First-Episode Mania Project. As of November 1, 1995, 123 bipolar manic or mixed subjects had reached their 6-month assessment after their original discharge date. Of those 123 subjects, 103 (83.7%) were bipolar manic and 20 (16.3%) were bipolar mixed. By the 6-month follow-up, 117 patients (95.1%) had been evaluated and 87 (70.7%) had completed a 2-year follow-up. Fewer than 8% of patients were lost to follow-up at 2 years.

One of the most interesting findings in these data is that the prevalence of comorbid substance abuse in this first-episode population was only 17%, in contrast to 41%–61% reported in multiple-episode populations (Keck et al. 1995; Regier et al. 1990). This finding may suggest that in most patients, the onset of mania precedes the onset of the SUD. A limitation about the generalizability of this observation is that it occurred in a population for whom the first episode led to hospitalization, and the same prevalence might not apply to populations in which first manic episodes were treated on an outpatient basis. However, one study examining the chronology of comorbid psychiatric disorders in patients with first-episode psychosis suggested that substance abuse was antecedent in most cases (Strakowski et al. 1995). Whether SUD also predates bipolar disorder in a high percentage of cases needs to be studied further.

Preventive Medicine and Bipolar Disorder

The medical profession is trained to treat illnesses and to prevent them from occurring. In bipolar disorder, we should aim to prevent the development of a comorbid SUD in order to improve the outcome of the bipolar condition. In fact, Kessler et al. (1994) coined an elegant term with applicability to psychiatry: the *secondary prevention of the primary condition*. This term would apply to bipolar disorder with SUD in that substance abuse is a known risk factor for poor outcome in mania. If one can secondarily prevent the development of an SUD, then one might prevent an overall worsening of outcome in the bipolar (primary) illness. Because individuals with comorbid conditions use more medical services than those without comorbidity, a strategy to reduce health care costs would involve reducing comorbidity in the mentally ill.

The question of how to prevent the development of SUD is complex. A reasonable approach is to identify risk factors. Studies have shown that mixed episodes are correlated with comorbid substance use. Again, little is known about whether patients who have mixed episodes are prone to the use of drugs or, for that matter, if the use of drugs will change the symptoms, such that otherwise purely manic patients would appear to have mixed symptoms. In the McLean-Harvard First-Episode Mania Project, our group found that 60% of patients with mixed mania had comorbid substance use, compared with only 27.2% of those with pure mania ($P = .004$). SUD comorbidity was highly associated with mixed episodes. Drug abuse or dependence was present in 20% of the mixed mania group, compared with 10.7% of the pure mania group. Therefore, even in a first-episode population, patients with mixed mania appear to have a higher prevalence of comorbid substance abuse. Patients with mixed mania were also older than those with pure mania (33 versus 28 years, $P = .012$).

Another important finding was that in the first-episode mania group, women were more likely than men to have substance abuse problems. This finding is in contrast to a higher rate of bipolar alcoholism among men than women, as reported in the studies by Winokur and colleagues (see Chapter 10 in this volume). The gender differences observed between the McLean-Harvard First-Episode Mania Project SUD bipolar patients and those in Winokur's sample may bear on possible changes in the epidemiology of SUD after repeated affective episodes in bipolar disorder.

The mixed mania group also experienced poorer psychosocial outcome at the 2-year follow-up. Only 33% of the mixed group were able to live independently, compared with 81.8% of the pure mania

group. The presence of drug abuse comorbidity led to a lower probability of recovery at 2 years. As depicted by the survival curve shown
in Figure 9–1, 2 years after discharge, 98.5% of those without drug
abuse comorbidity had recovered, compared with 85.7% of those
with drug abuse comorbidity ($P = .04$). The median time to recovery
for those without drug abuse was 43 days, compared with 55 days in
those with drug abuse comorbidity. When looking at outcome, our
group found, not surprisingly, that manic patients with SUD
comorbidity had a lower probability of recovery by 6 months than
did those without SUD comorbidity.

The survival curve shown in Figure 9–1 is a useful tool for educating patients and their families about the effect of substance abuse
on the course of bipolar disorder. The survival curve shows in its

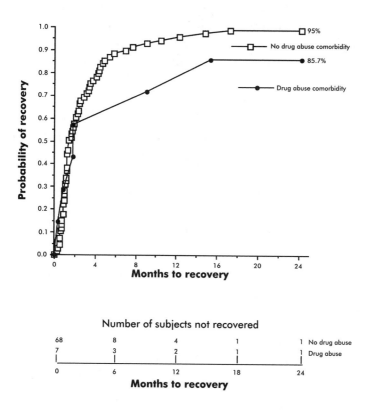

Figure 9–1. McLean-Harvard First-Episode Mania Project. Effects of
drug abuse comorbidity on recovery in first-episode mania.

horizontal axis a time line covering 24 months. The vertical line represents the probability of recovery. Figure 9–1 illustrates convincingly that patients who abuse alcohol or drugs are less likely to recover by 6 months or will take a longer time to recover than those who do not abuse alcohol or drugs.

Survival curves have become especially useful for health services research with a focus on how fast patients improve, how quickly they can be discharged from the hospital, and what may be the short-term risk of rehospitalization. In terms of rehospitalization, several studies have shown that SUD comorbidity will also cause relapse (Tohen et al. 1990, 1992). Substance abuse not only prolongs the time to recovery, but also decreases the time to relapse in patients who have recovered. In the McLean-Harvard First-Episode Mania Project, patients who abused drugs were more likely to have a relapse than were those who did not.

Our group also found that patients with SUD comorbidity were less likely to be compliant with pharmacological treatment than were those without SUD comorbidity. Half of those with SUD comorbidity were not taking psychotropic medication 2 years after discharge, compared with only 22% of those without SUD comorbidity. One must bear in mind that this is a naturalistic study, in which the data reflect not only the course of illness under ordinary conditions but also the physicians' prescribing behaviors. It is equally possible that treating physicians elected to stop their patients' medication for unclear reasons (e.g., toxicities) in those patients with SUD comorbidity. This latter explanation, however, appears rather unlikely.

Preventive Measures

Patients with concurrent substance abuse, including alcoholism, respond relatively poorly to lithium (Albanese et al. 1994). Because the epidemiological studies mentioned earlier in this chapter have shown that concurrent substance abuse is quite prevalent, careful attention must be paid to the possibility of occult substance abuse during the initial evaluation and at times of breakthrough episodes. If comorbidity accounts for one of the major reasons behind heavy service utilization, it becomes all the more important to address issues of substance abuse in bipolar patients and to practice preventive medicine. At McLean Hospital, our group obtained a grant from the National Institute of Drug Abuse (NIDA) (R. Weiss, principal investigator) to develop a manual for clinicians on how to conduct group psychotherapy in patients with bipolar disorder and comorbid substance use. We have speculated that educating patients about the risks of alcohol and drug use will affect the outcome of their disorders.

In order to understand the association between bipolar disorder and SUD, it is important to know the temporal sequence of onset, and in order to identify the onset sequence, longitudinal studies must start at the onset of the illness. Risk factors must also be identified. As discussed earlier in this chapter, we found that the presence of mixed symptoms is associated with SUD comorbidity. When a clinician attempts to predict outcome, for example, it may be useful for the clinician to consider which bipolar patients are at highest risk for developing substance use comorbidity. We found that women with mixed conditions are more likely to develop comorbid SUD than are men. An example of secondary prevention of the primary disorder occurs when one attempts to prevent or otherwise aggressively treat the substance abuse condition, which is likely to improve the outcome of the bipolar condition. The comorbid condition may be an indicator of global severity in bipolar disorder. Substance abuse per se may not worsen the outcome of bipolar disorder, but rather those bipolar patients with a more severe type of illness may have comorbid substance abuse. In addition to secondary prevention, treatment of SUD and bipolar disorder should proceed concurrently. The treatment of one disorder may affect the treatment of the other, as may be the case with anticonvulsant mood stabilizers such as valproate (Brady and Lydiard 1992; Sonne and Brady, in press).

Future Directions

SUD comorbidity needs to be seen as a time-varying covariate, which means that patients are not always abusing drugs or alcohol. Instead, it is a dynamic process that "turns on and off." The amount of time patients are using alcohol or drugs must be determined, as must the quantity of drugs being abused. Also, in patients who already have substance abuse problems, are those who relapse to substance abuse at a higher risk for relapse of their bipolar disorders? Clinicians must focus on preventive measures and treatment interventions in order to decrease the use of health services. Moreover, poor outcome for bipolar patients may be minimized greatly when clinicians attend carefully to modifiable risk factors for poor outcome, such as comorbid substance abuse.

References

Albanese M, Bartel R, Bruno R: Comparison of measures used to determine substance abuse in an inpatient psychiatric population. Am J Psychiatry 151:1077–1078, 1994

Black DW, Winokur G, Bell S, et al: Comorbidity and immediate outcome in the treatment of mania. Arch Gen Psychiatry 45:232–236, 1988

Brady KT, Lydiard RB: Bipolar affective disorder and substance abuse. J Clin Psychopharmacol (suppl 12):17S–22S, 1992

Bratfos O, Haug JO: The course of manic-depressive psychosis. Acta Psychiatr Scand 44:89–112, 1968

Feinman JA, Dunner DL: The effect of alcohol and substance abuse on the course of bipolar affective disorder. J Affect Disord 37:43–49, 1996

Fleiss JL, Dunner DL, Stallone F, et al: The life table; a method for analyzing longitudinal studies. Arch Gen Psychiatry 33:107–112, 1976

Hasin DS, Endicott J, Keller MB: RDC alcoholism in patients with major affective syndromes: two-year course. Am J Psychiatry 146:318–323, 1989

Hastings DWL: Follow-up results in psychiatric illness. Am J Psychiatry 114:1057–1060, 1958

Hesselbrock MN, Meyer RE, Keener JJ: Psychopathology in hospitalized alcoholics. Arch Gen Psychiatry 42:1050–1055, 1985

Himmelhoch JM, Garfinkel ME: Mixed mania: diagnosis and treatment. Psychopharmacol Bull 22:613–620, 1986

Himmelhoch JM, Mulla D, Neil JF, et al: Incidence and significance of mixed affective states in a bipolar population. Arch Gen Psychiatry 33:1062–1066, 1976

Hirschfeld RMA, Clayton PJ, Cohen I, et al: Practice guideline for the treatment of patients with bipolar disorder. Am J Psychiatry 151 (suppl 12): 1–36, 1994

Jamison KR, Akiskal HS: Medication compliance in patients with bipolar disorder. Psychiatr Clin North Am 6:175–192, 1983

Keck PE Jr, McElroy SL, Strakowski SM, et al: Outcome and comorbidity in first- compared with multiple-episode mania. J Nerv Ment Dis 183: 320–324, 1995

Keller MB, Lavori PW, Coryell W, et al: Differential outcome of pure manic, mixed/cycling, and pure depressive episodes in patients with bipolar illness. JAMA 255:3138–3142, 1986

Keller MB, Lavori PW, Friedman B, et al: The longitudinal interval follow-up evaluation (LIFE): a comprehensive method for assessing outcome in prospective longitudinal studies. Arch Gen Psychiatry 44:540–548, 1987

Kessler RC, McGonagle KA, Zhao S, et al: Lifetime and 12-month prevalence of DSM-III-R psychiatric disorders in the United States: results from the National Comorbidity Survey. Arch Gen Psychiatry 51:8–19, 1994

Khantzian EJ: The self-medication hypothesis of addictive disorders: focus on heroin and cocaine dependence. Am J Psychiatry 142:1259–1264, 1985

Kraepelin E: Manic-Depressive Insanity and Paranoia (1921). Translated by Barclay RM. Edited by Robertson GM. Edinburgh, Scotland, Livingstone. Reprint, New York, Arno Press, 1976

McElroy SL, Keck PE Jr, Pope HG Jr, et al: Clinical implications of the diagnosis of dysphoric or mixed mania. Am J Psychiatry 149:1633–1644, 1992

McElroy SL, Strakowski SM, Keck PE Jr, et al: Differences and similarities in mixed and pure mania. Compr Psychiatry 36:187–194, 1995

O'Sullivan K, Rynne C, Miller J, et al: A follow-up study on alcoholics with and without co-existing affective disorder. Br J Psychiatry 152:813–819, 1988

Post RM: Transduction of psychosocial stress into the neurobiology of treatment of affective disorder. Am J Psychiatry 149:999–1010, 1992

Post RM, Weiss SRB: Sensitization, kindling, and anticonvulsants in mania. J Clin Psychiatry 50 (suppl 12):23–30, 1989

Post RM, Ballenger JC, Rey AC, et al: Slow and rapid onset of manic episodes: implications for underlying biology. Psychiatry Res 4:229–237, 1981

Regier DA, Farmer ME, Rae DS, et al: Comorbidity of mental disorders with alcohol and other drug abuse: results from the Epidemiologic Catchment Area (ECA) study. JAMA 264:2511–2518, 1990

Robins LN, Helzer JE, Weissman MM, et al: Lifetime prevalence of specific psychiatric disorders in three sites. Arch Gen Psychiatry 41:949–958, 1984

Shobe FO, Brion P: Long term prognosis in manic-depressive illness. Arch Gen Psychiatry 24:334–337, 1971

Sonne SC, Brady KT: Bipolar disorder and substance abuse, in Comorbidity in Affective Disorders. Edited by Tohen M. New York, Marcel Dekker (in press)

Sonne SC, Brady KT, Morton WA: Substance abuse and bipolar affective disorder. J Nerv Ment Dis 182:349–352, 1994

Strakowski SM, Tohen M, Stoll AL, et al: Comorbidity in mania at first hospitalization. Am J Psychiatry 149:554–556, 1992

Strakowski SM, Keck PE Jr, McElroy SL, et al: Chronology of comorbid and principal syndromes in first-episode psychosis. Compr Psychiatry 36: 106–112, 1995

Tohen M, Waternaux CM, Tsuang MT, et al: Four-year follow-up of 24 first episode manic patients. J Affect Disord 19:79–86, 1990a

Tohen M, Waternaux CM, Tsuang MT, et al: Outcome in mania: a four year prospective study utilizing survival analysis. Arch Gen Psychiatry 47: 1106–1111, 1990b

Tohen M, Stoll AL, Strakowski SM, et al: The McLean First-Episode Psychosis Project: six month recovery and recurrence outcome. Schizophrenia Bull 18:273–282, 1992

Tohen M, Zarate CA Jr, Zarate SB, et al: The McLean/Harvard First-Episode Mania Project: pharmacologic treatment and outcome. Psychiatric Annals 26:S444–S448, 1996

Tohen M, Greenfield S, Weiss RD, et al: The effect of comorbid substance use disorders on the course of bipolar disorder: a review. Harv Rev Psychiatry 6:133–141, 1998

Weiss RD, Mirin SM: Substance abuse as an attempt at self-medication. Psychiatric Medicine 3:357–367, 1987

Weiss RD, Greenfield SF, Najavits LM, et al: Medication noncompliance among patients with bipolar disorder and substance use disorder. J Clin Psychiatry 59:172–174, 1998

Zis AP, Goodwin F: Major affective disorder as a recurrent illness: a critical review. Arch Gen Psychiatry 36:835–839, 1979

CHAPTER 10

Alcoholism in Bipolar Disorder

George Winokur, M.D.

Substance abuse, as described by Tohen and Zarate (Chapter 9, in this volume), is a common feature among patients with bipolar illness. In this chapter, I focus in greater depth on the phenomenology of alcoholism in bipolar disorder. Special attention to the relationship between these two illnesses is warranted based on clinical, genetic, and psychosocial empirical findings and on the unique problems that arise in the treatment of these disorders when they occur simultaneously.

Bipolar disorder and alcoholism occur together more often than would be expected by chance. Helzer and Pryzbeck (1988) presented evidence from the National Institute of Mental Health (NIMH) Epidemiologic Catchment Area (ECA) study that mania and alcoholism occur together 6.2 times as frequently as would be expected by chance. Our research group conducted a clinical study comparing male bipolar patients and control subjects (Winokur et al. 1995). Of the male control subjects, 16% had alcoholism, whereas 73% of the male bipolar patients had a diagnosis of alcoholism in addition to their diagnosis of mania or schizoaffective mania. The odds ratio for the comparison of alcoholism in these two groups was 14.56 ($P < .0001$). These data suggest that the link between alcoholism and mania is high. One possible explanation for the strong association between alcoholism and bipolar disorder involves the concept of *assortative mating*. This possibility suggests that bipolar patients are more likely than chance to marry people who have alcoholism.

Another possibility is that alcoholism may occur secondary to the recklessness associated with manic episodes. For example, Mirin et al. (1988) suggested that many bipolar patients use alcohol, presumably once an episode has begun, as part of the manic syndrome. Our research group at the University of Iowa found that alcoholism predated the mania in approximately half the cases studied, but in the remaining half, alcoholism arose secondary to the mania in temporal fashion (Winokur et al. 1995). Among the patients for whom alcoholism may be secondary to mania, an expansive lifestyle, common among many bipolar patients, may ultimately lead to alcoholism. Current methodologies make it difficult to subject this assumption to the null hypothesis.

Finally, alcoholism could exist independently and could precipitate mania. This possibility turns out to be quite interesting.

The Role of Alcoholism in Bipolar Disorder

Table 10–1 presents data from a study conducted by our research group on alcoholism and bipolar disorder based on a Veterans Ad-

Table 10–1. Comparison of alcoholic bipolar patients with nonalcoholic bipolar patients

	Alcoholic bipolar patients ($n = 14$)	Nonalcoholic bipolar patients ($n = 29$)	P value
Family history of psychiatric hospitalization	0%	41%	.003
Family history of alcoholism	21%	15%	NS
Siblings hospitalized for mental illness	0%	25%	.06
Mental illness in father	0%	28%	.03
Head injury and/or seizure disorder	50%	17%	.03
No. of jobs during 5-year follow-up (mean ± SD)	4.0 ± 2.9	2.0 ± 1.5	.006
Drug use	71%	32%	.02

Note. NS = not statistically significant.

ministration population (Winokur et al. 1993). We assessed 14 alcoholic bipolar patients and 29 nonalcoholic bipolar patients on a number of clinical features. We found that a family history of psychiatric hospitalization was more frequent in the nonalcoholic patients than in the alcoholic patients. Similarly, more siblings were hospitalized for mental illness and the rate of paternal mental illness was higher in the nonalcoholic patients than in the alcoholic patients. A limitation of the findings is that precise psychiatric diagnoses among family members were not obtainable for all subjects, and the presence of nonspecific psychiatric illness lacks informativeness. However, if the alcoholic bipolar patients had less family history of bipolar disorder, these results would suggest that alcoholism might be an etiological factor for bipolarity.

We also found that head injury and/or seizures were more frequent in the alcoholic bipolar patients. Head injury or seizures might precipitate mania. However, alcoholic bipolar patients might be more likely to have a head injury or seizure because of the alcoholism; therefore, instead of the head injury causing mania, it may simply be a consequence of the bipolar patient's alcohol abuse and increased likelihood of getting hurt.

With regard to occupational performance, alcoholic bipolar patients had significantly poorer work functioning than did nonalcoholic bipolar patients. Similarly, other drug use was higher in bipolar alcoholic patients, as one might expect.

We evaluated data from a large study involving 70 patients with bipolar disorder and alcoholism and 161 patients with bipolar disorder only (Winokur et al. 1995). These patients had been admitted to the NIMH Collaborative Depression Study at five centers: Washington University, the University of Iowa, Rush Medical College, Columbia University, and Harvard University. Our evaluation did not take into account an extensive follow-up during which some of the index patients who were bipolar became alcoholic and some patients who were unipolar became bipolar. Regardless, this study probably represents the largest sample of bipolar patients with known alcoholism ever to have been systematically studied as a group. Table 10–2 presents information comparing the bipolar patients with or without alcoholism on a number of major clinical variables. The most striking difference between the two groups is that an

Table 10–2.   Clinical, follow-up, and family data on alcoholic bipolar patients versus nonalcoholic bipolar patients

	Alcoholic bipolar patients ($n = 70$)	Nonalcoholic bipolar patients ($n = 161$)	P value
Male	71%	37%	.0001
Manic at intake	74%	70%	NS
Recovered	90%	91%	NS
Episodes/year during 5-year follow-up (mean)	0.05	0.05	NS
Family history of bipolar disorder	15%	13%	NS
Family history of unipolar depression	74%	63%	NS
Family history of alcoholism	21%	15%	NS

Note.   NS = not statistically significant.

alcoholic bipolar patient was far more likely to have been male than was a nonalcoholic bipolar patient. We found no significant differences in any of the other variables. It is interesting that the number of episodes per year during a 5-year follow-up was the same for both groups. This finding was unexpected, because patients with two diagnoses often tend to have more severe illness than do those with only one diagnosis. We found no significant differences in psychosis, recovery, or number of weeks of hospitalization, nor did we find significant differences between the alcoholic and the nonalcoholic bipolar patients in their family histories of bipolarity, unipolar depression, or alcoholism.

In some cases, alcoholism preceded bipolarity. We termed these patients *primary alcoholic patients.* If the bipolar illness preceded the alcoholism, we termed these patients *primary bipolar patients.* About half of this group of 70 patients had primary alcoholism, and the other half had primary bipolar disorder. Six patients were left out of the groupings because they had probable, not definite, alcoholism. The primary alcoholic patients, by definition, had an earlier age at onset of alcoholism than did the primary bipolar patients. Similarly, the primary bipolar patients had an earlier age at onset of affective illness than did the primary alcoholic patients. Sex ratio differed between the two groups: 71% of the primary alcoholic patients were male, whereas only 27% of the primary bipolar patients were male ($P < .0001$).

Table 10–3 presents other clinical differences between the primary alcoholic patients and the primary bipolar patients. The symptoms of alcoholism were quite similar in both groups. However, after recovery from the bipolar episode, the patients with primary alcoholism had fewer episodes in a 5-year follow-up than did the patients with primary bipolar disorder. The median time to first relapse was shorter for the subgroup with primary bipolar disorder (49 weeks) than for the primary alcoholism group (73 weeks) (Wilcoxon $\chi^2 = 5.62$, df $= 1$, $P < .02$). The patients with primary bipolar disorder were more likely to be chronically ill (17%) (i.e., to not have recovered from the index episode during a 5-year follow-up period) than were the patients with primary alcoholism (3%). This difference did not reach statistical significance, however, according to Fisher's exact test ($P = .09$).

Strikingly, when alcoholism preceded the emergence of bipolar symptoms, the overall course of illness was more benign. This observation can be interpreted to support the possibility that abusive

Table 10–3. Primary alcoholism versus primary bipolar disorder

	Primary alcoholism ($n = 34$)	Primary bipolar disorder ($n = 20$)	P value
Blackouts	53%	70%	NS
Tremors	32%	30%	NS
Delirium tremens	9%	10%	NS
Seizures	3%	3%	NS
Mental competency	15%	20%	NS
Family history of alcoholism	19%	29%	NS
Episodes after recovery during follow-up (mean ± SD)	155 ± 1.48	2.68 ± 2.38	.03

Note. NS = not statistically significant.

drinking precipitates a bipolar episode. It would be consistent with the idea that bipolar disorder in patients who also have alcoholism is somewhat less likely to become manifest in the absence of an evocative stressor and that an added stress such as abusive drinking might precipitate an affective episode.

We followed up this alcoholic bipolar cohort for 5 years and compared it with a group of patients who entered the Collaborative Depression Study and had a diagnosis of primary alcoholism with secondary depression. Table 10–4 presents the course of alcoholism in these two groups. By the end of 5 years, only 5% of the bipolar patients continued to have alcoholism, but 25% of the primary alcoholic patients continued to have this problem. Alcoholism in bipolar disorder improves rather dramatically over time. This finding is supported by preliminary data from a 10-year follow-up study of a related cohort. Among index bipolar patients, 30% had alcoholism. We followed up 131 bipolar patients for 10 years; of these patients, only 1 (<1%) had alcoholism at follow-up, indicating that alcoholism in primary bipolar patients diminishes considerably over time (Winokur et al. 1994, 1996).

To summarize, data support the possibility that alcoholism plays a role in precipitating mania. Alcoholism in bipolar disorder is common, observed in about 30% of cases of bipolar disorder. It is associated mainly with bipolar disease in men. The alcoholic bipolar patient does not differ from the nonalcoholic bipolar patient in terms of their clinical courses. However, if the alcoholism precedes the bipolar illness, such an individual is less likely to have episodes

Table 10–4. Course of alcoholism

	Primary alcoholism ($n = 70$)	Primary alcoholism and secondary depression ($n = 93$)	P value
Alcoholic at 2-year follow-up	23%	32%	.19
Alcoholic at 5-year follow-up	5%	25%	.003

in the future than is the individual whose bipolar illness succeeds the alcoholism. This observation also suggests that alcoholism may cause mania in someone who is predisposed to develop bipolar illness. Thus, for individuals who are biologically vulnerable to bipolar illness, alcoholism may be an important trigger—similar to antidepressants, sleep deprivation, or changing time zones—in evoking the diathesis for mania (see also Goldberg and Keck, Chapter 15, in this volume).

Familial Alcoholism and Bipolar Disorder

Links in the genetic vulnerability for bipolar illness and for alcoholism can be seen from family history data. Research in the field suggests that a family history of alcoholism tends to be higher among alcoholic bipolar patients than among nonalcoholic bipolar patients. This observation would suggest that bipolar illness and alcoholism are transmitted independently in the manic-depressive patient who has alcoholism (Dunner et al. 1979; Morrison 1975). The morbid risk for affective disorder in the relatives of alcoholic bipolar patients, however, was similar to the morbid risk in the families of nonalcoholic bipolar patients. These two studies do not indicate whether the alcoholism in the bipolar proband was chronologically primary or secondary; family members with independent alcoholism also were not separated from family members with bipolar illness. *Independent alcoholism* would be defined as alcoholism that exists in a person who does not have bipolar disease. This differentiation turns out to be an absolute necessity, because some of the alcoholism in bipolar illness could simply be part of the extravagant lifestyle of the bipolar patient who indulges in excessive behavior in many spheres.

To obtain a reasonable assessment of the role of familial alcoholism, bipolar subjects who have alcoholism must be eliminated from the analyses because alcoholism is overrepresented in bipolar patients. This methodological maneuver in a family study specifically eliminates those cases in which alcoholism is simply associated with bipolar illness itself.

Our group undertook a more precise, systematic analysis of alcoholism and bipolar illness in first-degree relatives of bipolar patients in a follow-up study of alcoholic versus nonalcoholic bipolar patients (Winokur et al. 1994). We evaluated the presence of alcoholism in three groups: 1) a group of patients with bipolar disorder and alcoholism, 2) a group of patients with bipolar disorder only, and 3) a group of comparison or control subjects. Figure 10–1 presents the life table associated with this analysis. Alcoholism decreased systematically in family members when comparing across alcoholic bipolar patients to nonalcoholic bipolar patients to the control subjects. However, this finding was only marginally significant ($P = .07$). Certainly, more familial alcoholism was seen in the bipolar patients with alcoholism than in the bipolar patients without alcoholism. Notably, both bipolar groups showed a higher proportion of family members who had independent alcoholism than was seen in the comparison group.[1]

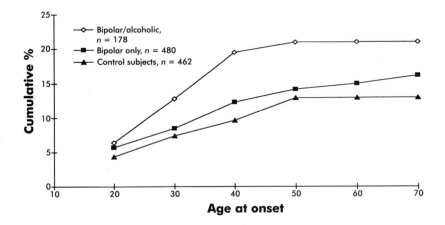

Figure 10–1.   Age to development of alcoholism in personally examined relatives of bipolar patients and control subjects. Relatives with only alcoholism were counted; bipolar relatives who were alcoholic were not counted. (Wilcoxon $\chi^2 = 5.4$, df = 2, $P < .07$)

_____

[1]Editor's note: Relatedly, a subsequent study by Feinman and Dunner (1996) found that *early age at onset* was more common among bipolar patients with comorbid substance abuse than among bipolar patients without substance abuse/dependence or among primary substance abuse/dependence patients who subsequently developed bipolar disorder.

We further explored the relationship between familial alcoholism and bipolar illness with a logistic regression analysis. Table 10–5 shows that the major significant difference between bipolar probands with and without alcoholism was sex: subjects with bipolar disorder and alcoholism were more likely to be male ($P = .0002$). Notably, no significant difference existed in familial alcoholism and bipolar disorder, which is consistent with the life table shown in Figure 10–1. The data in this logistic regression are derived from the presence or absence of the illness for an entire family, rather than for first-degree family members. Once more, a hierarchy exists: if a family member had bipolar illness, neither unipolar illness nor alcoholism was counted. If a relative had unipolar illness, alcoholism in the relative was not counted. Thus, the alcoholism in the logistic regression is alcoholism that stands alone rather than alcoholism related (possibly in a secondary fashion) to either mania or depression. Again, a hierarchy is needed here because if alcoholism were the result of bipolar illness itself, as well as the result of a genetic or familial contribution, it would not be possible to determine the cause of the association.

The data shown in Figure 10–1 and Table 10–5 are, strictly speaking, opposed to the *comorbidity* concept of two diseases. If a patient had two diseases, alcoholism and bipolar illness, a higher degree of alcoholism should be observed in family members. One would not necessarily find a higher degree of bipolar illness in the family members. In fact, no difference in the frequency of bipolar illness existed between the alcoholic bipolar patients and the nonalcoholic bipolar patients. The data presented here thus favor the concept of *cosyn-*

Table 10–5.   Results of logistic regression on sex and presence of specific illness in patients with bipolar disorder and alcoholism versus patients with bipolar disorder only

Variable	P value
Sex	.0002
Familial bipolar illness	.83
Familial unipolar illness	.19
Familial alcoholism	.15

dromality rather than comorbidity. *Comorbidity,* as it is defined, means that the individual has two diseases. For example, an individual could have pneumonia and also have polycystic kidney disease. *Cosyndromality* means that an individual in the course of an illness may have a syndrome that is very common in that illness but not necessarily a separate illness. An example would be alcoholism and secondary depression. Most of the literature on depression associated with alcoholism supports the idea that depression in alcoholic patients usually occurs secondary to the alcoholism. This instance illustrates cosyndromality because the occurrence of a depressive syndrome frequently complicates the course of alcoholism. Data supporting the hypothesis that alcoholism and bipolar illness are separately transmitted diseases reach only a trend level of significance. Therefore, alcoholism and bipolar illness appear to be cosyndromic rather than two separate disease entities.

If independent alcoholism were seen more frequently in the families of alcoholic bipolar patients, it would suggest that two diseases were present, which would support the concept of comorbidity. If alcoholism were more common in family members of nonalcoholic bipolar patients, it would suggest that a familial background of alcoholism might identify a gene relevant to the development of bipolar illness. In fact, Winokur and Reich (1970) noted this possibility. They evaluated 61 manic probands; 10 of the fathers (reflecting 16% of the patients) manifested alcoholism, and 25 of the manic probands had a family history of alcoholism. Nine of them had alcoholism on both sides of the family, and 16 had alcoholism on only one side of the family. No significant difference existed between paternal and maternal side of the family in terms of how much alcoholism was observed. Alcoholism occurred excessively among relatives of patients who manifested manic-depressive disease. These data suggested that alcoholism was a manifestation of a familial factor necessary, but not in itself sufficient, for manias to occur within the family. These initial findings indicated that alcoholism evolved independently of affective disorder in the families of manic probands; thus, alcoholism appeared to be the manifestation of a trait separate from an affective disorder itself. This conclusion led to the concept that a second genetic or familial factor related to alcoholism might contribute to the development of bipolar illness.

Data presented in Figure 10–1 and Table 10–5 do not support the idea that a separate genetic factor related to alcoholism is involved to produce bipolar illness. This question may be reevaluated, however. Because the follow-up is lengthy, some of the bipolar patients will develop alcoholism over time, and some of the unipolar patients will eventually convert to bipolar disorder. Of these patients, some may show alcoholism. Thus, the Collaborative Depression Study provides a broad database from which to assess whether independent alcoholism is related to the development of alcoholism in bipolar patients and whether alcoholism may contribute to a multifactorial background in bipolar illness.

Several other points warrant consideration. Bipolar II illness was eliminated from these evaluations because bipolar II illness is a diagnosis of questionable reliability over time (see Coryell, Chapter 12, in this volume) and because the genetics of bipolar II disorder show a strong association between probands and their first-degree relatives for hypomania (i.e., comparatively few bipolar I relatives are found among bipolar II probands) (Coryell et al. 1984; Rice et al. 1986). Bipolar II illness therefore has a familial relationship to bipolar II illness but not necessarily to bipolar I illness. Thus, at least from the perspective of heredity, many or most bipolar II patients may not be part of a homogeneous bipolar category.

Finally, the question of treatment remains. The patients in these studies were seen in tertiary-care centers and received considerable antimanic therapy. In most instances, this therapy was meaningful in terms of the course of bipolar illness itself. In regard to alcoholism per se, the prognosis generally appears best when the alcoholism is associated with bipolar illness. As noted earlier in this chapter, after 10 years of follow-up, only 1 of 131 bipolar patients continued to be actively alcoholic, which seems to indicate that the alcoholism in bipolar illness diminishes over time.

A Historical Case

The association between alcoholism and bipolar illness is not without its subtleties. Stanley (1995) presented a short account of the author Jack London's alcoholism and affective problems. London was known to have periods of enormous energy, during which time he hardly slept and devoted many hours to work or study. Stanley suggests that Jack London may have had bipolar illness.

According to London's own memoirs, by age 17 he drank every day, had morning tremors and gastrointestinal problems, and needed to drink in the morning in order to begin the day. He went away to sea and for 51 days did not drink and denied having any desire for alcohol, but when he reached shore, he resumed drinking heavily. Returning home, he entered night school and abstained from alcohol for 1½ years. During this time, he reported studying up to 19 hours daily for 3 months. Could London have been in the midst of a manic episode? Might such an episode have been triggered by his drinking?

London finished school and resumed drinking heavily, but after a short period he started to write and did so in a frenzied manner. Is it possible that his short bout of alcoholism brought on another manic episode? It is unknown whether he had a family history of alcoholism; if he did, and although this is speculation, alcoholism might have not only precipitated a manic episode but predisposed him to bipolar illness. These possibilities are not mutually exclusive, but they represent one interpretation of his behavior.

Summary

Compelling data suggest that alcoholism and bipolar illness co-occur far more often than would be expected by chance alone. Family history studies of bipolar patients with or without alcoholism suggest considerable overlap in the inheritance patterns of these two disorders, suggesting that they may be cosyndromal manifestations of the same underlying disease process. Bipolar patients with alcoholism may have greater work impairment and poorer psychosocial functioning. However, in contrast to patients with pure alcoholism, active alcohol abuse itself appears to diminish over time when it is associated with bipolar illness. Importantly, active alcohol abuse may precipitate manias among individuals with a diathesis or vulnerability to bipolar illness.

References

Coryell W, Endicott J, Reich T, et al: A family study of bipolar II disorder. Br J Psychiatry 145:49–54, 1984

Dunner D, Hensch B, Fieve R: Bipolar illness: factors in drinking behavior. Am J Psychiatry 136:583–585, 1979

Feinman JA, Dunner DL: The effect of alcohol and substance abuse on the course of bipolar affective disorder. J Affect Disord 37:43–49, 1996

Helzer J, Pryzbeck T: The co-occurrence of alcoholism with other psychiatric disorders in the general population and its impact on treatment. J Stud Alcohol 49:219–224, 1988

Mirin SM, Weiss RD, Michael J, et al: Psychopathology in substance abusers: diagnosis and treatment. Am J Drug Alcohol Abuse 14:139–157, 1988

Morrison J: The family histories of manic-depressive patients with and without alcoholism. J Nerv Ment Dis 160:227–229, 1975

Rice J, McDonald-Scott P, Endicott J, et al: The stability of diagnosis with an application to bipolar II disorder. Psychiatry Res 19:285–296, 1986

Stanley WJ: "John Barleycorn"; Jack London's "Alcoholic Memoirs." Psychiatric Bulletin 19:638–639, 1995

Winokur G, Reich T: Two genetic factors in manic-depressive disease. Compr Psychiatry 11:93–99, 1970

Winokur G, Cook B, Liskow B, et al: Alcoholism in manic depressive (bipolar) patients. J Stud Alcohol 54:574–576, 1993

Winokur G, Coryell W, Akiskal H, et al: Manic-depressive (bipolar) disorder: the course in light of a prospective ten year follow-up of 131 patients. Acta Psychiatr Scand 89:102–110, 1994

Winokur G, Coryell W, Akiskal H, et al: Alcoholism in manic-depressive (bipolar) illness: familial illness, course of illness, and the primary-secondary distinction. Am J Psychiatry 152:365–372, 1995

Winokur G, Coryell W, Endicott J, et al: Familial alcoholism in manic-depressive (bipolar) disease. Am J Med Genet 67:197–201, 1996

CHAPTER 11

Rapid-Cycling Bipolar Affective Disorder

David L. Dunner, M.D.

*I*n this chapter, I review the concept and history of rapid cycling as a course modifier for bipolar affective disorder and discuss its addition to the nomenclature in DSM-IV (American Psychiatric Association 1994). I also discuss theories relating to the etiology of rapid cycling and review treatments that have been suggested for rapid cycling.

History

Kraepelin (1921/1976) coined the term *manic depressive,* and Falret (1890) was the first to highlight the cycling nature of bipolar affective disorder when he coined the term *la folie circulaire.* In the 1960s, research into bipolar disorder focused on behavioral and biochemical effects of mania and depression, and investigators attempted to find patients who had a high frequency of mood changes (Murphy et al. 1971). Several research groups studied *24-hour rapid cyclers,* patients whose mood state alternated from depression to mania in a stable fashion (Bunney et al. 1965; Jenner et al. 1967). The purpose of studying these patients was to identify biological differences between mania and depression and to study the *switch* process from depression to mania (Bunney et al. 1972).

The modern concept of rapid cycling derived from patients who did not respond to treatment with lithium carbonate. Stancer and colleagues (1970) described some patients who had responded poorly to lithium maintenance treatment. Dunner and Fieve (1974) provided the most frequently cited definition of rapid cycling. This research came about through our attempt to investigate the success and the failure of lithium maintenance. At the time, lithium's long-term effects were not well established or highly regarded. Thus, considerable research efforts attempted to show that lithium treatment was effective, not only for acute mania but also for prevention of future attacks of mania and depression in bipolar patients. For this research, we reviewed data from patients treated with maintenance lithium and found that these patients tended to have breakthrough episodes. We selected patients attending the Lithium Clinic at the New York Psychiatric Institute for further analysis. We reviewed their charts and abstracted data for several variables. The clinical histories of 55 such patients prior to lithium treatment seemed to predict early lithium treatment failure. Those patients who had many affective episodes did not do as well as those who had few episodes. These data suggested that patients who had four or more episodes per year seemed to account for most of the early (within 6 months) lithium maintenance failures. Patients who had few episodes per year did better, and some remained well throughout the period of follow-up (up to 24 months). Patients were termed *rapid cyclers* if they had four or more episodes in the year prior to lithium treatment. Such patients accounted for 50% of the overall group of patients who failed to stay well while taking lithium (Dunner and Fieve 1974).

At that time, the notion of bipolar cycles was not well established; thus, episodes rather than cycles were counted. An *episode* is a period of depression or a period of mania or hypomania, whereas a *cycle* is an episode of depression followed by a period of mania or hypomania (or an episode of mania or hypomania followed by depression). Perhaps it would have been better to express the frequency of attacks as cycles rather than episodes, because treatment approaches for stabilization of rapid cycling seem to be more effective if mania (and the switch from depression to mania) is prevented rather than treatment being aimed at individual episodes.

Dunner and Fieve (1974) set the definition of rapid cycling at four or more episodes per year, and this definition has been cited subsequently by most investigators. Prien et al. (1974) confirmed the high failure rate of rapid cycling in a maintenance study in which patients with frequent attacks tended not to do as well on maintenance lithium treatment as did other patients.

Several studies determining the frequencies of affective attacks in bipolar patients prior to lithium treatment or during placebo treatment of bipolar disorder suggested that the natural history of bipolar disorder involves about four episodes in 10 years (Dunner et al. 1979; Winokur et al. 1969). Approximately 80% of these episodes involve mania and rehospitalization. Thus, although a range in episode frequency exists within the spectrum of bipolar disorder, the episode frequency is on average about 0.4 episodes per patient year. In contrast, rapid cycling involves an episode frequency 10 times higher than that, or four or more episodes per patient year.

Clinical Characteristics of Rapid Cyclers

Research on rapid cycling was somewhat easier to accomplish in the 1970s than it was later because lithium was not a well-established and widely used treatment until after the 1970s. Thus, in order to be treated with lithium, patients went to academic centers or to the few private clinicians who offered lithium treatment. Affective or mood disorder centers or lithium clinics were common within academic departments of psychiatry. These centers often treated several hundred patients, who were also available for research. Because rapid cycling occurs in approximately 15% of such clinic populations (Dunner et al. 1977), the chance of an individual clinician having sufficient rapid-cycling patients for research purposes was low in comparison to the lithium centers, which had sufficient numbers of rapid-cycling patients to develop a database related to them. After lithium treatment became established and widely utilized, patients no longer needed to attend such centers and instead were treated by psychiatrists and family physicians.

An initial question was whether rapid-cycling patients differed from non-rapid-cycling patients. In general, the two groups are very similar. Most studies show that more rapid-cycling patients are women than men. The overall male-to-female ratio for bipolar disorder is about equal, but 70%–90% of rapid-cycling patients are women, according to almost all samples (Alarcon 1985; Dunner and Fieve 1974; Dunner et al. 1977; Wehr et al. 1988). Furthermore, the percentage of women seems to increase further with increasing cycle frequencies (Bauer and Whybrow 1991).[1]

One notable finding is that most rapid-cycling patients are bipolar rather than unipolar. In fact, it is unusual to find unipolar patients who have multiple episodes per year who do not also have a history of hypomania (Bauer and Whybrow 1991; Zisook 1988). A clinical implication of this finding is that if a clinician is evaluating a patient who has multiple depressive episodes in 1 year, the clinician should inquire about a history of brief hypomanic mood swings, because they are likely to be present. Furthermore, making a diagnosis of rapid-cycling bipolar disorder versus unipolar recurrent depression has many treatment implications (e.g., the use of lithium versus antidepressant pharmacotherapy for maintenance).

Other studies have compared clinical factors among rapid-cycling and non-rapid-cycling patients. The two groups do not differ by age at onset of illness, history of hospitalization for mania (bipolar I versus bipolar II), suicide attempt history, or family history (Alarcon 1985; Coryell et al. 1992; Dunner et al. 1977; Wehr et al. 1988; Wu and Dunner 1993). In a family study of bipolar patients, Nurnberger et al. (1988) interviewed relatives of rapid-cycling and non-rapid-cycling patients. They found a similar morbid risk for mania among relatives for both groups. Furthermore, rapid cycling also occurred in the families of both groups. These clinical and family data suggest that rapid-cycling patients are not clinically different from non-rapid-cycling patients in terms of symptoms. The major differences are a higher frequency of episodes and a greater tendency for women than men to have this rapid-cycling form of illness.

In terms of cycle frequency, most rapid cyclers are at the minimal end of the criteria for rapid cycling; that is, they have four episodes per year (Dunner et al. 1977). As the cycle frequency increases, the number of patients within a clinical population who experience rapid cycling decreases proportionally.

Laboratory findings have generally not been able to differentiate rapid-cycling from non-rapid-cycling patients, with the exception of

---

[1]For additional discussion of the increased risk for rapid cycling in women versus men, see Leibenluft (1996).

thyroid function tests. Several studies (Cho et al. 1978; Cowdry et al. 1983; Nurnberger et al. 1988), but not all (Bauer et al. 1990; Wehr et al. 1988), have suggested that rapid-cycling patients, particularly women rapid cyclers, tend to have thyroid sensitivity to lithium treatment or a history of thyroid disease before lithium treatment (Joffe et al. 1988).

Some reports indicate that rapid cycling can be induced by treatment with tricyclic antidepressants (TCAs) (Wehr and Goodwin 1979). However, most bipolar patients have a history of antidepressant treatment for their depressive phases, and only a limited number (about 15%) of such patients become rapid cyclers. Bauer et al. (1990) compared patients whose rapid cycling occurred during treatment with TCAs with patients who were spontaneous rapid cyclers, and they failed to find differences in thyroid status, treatment outcome, or clinical characteristics. Furthermore, rapid cycling can appear intermittently (Coryell et al. 1992; Post et al. 1986; Roy-Byrne et al. 1985; Wehr et al. 1988), suggesting that investigators should find few differences between rapid-cycling and non-rapid-cycling patients.

In summary, rapid cycling was defined clinically as a form of bipolar disorder in which patients had a high rate of early lithium treatment failure and had multiple affective episodes before being started on lithium. Except for the increased likelihood for such patients to be women than men, as compared with other bipolar affective disorder patients, no clinical or family differences have been found. In some instances, rapid cycling occurs during antidepressant pharmacotherapy. Laboratory studies have indicated alterations in thyroid function in some rapid-cycling patients, suggesting the possibility that the combination of having a tendency toward bipolar disorder, being a woman, being treated with a TCA, and having an underlying thyroid dysfunction are predisposing factors for the rapid-cycling condition.

The fact that rapid cyclers and other bipolar patients have similar family histories for mania casts doubt on the hypotheses linking family history as a predictor of lithium maintenance response (Mendlewicz et al. 1972). Furthermore, an inherent illogic exists in this hypothesis. Family history can change from negative to positive if a relative becomes manic. Similarly, lithium response can change if a patient's first breakthrough episode of hypomania or depression occurs during lithium treatment (Fleiss et al. 1978). Thus, both variables are apt to change and in a direction to obscure any relationship between family history and lithium maintenance response.

Rapid Cycling in DSM-III and DSM-III-R

In DSM-III (American Psychiatric Association 1980), the criteria for mania included a 1-week or greater duration of symptoms, and the criteria for major depression included 2 weeks or greater duration of symptoms. Hypomania with depression (bipolar II) was listed as atypical bipolar disorder. Rapid cycling was not mentioned in DSM-III.

DSM-III-R (American Psychiatric Association 1987) eliminated duration criteria for mania, leading to some degree of confusion regarding the maximal cycle frequency associated with rapid cycling and obscuring the definitions of cyclothymic disorder, mixed mania, and rapid cycling. Some authors have described rapid-cycling patients who have hundreds of episodes per year (Calabrese and Delucchi 1989, 1990) or within-a-day cycles of depression and mania. Furthermore, others have described a cyclic form of depression called *recurrent brief depression* (Angst et al. 1990). Such patients meet criteria for major depression except for duration (the depressions last less than 2 weeks) and have multiple annual depressive periods without hypomania.

Rapid Cycling in DSM-IV

The decision to include rapid cycling in DSM-IV was made after duration criteria were defined for hypomania and mania. In determining the duration of hypomania, the original criteria described by Dunner et al. (1976a) were based on an observation of "normal" women in a study of premenstrual depression. These women described less than 2-day periods of hypomanic symptoms premenstrually. In determining the minimal duration of hypomanic symptoms for the bipolar II definition, our group suggested the criterion of 3 days or more, because women with no psychiatric disorders experienced up to 2 days of such symptoms. The 3-day minimal duration criterion has never been validated, and, indeed, most bipolar II patients have considerably longer periods of hypomania.

For ICD-10 (World Health Organization 1992), a 4-day minimal duration for hypomania was selected, and the DSM-IV Mood Disorders Work Group agreed with the ICD-10 group because no data were available to determine whether 3 days or 4 days would be a better definition. The DSM-IV Mood Disorders Work Group also reinstated a minimal criterion of 1 week for the duration of mania (American Psychiatric Association 1993). Thus, in DSM-IV the criteria for rapid cycling would be at least 4 days of hypomania and 2 weeks of depression; in other words, 18 days for one cycle or no more than 20 cycles (40 episodes) per year. These criteria would also mean that patients who had more frequent cycles than stated or whose hypomanic or depressive episodes were shorter than 4 days or 14 days, respectively, would be termed *cyclothymic* and not rapid cyclers. Thus, some patients described in the literature and treatment studies as having several hundred episodes per year (*ultra-rapid cyclers*) would be reclassified as having cyclothymic disorder rather than bipolar disorder with rapid cycling. Because rapid cycling seems to be associated more frequently with bipolar disorder and rarely with unipolar disorder, the proposal for DSM-IV was that rapid cycling be a parenthetical modifier for bipolar disorder—Type I and Type II. Recurrent brief depressive disorder, accepted in ICD-10, was not accepted as a formal diagnosis in DSM-IV but was placed in an appendix with a notation that further study of this condition was needed.

In reviewing the criteria for rapid cycling for DSM-IV, Bauer and colleagues (1994) undertook a study to determine whether Dunner and Fieve's (1974) episode frequency of four episodes per year could be validated. The main clinical differentiation between rapid-cycling and non-rapid-cycling patients is the percentage of women. These investigators undertook a multicenter study to determine the relationship between episode frequency and sex ratio. Their study determined four episodes per year was the minimum episode frequency for rapid cyclers in that the ratio of women to men increased as the number of episodes per year increased above four.

In DSM-IV, mixed mania is differentiated from rapid cycling and from cyclothymic disorder. Mixed mania is a severe manic episode with an excessive mixture of depressive symptoms. Cyclothymic disorder is a chronic (2 years or greater) condition with highs and lows too brief to meet criteria for hypomanic episode and major depressive episode. Inconsistency in the definition of mixed mania in research settings has led to variability in the reported prevalence of this condition (McElroy et al. 1992; Swann 1995).

The DSM-IV criteria discussed earlier in this chapter provide a basis for clarifying the types of frequent mood cycling seen among bipolar and nonbipolar patients and also encourage further research in this area. Krauthammer and Klerman (1978) described "secondary" forms of mania, and in our clinical experience, patients with histories of significant head trauma and brain injury, multiple sclerosis, endocrine dysfunction, and substance abuse can exhibit rapidly fluctuating mood swings. The diagnostic criteria for borderline personality disorder include affective instability usually lasting a few hours and rarely a few days. Wolpert et al. (1990) reported an increase in cycle frequency and complexity of cycling among bipolar patients over a 25-year span. Wolpert and colleagues assessed cycle frequency and mood fluctuations in samples of bipolar patients from 1960, 1975, and 1985.

One factor that may account for the increase in cycle frequency (ultrarapid cycling) so frequently encountered in today's clinical settings is substance abuse. Our group reported that bipolar patients with histories of substance abuse were significantly more likely to exhibit within-a-day cycling than were bipolar patients who had no history of substance abuse (Feinman and Dunner 1996). Furthermore, clinicians may tend to overdiagnose as bipolar rapid cyclers patients who show periods of irritability. Adherence to DSM-IV criteria for bipolar disorder may be helpful in restricting the definition of rapid cycling.

Hypotheses Regarding the Etiology of Rapid Cycling

Three compelling hypotheses exist regarding the etiology of rapid cycling: 1) biological rhythm dysregulation, 2) behavioral sensitization and kindling, and 3) central nervous system thyroid dysregulation. Clinical data support each hypothesis.

Biological Rhythm Dysregulation

Goodwin and Jamison (1990) reviewed the notion of "free-running" biological rhythms as a basis for rapid cycling. Briefly, Halberg (1968) proposed that some circadian rhythms were not entrained on a 24-hour cycle but run free, going in and out of phase with other circadian rhythms synchronized with the 24-hour day-night cycle. Kripke and colleagues (1978, 1983) studied rapid cyclers and noted that five of seven patients had shorter-than-24-hour circadian rhythms. Wehr et al. (1985) also found abnormally short cycles in one bipolar patient studied in a time-free (isolation) condition. Studies showing induction of rapid cycling by use of TCAs in bipolar patients are also consistent with this hypothesis (Joffe et al. 1988), as animal studies indicate that the sleep-wake cycle can be lengthened by treatment with antidepressants (Wehr and Wirz-Justice 1982). The report that rapid cyclers had 48-hour sleep-wake cycles at the onset of the manic phase also supports the hypothesis of biological rhythm dysregulation (Wehr et al. 1982). This hypothesis posits that an abnormality in the sleep oscillator underlies frequent mood shifts.

Behavioral Sensitization and Kindling

Post and colleagues (Post 1986; Post and Weiss 1989; Post et al. 1984) have developed the hypothesis of behavioral sensitization and kindling as the basis of rapid cycling. This model proposes that repeated mood alterations to environmental stressors ultimately result in spontaneous and increasingly frequent episodes (see Post et al., Chapter 5, in this volume). Laboratory induction of seizures in animals by repeated electrical stimulation and the clinical effects of anticonvulsants (carbamazepine and valproate) on the course of rapid cycling provide interesting clinical parallels (Ballenger and Post 1980; Calabrese and Delucchi 1990).

Central Nervous System Thyroid Dysregulation

Bauer and Whybrow (1990) suggested that an alteration in central nervous system thyroid hormone, particularly in the function of thyroxine (T_4), is related to rapid cycling. They administered high doses of T_4 in combination with lithium to a few rapid-cycling bipolar patients and noted clinical improvement (Bauer and Whybrow 1990). Their report confirmed Stancer and Persad's (1982) study regarding positive effects of thyroid hormone supplements on mood stabilization in rapid-cycling patients.

Treatment Recommendations

In maintenance lithium treatment for bipolar disorder, manic and hypomanic episodes appear to be stabilized first and then patients experience recurrent depressive episodes with minimal hypomanic time (Coppen et al. 1971; Cundall et al. 1972; Prien et al. 1973; Stallone et al. 1973). Lithium's antidepressant maintenance effects become apparent only after long-term treatment. For example, antidepressant effects for lithium-treated bipolar II patients were shown after 3 years of treatment (Dunner et al. 1976b, 1982), whereas antimanic effects could be shown in bipolar I patients after 2 years of treatment (Stallone et al. 1973). A manic or hypomanic episode can be preceded by a depressive episode. Taking an antidepressant while switching from depression to hypomania may cause the cycle to continue, because postmanic or posthypomanic depressions are hypothesized to be a consequence of mood elevation (i.e., highs cause lows). The observation that cycling can be induced by TCA treatment supports this notion (Wehr and Goodwin 1979).

The first point in treatment is for the clinician to diagnose rapid cycling. Rapid cycling should be suspected in a patient who complains of recurrent major depressive episodes occurring several times a year. Such a patient should be evaluated carefully for a history of hypomanic episodes, which sometimes is not recognized by the patient but may be defined better by the patient's friends or significant other. These episodes can also be present in a patient who describes a chronic depression but who seems to have a several-day period of alleviation of depression (which turns out to be hypomania and not just normal mood as found in a dysthymic pattern).

My colleagues and I recommend that patients and their families become educated about the course of manic-depressive illness, rapid cycling, and lithium treatment by reading a book particularly designed for patients, namely *Moodswing* (Fieve 1975). We recommend this book to educate both patients and their families about the illness as well as about lithium treatment and lithium side effects. *Moodswing* also contains chapters about rapid cycling.

We also find it useful to have the patient keep a daily mood calendar so that the clinician and the patient can anticipate switches from depression to hypomania. If a goal of treatment is to stabilize moods, then the clinician must first stabilize the mood elevation component of the mood cycle. Some patients have a regularly occurring switch from depression to mania or hypomania, and determining the timing of this switch can be of value in terms of treatment planning. For example, if the time of the switch from depression to hypomania can be anticipated, higher doses of mood stabilizers and/or antimanic medications can be prescribed just prior to this switch to lessen the likelihood of hypomania (and thus prevent the posthypomanic depression).

Because of the hypothesis about biological rhythm alterations, we also recommend that patients structure their days (i.e., get up at the same time, go to bed at the same time, and eat their meals at the same time). As yet, no clear evidence indicates that this approach has any benefit, but certainly sleep disorders are common in mood disorders. Miklowitz and Frank (Chapter 4, in this volume) address the issue of maintaining sleep and social "hygiene" as an essential feature related to treatment course and outcome in bipolar patients. By attempting to regulate the patient's sleep, the clinician may provide some stability to the patient's biological rhythms. We also recommend a daily regular exercise program, as regular exercise tends to alleviate symptoms of hypomania and may have mild antidepressant effects.

In terms of laboratory assessment, we obtain a physical examination and a prelithium evaluation, including a thyroid screen and thyroid-stimulating hormone (TSH) screen. Any abnormalities in thyroid function need to be addressed with appropriate thyroid medication. We had been in the practice of obtaining thyroid antibodies but found a very low yield of positive responses and would instead prefer to monitor TSH during lithium treatment to determine if hypothyroidism occurs.

Not all antimanic medication is useful in mood stabilization. Three compounds—lithium carbonate, valproate, and carbamazepine—are the most useful for treatment of rapid cycling. We feel lithium alone should be the first pharmacological treatment for rapid cycling. Indeed, lithium alone seems to have a positive effect in many rapid-cycling patients (Dunner and Fieve 1974; Dunner et al. 1977; Kukopulos et al. 1980; Prien et al. 1984; Wehr et al. 1988). The mood-stabilizing effects of lithium are not immediately apparent. The patient should be encouraged to continue taking this medication for at least 6 months, and he or she should be monitored carefully for the possible emergence of hypothyroidism because this may occur during lithium treatment, especially among women rapid cyclers. Antidepressant pharmacotherapy should be avoided if possible in order not to enhance the switch process from depression to hypomania.

If the treatment is successful, the hypomanias are likely to be diminished considerably and the depressions will be little affected, at least over the initial few months of treatment. The presence of depression and the wish to avoid antidepressant pharmacotherapy creates certain problems. Exercise alone and structure to one's day do not necessarily adequately treat the depressive phase. Therefore, we also suggest that patients have psychotherapies designed for the treatment of mood disorder, particularly cognitive therapy or interpersonal psychotherapy. Also, if a patient continues to have hypomanic episodes and is cycling on a regular basis, it may be useful to increase the dose of lithium just prior to the anticipated switch to hypomania in order to attenuate the episode.

The role of antidepressants in bipolar disorder is highly controversial (see Goldberg and Kocsis, Chapter 7, in this volume). If antidepressant pharmacotherapy is needed, we would not recommend the TCAs but instead would recommend any of the selective serotonin reuptake inhibitors (SSRIs), bupropion, or other newer antidepressants. These latter medications, as noted in Chapter 7, seem to have a lower treatment-emergent hypomania effect than do TCAs. The short-half-life SSRIs, such as paroxetine and sertraline, may be of particular benefit because the clinician could more easily discontinue treatment if the patient switched suddenly to hypomania.

In general, however, we prefer not to treat patients with antidepressant pharmacotherapy. Often the depressive phase lasts only a few weeks, and most antidepressants take 2–4 weeks to exert their antidepressant effects. The typical rapid cycler is out of the depressive phase before the anticipated onset of the effect of antidepressant pharmacotherapy.

If the patient does not respond to lithium monotherapy, we suggest adding a second mood stabilizer, either carbamazepine or valproate. These medications have been used successfully in the stabilization of bipolar mood disorders (Calabrese and Delucchi 1990; Calabrese et al. 1997; Wehr et al. 1982), and some researchers advocate their use as first-line treatments instead of lithium. Other anticonvulsants with potential mood-stabilizing effects, such as lamotrigine, have been reported in preliminary open trials and case reports as useful in rapid-cycling bipolar patients (Fatemi et al. 1997; Labbate and Rubey 1997; see also Post et al., Chapter 5, in this volume). Our general approach is to add either carbamazepine or valproate (with no particular preference for either) to lithium rather than switching, because we have found better results clinically by adding rather than switching. A complicated but important research question to answer would be, "What is the best treatment strategy for rapid cycling?" Such research could develop a multicenter study and randomly assign rapid cyclers to lithium, valproate, or carbamazepine as the initial treatment and then to various combinations if treatment fails. In the absence of such data, clinicians must rely on clinical experience. It is important to monitor blood levels and indicated medical tests for these mood stabilizers.

A 6-month trial of combined therapy is our intent. If the patient does not respond, we would switch to lithium and to the other mood stabilizer. During this time, the clinician should monitor the patient's thyroid function, use antidepressants sparingly, consider cognitive therapy approaches, and probably keep lithium doses in the moderate range. We have not found that high doses of lithium are of much practical use because high lithium doses seem to be related to an increased rate of side effects.

Other agents that could be added in selected patients include benzodiazepines, particularly clonazepam. This medication was effective in the treatment of acute mania in a small controlled study (Chouinard 1987). We have also used antipsychotic medications such as thioridazine. The use of antipsychotic medications, although previously recommended, should be used with greater caution because bipolar patients seem to be at higher risk for the development of tardive dyskinesia than are other patients, and the use of antipsychotic medication has led to this disorder in some rapid cyclers. If an antipsychotic medication is prescribed, the lowest dose should be used, and the patient should be monitored frequently for tardive dyskinesia with the Abnormal Involuntary Movements Scale (AIMS). This scale is used widely to assess signs of movement disorders and tardive dyskinesia. The patient should also be informed about the possibility of tardive dyskinesia. Risperidone, olanzapine, or other atypical antipsychotics may have a reduced risk of tardive dyskinesia and may become the preferable antipsychotic. Clozapine has been reported to be effective (Calabrese et al. 1991).

Electroconvulsive treatment (ECT) has been proposed for medication-resistant rapid cyclers. Again, the principle seems to be that treatments effective in mania may be effective in rapid cycling. We suggest that lithium be discontinued prior to ECT because neurotoxicity has been reported when ECT was administered in the presence of lithium (Small et al. 1980).

We have encountered some patients who have very frequent bipolar mood shifts, often describing these shifts in terms of hours or days (1–2 days) rather than using the DSM-IV criteria. These patients have been called *truncated-episode patients* (Bauer et al. 1994) or ultrarapid cyclers. As noted earlier in this chapter, such patients may have histories of head trauma, extensive polysubstance abuse, or an underlying endocrine dysfunction. In general, such patients may be less likely to respond to lithium maintenance treatment alone, and we often opt for anticonvulsants as the primary treatment.

Summary

In summary, the treatment for rapid cycling involves educational, psychotherapeutic, and psychopharmacological approaches (Dunner et al. 1977; McElroy et al. 1992). Most patients will likely require long-term treatment to show beneficial effects.

References

Alarcon RD: Rapid cycling affective disorders: a clinical review. Compr Psychiatry 26:522–540, 1985

American Psychiatric Association: Diagnostic and Statistical Manual of Mental Disorders, 3rd Edition. Washington, DC, American Psychiatric Association, 1980

American Psychiatric Association: Diagnostic and Statistical Manual of Mental Disorders, 3rd Edition, Revised. Washington, DC, American Psychiatric Association, 1987

American Psychiatric Association: DSM-IV Draft Criteria. Washington, DC, American Psychiatric Association, 1993

American Psychiatric Association: Diagnostic and Statistical Manual of Mental Disorders, 4th Edition. Washington, DC, American Psychiatric Association, 1994

Angst J, Merikangas K, Scheidegger P, et al: Recurrent brief depression: a new subtype of affective disorder. J Affect Disord 19:87–98, 1990

Ballenger JC, Post RM: Carbamazepine in manic-depressive illness: a new treatment. Am J Psychiatry 137:782–790, 1980

Bauer MS, Whybrow PC: Rapid cycling bipolar affective disorder, II: treatment of refractory rapid cycling with high-dose levothyroroxine: a preliminary study. Arch Gen Psychiatry 47:435–440, 1990

Bauer M, Whybrow P: Rapid cycling bipolar disorder: clinical features, treatment and etiology, in Refractory Depression—Frontiers in Research and Treatment. Edited by Amsterdam J. New York, Raven, 1991, pp 191–208

Bauer MS, Whybrow PC, Winokur A: Rapid cycling bipolar affective disorder: I. association with grade I hypothyroidism. Arch Gen Psychiatry 47:427–432, 1990

Bauer MS, Calabrese J, Dunner DL, et al: Multi-site data reanalysis: validity of rapid cycling as a course modifier for bipolar disorder in DSM-IV. Am J Psychiatry 151:506–515, 1994

Bunney WE Jr, Hartman EL, Mason JW: Study of a patient with 48 hour manic-depressive cycles. Arch Gen Psychiatry 12:619–625, 1965

Bunney WE Jr, Murphy DL, Goodwin FK, et al: The "switch process" in manic-depressive illness, I: a systematic study of sequential behavior change. Arch Gen Psychiatry 27:295–302, 1972

Calabrese JR, Delucchi GA: Phenomenology of rapid cycling manic depression and its treatment with valproate. J Clin Psychiatry 50 (suppl):30–34, 1989

Calabrese JR, Delucchi GA: Spectrum of efficacy of valproate in 55 patients with rapid cycling bipolar disorder. Am J Psychiatry 147:431–444, 1990

Calabrese JR, Meltzer HY, Markovitz PJ: Clozapine prophylaxis in rapid-cycling bipolar disorder. J Clin Psychopharmacol 11:396–397, 1991

Calabrese JR, Fatemi SH, Woyshville MJ: Diagnosis and treatment of rapid-cycling bipolar disorder, in Current Psychiatric Therapy, 2nd Edition. Edited by Dunner DL. Philadelphia, PA, WB Saunders, 1997, pp 266–270

Cho JT, Bone S, Dunner DL, et al: The effect of lithium treatment on thyroid function in patients with primary affective disorder. Am J Psychiatry 136:115–116, 1978

Chouinard G: Clonazepam in acute maintenance treatment of bipolar affective disorder. J Clin Psychiatry 48 (suppl):29–36, 1987

Coppen A, Noguera R, Bailey J, et al: Prophylactic lithium in affective disorders: controlled trial. Lancet 2:275–279, 1971

Coryell W, Endicott J, Keller M: Rapid cycling affective disorder: demographics, diagnosis, family history, and course. Arch Gen Psychiatry 49:126–131, 1992

Cowdry RW, Wehr TA, Zis AP, et al: Thyroid abnormalities associated with rapid-cycling bipolar illness. Arch Gen Psychiatry 40:414–420, 1983

Cundall R, Brooks PW, Murray LG: A controlled evaluation of lithium prophylaxis in affective disorders. Psychol Med 2:308–311, 1972

Dunner DL: Rapid cycling bipolar manic depressive illness. Psychiatr Clin North Am 2:461–467, 1979

Dunner DL, Fieve RR: Clinical factors in lithium prophylactic failure. Arch Gen Psychiatry 30:229–233, 1974

Dunner DL, Gershon ES, Goodwin FK: Heritable factors in the severity of affective illness. Biol Psychiatry 11:31–42, 1976a

Dunner DL, Stallone F, Fieve RR: Lithium carbonate and affective disorders, V: a double-blind study of prophylaxis of depression in bipolar illness. Arch Gen Psychiatry 33:117–120, 1976b

Dunner DL, Patrick V, Fieve RR: Rapid cycling manic depressive patients. Compr Psychiatry 18:561–566, 1977

Dunner DL, Murphy D, Stallone F, et al: Episode frequency prior to lithium treatment in bipolar manic-depressive patients. Compr Psychiatry 20: 511–515, 1979

Dunner DL, Stallone F, Fieve RR: Prophylaxis with lithium carbonate: an update (letter). Arch Gen Psychiatry 39:1344–1345, 1982

Falret J: La folie circulaire ou folie a formes alterns, in Etudes Cliniques sur Les Maladies Mentales et Nerveuses. Paris, Librarie JB Bailliere et Fils, 1890

Fatemi SH, Rapport DJ, Calabrese JR, et al: Lamotrigine in rapid-cycling bipolar disorder. J Clin Psychiatry 58:522–527, 1997

Feinman J, Dunner DL: The effect of alcohol and substance abuse on the course of bipolar affective disorder. J Affect Disord 37:43–49, 1996

Fieve RR: Moodswing: The Third Revolution in Psychiatry, New York, William Morrow, 1975

Fleiss JL, Prien RF, Dunner DL, et al: Actuarial studies of the course of manic-depressive illness. Compr Psychiatry 19:355–362, 1978

Goodwin FK, Jamison KR: Manic-Depressive Illness. New York, Oxford University Press, 1990

Halberg G: Physiologic considerations underlying rhythometry, with special reference to emotional illness, in Cycles Biologiques et Psychiatrie Symposium Bel-Air III. Edited by DeAjuriaguerra J. Geneva, Switzerland, Masson Et Cie, 1968, pp 73–126

Jenner FA, Gjessing LR, Cox JR, et al: A manic-depressive psychotic with a persistent forty-eight hour cycle. Br J Psychiatry 113:895–910, 1967

Joffe RT, Kutcher S, MacDonald C: Thyroid function and bipolar affective disorder. Psychiatry Res 25:117–121, 1988

Kraepelin E: Manic-Depressive Insanity and Paranoia (1921). Translated by Barclay RM. Edited by Robertson GM. Edinburgh, Scotland, Livingstone. Reprint, New York, Arno Press, 1976

Krauthammer C, Klerman GL: Secondary mania: manic syndromes associated with antecedent physical illness or drugs. Arch Gen Psychiatry 35:1333–1339, 1978

Kripke DF: Phase advance theories for affective illnesses, in Circadian Rhythms in Psychiatry. Edited by Wehr TA, Goodwin FK. Pacific Grove, CA, Boxwood Press, 1983, pp 41–69

Kripke DF, Mullaney DJ, Atkinson M, et al: Circadian rhythm disorders in manic-depressives. Biol Psychiatry 13:335–351, 1978

Kukopulos A, Reginaldi D, Laddomada P, et al: Course of the manic-depressive cycle and changes caused by treatments. Pharmacopsychiatry 13:156–167, 1980

Labbate LA, Rubey RN: Lamotrigine for treatment-refractory bipolar disorder (letter). Am J Psychiatry 154:1317, 1997

Leibenluft E: Women with bipolar illness: clinical and research issues. Am J Psychiatry 153:163–173, 1996

McElroy SL, Keck PE Jr, Pope HG Jr, et al: Clinical and research implications of dysphoric or mixed mania or hypomania. Am J Psychiatry 149:1633–1644, 1992

Mendlewicz J, Fieve RR, Stallone F, et al: Genetic history as a predictor of lithium response in manic depressive illness. Lancet 1:599–600, 1972

Murphy DL, Goodwin FK, Bunney WE Jr: Clinical and pharmacological investigations of the psychology of affective disorders. International Pharmacopsychiatry 6:137–146, 1971

Nurnberger JI Jr, Guroff JJ, Hamovit J, et al: A family study of rapid-cycling bipolar illness. J Affect Disord 15:87–91, 1988

Post RM, Weiss SRB: Non-homologous animal models of affective illness: clinical relevance of sensitization and kindling, in Animal Models of Depression. Edited by Koob G, Ehlers C, Kupfer DJ. Boston, MA, Birkhauser, 1989, pp 30–54

Post RM, Putnam F, Contel NR, et al: Electroconvulsive seizures inhibit amygdala kindling: implications for mechanisms of action in affective illness. Epilepsia 25:234–239, 1984

Post RM, Rubinow DR, Ballenger JC: Conditioning and sensitization in the longitudinal course of affective illness. Br J Psychiatry 149:191–201, 1986

Prien RF, Caffey EM Jr, Klett CJ: Prophylactic efficacy of lithium carbonate in manic depressive illness. Arch Gen Psychiatry 28:337–341, 1973

Prien RF, Caffey EM Jr, Klett CJ: Factors associated with treatment success in lithium carbonate prophylaxis: report of the Veterans Administration and National Institute of Mental Health Collaborative Study Group. Arch Gen Psychiatry 31:189–192, 1974

Prien RF, Kupfer DJ, Mansky PA, et al: Drug therapy in the prevention of recurrences in unipolar and bipolar affective disorders: report of the NIMH Collaborative Study Group comparing lithium carbonate, imipramine, and a lithium carbonate-imipramine combination. Arch Gen Psychiatry 41:1096–1104, 1984

Roy-Byrne P, Post RM, Uhde TW, et al: The longitudinal course of recurrent affective illness: life chart data from research patients at the NIMH. Acta Psychiatr Scand 71 (suppl 317):1–34, 1985

Small JG, Kellams JJ, Milstein V, et al: Complications with electroconvulsive treatment combined with lithium. Biol Psychiatry 15:103–112, 1980

Stallone F, Shelley E, Mendlewicz J, et al: The use of lithium in affective disorders, III: a double blind study of prophylaxis in bipolar illness. Am J Psychiatry 130:1006–1010, 1973

Stancer H, Persad E: Treatment of intractable rapid-cycling manic-depressive disorder with levothyroxine: clinical observations. Arch Gen Psychiatry 39:311–312, 1982

Stancer HC, Furlong FW, Godse DD: A longitudinal investigation of lithium as a prophylactic agent for recurrent depression. Can Psychiatric Assoc J 15:29–40, 1970

Swann AC: Mixed or dysphoric manic states: psychopathology and treatment. J Clin Psychiatry 56 (suppl):6–10, 1995

Wehr TA, Goodwin FK: Rapid cycling in manic depressives induced by tricyclic antidepressants. Arch Gen Psychiatry 36:555–559, 1979

Wehr TA, Wirz-Justice A: Circadian rhythm mechanism in affective illness and in antidepressant drug action. Psychopsychiatry 15:31–39, 1982

Wehr TA, Goodwin FK, Wirz-Justice A, et al: 48 hour sleep-wake cycles in manic depressive illness: naturalistic observation and sleep-deprivation experiments. Arch Gen Psychiatry 39:559–565, 1982

Wehr TA, Sack DA, Duncan WC, et al: Sleep and circadian rhythms in affective patients isolated from external time cues. Psychiatry Res 15:327–339, 1985

Wehr TA, Sack DA, Rosenthal NE, et al: Rapid cycling affective disorder: contributing factors and treatment responses in 51 patients. Am J Psychiatry 145:179–184, 1988

Winokur G, Clayton PJ, Reich J: Manic Depressive Illness. St. Louis, MO, Mosby, 1969

Wolpert EA, Goldberg JF, Harrow M: Rapid cycling in unipolar and bipolar affective disorders. Am J Psychiatry 147:725–728, 1990

World Health Organization: International Statistical Classification of Diseases and Related Health Problems, 10th Revision. Geneva, Switzerland, World Health Organization, 1992

Wu LH, Dunner DL: Suicide attempts in rapid cycling bipolar patients. J Affect Disord 29:57–61, 1993

Zisook S: Cyclic 48-hour unipolar depression. J Nerv Mental Dis 176:53–56, 1988

Bipolar II Disorder: The Importance of Hypomania

William Coryell, M.D.

Researchers and clinicians have long been aware that manic symptoms appear at many levels of severity. Kraepelin (1921/1976, p. 61) provided separate descriptions of mania and hypomania but asserted, "From the slighter forms of mania here described, imperceptible transitions gradually lead to the morbid state of actual acute mania." A diagnostic distinction based on the severity of manic symptoms is a recent development, however, and essentially all of the underlying evidence has appeared in the past 20 years. Since then, data have accumulated in clear support of a separation between bipolar I and bipolar II disorders, and the distinction now has both theoretical and practical importance.

Diagnosis

The earliest proposals to subcategorize bipolar illness on the basis of symptom severity grew from efforts by Dunner and colleagues to classify subjects in biological studies (Dunner 1993). They limited their proposed distinctions to patients with primary affective disorders according to the criteria of Feighner et al. (1972) and assigned a label of bipolar I to individuals who had been hospitalized for mania. Those who had had maniclike symptoms, but who had been hospitalized only for depression, were designated as bipolar II, whereas those who had received outpatient treatment only were grouped as "bipolar other" (Dunner et al. 1976; Fieve et al. 1984).

Angst (1978) used a similar definition but did not explicitly limit its application to patients with primary affective disorder. The Research Diagnostic Criteria (RDC; Spitzer et al. 1978) likewise did not limit the separation of bipolar I and bipolar II disorders to patients with primary affective disorder. These criteria also extended the definition of mania to include those who had experienced "serious impairment," even if hospitalization had not occurred (Table 12–1). Neither DSM-III nor DSM-III-R (American Psychiatric Association 1980, 1987) provided operational criteria for bipolar II disorder. DSM-IV (American Psychiatric Association 1994) provided such criteria, but they appeared only relatively recently. Therefore, essentially all of the published studies have used the RDC or the definitions of Dunner et al. (1976) or Angst (1978). The differences in these definitions undoubtedly account for some of the inconsistencies in research findings.

The diagnosis of hypomania poses special difficulties. Episodes

---

Table 12–1.   Definitions for bipolar II disorder

Dunner et al. (1976): bipolar II
   Primary affective disorder (Feighner et al. 1972)
   Hospitalization for depression but never for manic symptoms
   Minimum of 2 days' duration for hypomanic symptoms
Angst (1978): Dm
   Hospitalization for depression (D) but never for manic symptoms (m)
Research Diagnostic Criteria (Spitzer et al. 1978): bipolar II
   Elevated, expansive, or irritable mood
   At least two additional manic symptoms
   Minimum of 1 week's duration (2 days for "probable")
   Does not meet criteria for mania (symptoms did not result in
      hospitalization or serious impairment, nor did they make
      meaningful conversation impossible)
DSM-IV (American Psychiatric Press 1994): bipolar II
   Elevated, expansive, or irritable mood
   At least three (four, if only irritable) additional manic symptoms
   Minimum of 4 days' duration
   Change is observable by others
   No "marked" impairment, hospitalization, or psychotic features

are often brief and, by definition, do not cause serious impairment. Hypomanic symptoms per se rarely lead to treatment, and clinicians rarely witness hypomanic syndromes directly. Clinicians must instead rely on the recollections of patients and informants.

Not surprisingly, the few reliability studies that have considered the bipolar II category yielded mixed results. Andreason et al. (1981) conducted a test-retest study of relatives and derived a kappa value of 0.67, indicating fair agreement between two independent raters. When Keller et al. (1981) applied the same design to actively ill patients, the lifetime diagnosis of hypomania was the least reliable of diagnoses, with a kappa value of 0.26. These studies were limited by low base rates for hypomania; three and four patients, respectively, were given a consensus diagnosis of bipolar II disorder. Rice et al. (1986) took a more rigorous approach and compared results of diagnostic interviews conducted 6 years apart. Both interviews took a lifetime perspective at the time of the first assessment. Only one of seven patients with a diagnosis of bipolar II disorder at the first interview was given that diagnosis at the second. Another three were first given the diagnosis at the second interview only. Notably, a positive diagnosis on either interview was associated with a family history of bipolarity. This finding indicated that the RDC, as applied with the Schedule for Affective Disorders and Schizophrenia—Lifetime Version (Endicott and Spitzer 1978), had high specificity but low sensitivity to bipolar II disorder.

Dunner and Tay (1993) described a reliability study specifically focused on polarity distinctions. Their study yielded a kappa value of 0.67 for agreement between an expert clinician who used a semistructured interview and a nonphysician interviewer who used the Structured Clinical Interview for DSM-III-R (Spitzer and Williams 1985). The expert assigned a bipolar II diagnosis substantially more often than did the less experienced interviewer. The authors concluded that interviewers may be insensitive to histories of hypomania if they limit probing or if they fail to direct questioning about hypomania to periods immediately before or after depressive episodes. Clinicians should routinely question their depressed patients about "high" periods that may have preceded or followed earlier depressive episodes.

Although a diagnosis of hypomania can be missed easily, it can also be misapplied in many circumstances. Chronic instability of mood is a cardinal feature of borderline personality disorder, and many patients with somatization disorder are highly suggestible. Either circumstance can result in false-positive assessments of hypomanic symptoms. Whenever a diagnosis of bipolar II disorder is being considered, and particularly when signs and symptoms of other nonaffective disorders are present, the interviewer should determine whether individuals other than the patient regularly notice the symptoms comprising suspected hypomanic periods. For example, do spouses or friends observe pressured speech, hyperactivity, or euphoria? DSM-IV specifies that hypomanic symptoms be observable by others, but earlier definitions did not include this provision.

Family History

Family studies constitute a powerful and often-used approach to diagnostic validity (Feighner et al. 1972). Illnesses among relatives can be ascertained either indirectly, through the interview of a proband (*family history method*), or directly, through the interview of relatives themselves (*family study method*). The latter method is necessary to test the separation of bipolar I and bipolar II disorders because hypomanic episodes are often too ephemeral to be assessed meaningfully with the family history method.

Table 12–2 summarizes results from the five family studies that separated bipolar I and bipolar II disorders in both probands and relatives. Several highly regular patterns are apparent:

- In all five studies, bipolar II disorder is most prevalent in the relatives of bipolar II probands.
- In all five studies, bipolar I disorder is less prevalent in the relatives of bipolar II probands than in the relatives of bipolar I probands.
- In the four studies that included nonbipolar major depressive disorder probands, rates of bipolar I illness were higher among the relatives of bipolar II probands than among the relatives of nonbipolar major depressive disorder probands.
- In all five studies, rates of major affective disorder (bipolar I

Table 12–2. Family studies of bipolar II disorder

Proband diagnosis	Fieve et al. (1984)	Gershon et al. (1982)	Coryell et al. (1984)	Heun & Maier (1993b)	Simpson et al. (1993)
Morbid risks for bipolar I disorder					
Bipolar I	3.6	4.5	2.9	3.6	15.5
Bipolar II	0.7	2.6	0.9	3.5	2.1
Nonbipolar	0.4	1.5	0.2	1.0	NA
Morbid risks for bipolar II disorder					
Bipolar I	1.4	4.1	2.5	1.8	22.4
Bipolar II	4.2	4.5	9.8	6.1	40.4
Nonbipolar	1.1	1.5	2.6	0.3	NA
Morbid risks for nonbipolar major depressive disorder					
Bipolar I	7.4	14.0	22.7	16.3	15.5
Bipolar II	11.1	17.3	21.4	18.3	19.1
Nonbipolar	8.7	16.6	29.4	19.0	NA
Morbid risks for bipolar I, bipolar II, and nonbipolar major depressive disorders					
Bipolar I	14.9	22.6	28.1	21.7	37.9
Bipolar II	18.5	24.2	32.1	27.9	42.5
Nonbipolar	10.2	19.6	32.2	20.3	NA

Note.   NA = This study did not include nonbipolar probands.

disorder plus bipolar II disorder plus nonbipolar major depressive disorder) are higher among the relatives of bipolar II probands than among the relatives of bipolar I probands.

Several conclusions follow from these patterns. One is that the spectrum view of bipolar I, bipolar II, and nonbipolar illnesses is untenable. This would predict a stepwise increase in familial loading for affective disorder with the highest rates of major affective disorder among the relatives of bipolar I probands. None of the studies showed this relationship.

Another conclusion is that bipolar II merits a degree of diagnostic autonomy in that it appears to "breed true" (i.e., it is found chiefly among the relatives of bipolar II probands). This conclusion is further supported by descriptions of several large pedigrees highly loaded for bipolar II illness. One pedigree included 11 individuals with definite affective disorder, and of these patients, 10 had bipolar II disorder (DePaulo et al. 1990). In the other pedigree, all 6 ill family members had bipolar II disorder (Heun and Maier 1993a).

Although family studies have revealed clear differences between bipolar I and bipolar II disorders, they have also indicated some similarities. In particular, the association between bipolar illness in probands and high levels of achievement and creativity in relatives (Andreason 1987; Richards et al. 1988; Woodruff et al. 1971) also extends to bipolar II illness (Coryell et al. 1989a; Verdoux and Bourgeois 1995).

Demographics and Phenomenology

Comparisons have regularly revealed that bipolar II disorder has, on average, an earlier age at onset than does nonbipolar disorder (Akiskal et al. 1995; Angst 1986; Cassano et al. 1992; Coryell et al. 1985, 1995; McMahon et al. 1994). Some studies found a significantly higher proportion of males among patients with bipolar II illness than among those with nonbipolar major depression (Cassano et al. 1992; Fieve et al. 1984), but many studies found no clear differences in sex ratios between these two groups.

By definition, symptoms of hypomania differ quantitatively from those of mania. No clear qualitative differences appear to exist between manic and hypomanic syndromes, but this possibility has not been explored fully.

In two studies, bipolar II patients were more likely than nonbipolar major depressive disorder patients to have a history of suicide attempts (Endicott et al. 1985; Kupfer et al. 1988a). Stallone et al. (1980) are often cited as showing a higher suicide attempt rate among bipolar II patients, but in their study, an increased risk for suicide attempts was confined to "bipolar other" patients, those who had not been hospitalized. When "bipolar other" patients are combined with those designated as bipolar II, the resulting group has a suicide attempt rate identical to that for nonbipolar major depression patients. Moreover, large-scale prospective studies have not reported increased risks for either attempted or completed suicide among bipolar II patients (Angst 1978; Coryell et al. 1989b; Wicki and Angst 1991).

Few other depressive symptoms have consistently distinguished bipolar II patients from either bipolar I or nonbipolar patients. According to two studies, bipolar II depression is more likely than nonbipolar depression to feature psychomotor retardation (Andreason et al. 1988; Dunner 1983), and according to two other studies, bipolar II patients are more likely to exhibit schizotypal features (Coryell et al. 1985; Endicott et al. 1985).

Other demographic and phenomenological differences between bipolar II and nonbipolar groups have been reported but generally only by single studies. Differences between bipolar I and bipolar II groups in depressive symptoms have been reported only sporadically.

Natural History

Many studies have observed that bipolar I patients have higher recurrence rates during follow-up than do nonbipolar major depression patients (reviewed in Coryell and Winokur 1992). Bipolar I and bipolar II disorders resemble each other in this respect. Individuals with bipolar II disorder also recall more depressive episodes in retrospective assessments than do individuals with nonbipolar depression (Angst 1978; Coryell et al. 1985, 1989b; Giles et al. 1986). In a large, prospective follow-up study, bipolar II patients had a significantly shorter time to relapse than did nonbipolar patients (Coryell et al. 1989b). Bipolar I, bipolar II, and nonbipolar patients experience, on average, 2.4, 2.4, and 1.5 new major depressive episodes, respectively, over a 5-year period ($F = 14.2$, df $= 2.556$, $P = .0001$). Multiple relapses occurred in 29 of 64 (45.3%) of the bipolar II patients, in 21 of 53 (39.6%) of the bipolar I patients, and in 127 of 442 (28.7%) of the nonbipolar patients ($\chi^2 = 10.2$, df $= 4$, $P < .01$). Despite their greater proclivity to relapse, bipolar II patients were not more likely than nonbipolar major depression patients to be hospitalized multiple times, nor did they make more suicide attempts, serious or otherwise. Bipolar II patients were significantly more likely to experience work impairment after 5 years than were nonbipolar patients, but the two groups did not differ on a number of other psychosocial outcome variables.

Not surprisingly, bipolar I patients were more likely to be rehospitalized than were bipolar II patients; 27 (50.9%) of the bipolar I patients and 20 (31.3%) of the bipolar II patients were hospitalized multiple times in the 5-year follow-up period. Nevertheless, none of the psychosocial measures indicated more impairment in the bipolar I group.

Bipolar I and bipolar II patients also share a liability to rapid cycling. Such a course, often defined as four or more episodes or *switches* in 1 year, is very rare in nonbipolar major depression but relatively common in both bipolar I and bipolar II conditions. In the three largest series of rapid-cycling patients described so far, 24.4% (Coryell et al. 1992), 47.1% (Wehr et al. 1988), and 40.5% (Maj et al. 1994) had received a bipolar II diagnosis. These observations are consistent with the overall higher rates of recurrence by which bipolar I and bipolar II disorders resemble each other and differ from nonbipolar major depression (see also Dunner, Chapter 11, in this volume).

The designations of bipolar I, bipolar II, and nonbipolar disorders have prognostic significance that is fundamental to diagnostic validity. Of those patients who completed 10 years of follow-up, only 5% of those who began as nonbipolar developed one or more hypomanias, and only 5% developed mania (Coryell et al. 1995). The features that predicted a switch from nonbipolar to bipolar II disorder did not overlap with the predictors of a switch to bipolar I disorder. The former switch was associated with younger age and chronicity, whereas those who would manifest bipolar I disorder were more likely to have been psychotic and to have a family history of mania.

The likelihood that patients who began the study with a bipolar II diagnosis would develop mania in the next decade also was low. Of the 67 who were followed up for 10 years, only 5 (7.5%) developed mania. However, a survival analysis, which included those who failed to complete follow-up, indicated that as many as 15% of patients with a bipolar II diagnosis may eventually develop mania. This estimate is consistent with the family study data mentioned earlier in this chapter in suggesting that a small subset of bipolar II probands may, in fact, have bipolar I illness.

Finally, those patients who had received a bipolar I diagnosis when follow-up began rarely exhibited a course suggestive of bipolar II disorder. Only 11 of 152 patients had hypomanic episodes without additional periods of mania. Thus, close surveillance over a 10-year period revealed that the distinction between bipolar II disorder and both nonbipolar and bipolar I groups is a stable one. This observation complements the patterns seen in family studies.

A large lithium discontinuation study provided further evidence for the diagnostic stability of bipolar I and bipolar II disorders (Faedda et al. 1993). Fifteen of 26 bipolar II patients (57.7%) developed recurrences after lithium discontinuation, but none developed manic episodes. In contrast, 20 of 38 bipolar I patients (52.6%) developed mania as their first recurrence after lithium discontinuation. The difference in risk for mania after lithium discontinuation was highly significant ($\chi^2 = 19.9$, df $= 1$, $P < .001$).

Treatment

As shown earlier in this chapter, family study data distinguish bipolar II disorder from both nonbipolar and bipolar I disorders, and patients with bipolar II disorder are likely to retain this diagnosis over time. Nevertheless, important similarities between bipolar I and bipolar II groups include an increased likelihood of recurrence and of a rapid-cycling course. Together, these findings leave open the question of whether bipolar I and bipolar II disorders will show equivalent responses to treatment, either acute or prophylactic.

The acute treatment of hypomania is rarely a clinical problem because patients so infrequently seek treatment while hypomanic. The acute treatment of depression in patients with a history of hypomania is a much more common, and frequently difficult, problem.

The balance of relevant studies indicate that lithium has better antidepressant efficacy in bipolar depression than in unipolar depression (Baron et al. 1975; Goodwin et al. 1972; Kupfer and Spiker 1981; Noyes et al. 1974). Unfortunately, although several of these studies explicitly included patients with bipolar II disorder, none isolated this group in the results. Presumably, a difference in response rates between bipolar I and bipolar II patients would have been noted, had it existed. Tondo et al. (1998) recently made such a comparison with a cohort of 188 bipolar I and 129 bipolar II patients. In this retrospective study, lithium's effects on manic and hypomanic recurrences appeared larger in the bipolar II group, although the two groups experienced similar reductions in depressive episodes.

At least some evidence indicates that tricyclic antidepressants (TCAs) are less effective in the treatment of bipolar I depression than nonbipolar depression (Kupfer and Spiker 1981), although other studies have failed to associate bipolarity with a poor TCA response (Katz et al. 1987). Notably, Kupfer and Spiker (1981) found that TCA response was particularly unlikely among bipolar II patients. Moreover, Himmelhoch et al. (1991) randomly assigned 56 bipolar patients to tranylcypromine or imipramine and found clearly better outcomes with the former medication. The advantage of monoamine oxidase inhibitors (MAOIs) over TCAs was as large for bipolar II patients as for bipolar I patients. The use of MAOIs for depression in bipolar I and bipolar II patients is discussed further in this volume by Himmelhoch, Chapter 13, and Goldberg and Keck, Chapter 15.

How efficacious are the selective serotonin reuptake inhibitors (SSRIs) in the treatment of bipolar depression? Data pertaining to this question are also surprisingly scarce. Cohn et al. (1989) randomly assigned 89 patients with DSM-III bipolar depression to fluoxetine, imipramine, or placebo. Those who took fluoxetine had significantly better outcomes than did those who took either imipramine or placebo. Notably, the differential between fluoxetine and placebo was larger than that seen in most studies of unipolar depression; 18 of 21 patients (85.7%) who took fluoxetine for at least 3 weeks were considered responders, compared with 5 of 13 patients (38.5%) who took placebo ($\chi^2 = 8.2$, df = 1, $P = .004$). Unfortunately, the sample did not specifically include patients with bipolar II disorder. To this study, though, can be added an open trial of fluoxetine in bipolar II patients (Simpson and DePaulo 1991). Despite preexisting chronicity (mean episode duration of 5.3 years), all but 1 of the 16 patients had fair to very good outcomes. In summary, even though the relevant studies are few, they feature consistencies indicating that a history of mania or hypomania portends a relatively poor response to TCAs and a better response to SSRIs and MAOIs.

There appear to be only two placebo-controlled trials of lithium prophylaxis in bipolar II illness (Dunner et al. 1982; Kane et al. 1982). In both studies, lithium treatment was associated with a significantly better outcome, although in both studies, significance levels were only modest, in part because of small sample sizes. Notably, Dunner et al. (1982) found that significant differences did not emerge until 33 months had passed. The authors concluded that the benefit of maintenance therapy may require several years to manifest itself fully.

Lithium discontinuation offers another way to assess prophylactic efficacy. One study of lithium discontinuation compared bipolar I and bipolar II groups (Faedda et al. 1993) and found that relapses into depression after lithium discontinuation were more common among bipolar II patients at a trend level of significance. Given that risks for depression are similar for bipolar I and bipolar II patients in long-term, naturalistic studies (Coryell et al. 1989b), this finding indicates that lithium exerts at least as much protection for bipolar II patients as for bipolar I patients.

It is now widely assumed that essentially any of the established antidepressants can induce mania, particularly in patients with known bipolar disorder (see Goldberg and Kocsis, Chapter 7, in this volume). This assumption is puzzling given that no comparison between any antidepressant and placebo (Prien et al. 1973) or between lithium with an antidepressant and lithium without an antidepressant (Prien et al. 1984; Quitkin et al. 1981) has shown a significant difference in the risk for new manic episodes. Nor did Peet's (1994) meta-analysis find significantly higher rates of manic recurrences in bipolar patients given TCAs than in those given placebo, though a trend existed in that direction. In that same analysis, though, mania was less likely after SSRI therapy than after TCA therapy: 9 of 242 patients (3.7%) taking SSRIs developed mania, compared with 14 of 125 patients (11.2%) taking TCAs ($\chi^2 = 7.9$, df = 1, $P < .005$). Whether SSRI treatment offers the same advantage over TCA treatment for bipolar II depression is unknown, although several open studies suggest that SSRIs can be used safely in these patients. Kupfer et al. (1988b) described a continuation phase in which 24 patients with bipolar II illness received a combination of imipramine and interpersonal psychotherapy. One patient developed hypomania, but none developed mania. Likewise, in Simpson and DePaulo's study (1991), none of the 16 bipolar II patients taking fluoxetine developed mania, even though the mean treatment duration was 13.6 months.

Haykal and Akiskal (1990) used bupropion to treat rapid-cycling bipolar II disorder in six patients and described encouraging results with no switches into mania. Sachs et al. (1994) randomly assigned bipolar patients to bupropion or desipramine and reported a higher switch rate with the latter medication. Half the patients (5 of 10) developed mania or hypomania during an acute 8-week phase or during a crossover phase; in contrast, only 1 of 9 patients taking bupropion developed mania or hypomania (Fisher's exact test, $P = .08$).

Antidepressants are widely suspected to provoke rapid cycling (Altshuler et al. 1995; Kukopulos et al. 1980, 1983; Wehr and Goodwin 1979, 1987; Wehr et al. 1988). This perception arose from naturalistic studies in which rapid cycling appeared to develop with the use of antidepressants and to resolve when their use ceased. However, analyses from the Collaborative Depression Study (Coryell 1993; Coryell et al. 1992) showed that both depression and antidepressant treatment tend to precede periods of rapid cycling and that, in regression analyses, the existence of depression rather than the use of antidepressants is significantly related to subsequent rapid cycling. Thus, the often ignored fact that depression leads to antidepressant treatment promotes a *post hoc, ergo propter hoc* conclusion that antidepressant treatment causes rapid cycling.

A study with vigor sufficient to settle this question is unlikely because it would require that treatment, other than ongoing thymoleptic medication, be withheld for an extended period. Uncertainty will persist, and, in that context, a trial with thymoleptics alone would be a reasonable option for bipolar patients who persist in a rapid-cycling course while taking antidepressants. Optimization of the thymoleptic regimen would include careful attention to lithium levels and the use of combinations, in particular, lithium with either of the widely used anticonvulsants, carbamazepine or valproate.

Among nonpharmacological options for the treatment of depression, phototherapy may have particular relevance for bipolar II disorder. This disorder appears to be overrepresented in samples of patients with seasonal affective disorder (SAD), the pattern for which light therapy is customarily recommended (Rosenthal et al. 1984; Thompson and Isaacs 1988; Wirz-Justice et al. 1986). Although the bulk of research on phototherapy has focused on SAD, evidence indicates that it is effective also in nonseasonal depression (Lam et al. 1989). The question of whether a history of hypomania may itself predict response to light therapy has not been explored. In any event, a history of hypomania should at least alert clinicians to the possibility of a seasonal pattern, as this possibility may broaden the array of effective treatment options.

Summary

Although the distinction between bipolar I and bipolar II disorders is a recent one, interest in this area has grown rapidly and a substantial literature has developed. In comparison to nonbipolar disorder, both bipolar I and bipolar II disorders feature an earlier age at onset, a higher likelihood of psychomotor retardation, higher recurrence rates, and an increased risk for rapid cycling. In these respects, bipolar I and bipolar II disorders resemble each other. In other respects, the disorders are distinct. Family studies show that morbid risks for bipolar II disorder are highest for the relatives of bipolar II probands; follow-up studies show that bipolar II patients rarely develop manic episodes. Apparently, bipolar I and bipolar II disorders share a relatively poor response to TCAs and better responses to MAOIs and SSRIs. The scant evidence available suggests that lithium has prophylactic effects for bipolar II depression.

References

Akiskal HS, Maser JD, Zeller PF, et al: Switching from "unipolar" to bipolar II: an 11-year prospective study of clinical and temperamental predictors in 559 patients. Arch Gen Psychiatry 52:114–123, 1995

Altshuler LL, Post RM, Leverich GS, et al: Antidepressant-induced mania and cycle acceleration: a controversy revisited. Am J Psychiatry 152: 1130–1138, 1995

American Psychiatric Association: Diagnostic and Statistical Manual of Mental Disorders, 3rd Edition. Washington, DC, American Psychiatric Association, 1980

American Psychiatric Association: Diagnostic and Statistical Manual of Mental Disorders, 3rd Edition, Revised. Washington, DC, American Psychiatric Association, 1987

American Psychiatric Association: Diagnostic and Statistical Manual of Mental Disorders, 4th Edition. Washington, DC, American Psychiatric Association, 1994

Andreason NC: Creativity and mental illness: prevalence rates in writers and their first-degree relatives. Am J Psychiatry 144:1288–1292, 1987

Andreason NC, Grove WM, Shapiro RW, et al: Reliability of lifetime diagnoses: a multicenter collaborative perspective. Arch Gen Psychiatry 38:400–405, 1981

Andreason NC, Grove WM, Endicott J, et al: The phenomenology of depression. Psychiatry and Psychobiology 3:1–10, 1988

Angst J: The course of affective disorders, II: typology of bipolar manic-depressive illness. Archives of Psychiatry and Neurological Sciences 226:65–73, 1978

Angst J: The course of major depression, atypical bipolar disorder, and bipolar disorder, in New Results in Depression Research. Edited by Hippius H, Klerman GL, Matussek N. Berlin/Heidelberg, Springer-Verlag, 1986, pp 26–35

Baron M, Gershon ES, Rudy V, et al: Lithium carbonate response in depression. Arch Gen Psychiatry 32:1107–1111, 1975

Cassano GB, Akiskal HS, Savino M, et al: Proposed subtypes of bipolar II and related disorders: with hypomanic episodes (or cyclothymia) and with hyperthymic temperament. J Affect Disord 26:127–140, 1992

Cohn JB, Collins G, Ashbrook E, et al: A comparison of fluoxetine, imipramine and placebo in patients with bipolar depressive disorder. Int Clin Psychopharmacol 4:313–322, 1989

Coryell W: Can antidepressants induce rapid cycling? (letter) Arch Gen Psychiatry 50:497–498, 1993

Coryell W, Winokur G: Course and outcome, in Handbook of Affective Disorders, 2nd Edition. Edited by Paykel E. London, Churchill Livingstone, 1992, pp 89–108

Coryell W, Endicott J, Reich T, et al: A family study of bipolar II disorder. Br J Psychiatry 145:49–54, 1984

Coryell W, Endicott J, Andreason N, et al: A comparison of bipolar I, bipolar II and nonbipolar major depression among the relatives of affectively ill probands. Am J Psychiatry 142:817–821, 1985

Coryell W, Endicott J, Keller M, et al: Bipolar affective disorder and high achievement: a familial association. Am J Psychiatry 146:983–988, 1989a

Coryell W, Keller M, Endicott J, et al: Bipolar II illness: course and outcome over a five-year period. Psychol Med 19:129–141, 1989b

Coryell W, Endicott J, Keller M: Rapid cycling affective disorder: demographics, diagnosis, family history and course. Arch Gen Psychiatry 49:126–131, 1992

Coryell W, Endicott J, Maser J, et al: Long-term stability of polarity distinctions in the affective disorders. Am J Psychiatry 152:385–390, 1995

DePaulo DR, Simpson SG, Gayle JO, et al: Bipolar II disorder in six sisters. J Affect Disord 19:259–264, 1990

Dunner DL: Subtypes of bipolar affective disorder with particular regard to bipolar II. Psychiatric Developments 1:75–86, 1983

Dunner DL: A review of the diagnostic status of "bipolar II" for the DSM-IV Work Group on Mood Disorders. Depression 1:2–10, 1993

Dunner DL, Tay LK: Diagnostic reliability of the history of hypomania in bipolar II patients and patients with major depression. Compr Psychiatry 34:303–307, 1993

Dunner DL, Dwyer T, Fieve RR: Depressive symptoms in patients with unipolar and bipolar affective disorder. Compr Psychiatry 27:447–451, 1976

Dunner DL, Stallone F, Fieve RR: Prophylaxis with lithium carbonate: an update. Arch Gen Psychiatry 39:1344–1345, 1982

Endicott J, Spitzer RL: A diagnostic interview: the Schedule for Affective Disorders and Schizophrenia. Arch Gen Psychiatry 35:837–844, 1978

Endicott J, Nee J, Andreason N, et al: Bipolar II: combine or keep separate? J Affect Disord 8:17–28, 1985

Faedda GL, Tondo L, Baldessarini RJ, et al: Outcome after rapid versus gradual discontinuation of lithium treatment in bipolar disorders. Arch Gen Psychiatry 50:448–455, 1993

Feighner J, Robins E, Guze S, et al: Diagnostic criteria for use in psychiatric research. Arch Gen Psychiatry 26:57–63, 1972

Fieve RR, Go R, Dunner DL, et al: Search for biological/genetic markers in a long-term epidemiological and morbid risk study of affective disorders. J Psychiatry Res 18:425–445, 1984

Gershon ES, Hamovit J, Guroff JJ, et al: A family study of schizoaffective, bipolar I, bipolar II, unipolar and normal control probands. Arch Gen Psychiatry 39:1157–1167, 1982

Giles DE, Rush AJ, Roffwarg HP: Sleep parameters in bipolar I, bipolar II and unipolar depression. Biol Psychiatry 21:1340–1343, 1986

Goodwin FK, Murphy DL, Dunner DL, et al: Lithium response in unipolar vs. bipolar depression. Am J Psychiatry 129:44–47, 1972

Haykal RF, Akiskal HS: Bupropion as a promising approach to rapid cycling bipolar II patients. J Clin Psychiatry 51:450–455, 1990

Heun R, Maier W: Bipolar II disorders in six first-degree relatives. Biol Psychiatry 34:274–276, 1993a

Heun R, Maier W: The distinction of bipolar II disorder from bipolar I disorder and recurrent unipolar depression: results of a controlled family study. Acta Psychiatr Scand 87:279–284, 1993b

Himmelhoch JM, Thase ME, Mallinger AG, et al: Tranylcypromine versus imipramine in anergic bipolar depression. Am J Psychiatry 148:910–916, 1991

Kane JM, Quitkin FM, Rifkin A, et al: Lithium carbonate and imipramine in the prophylaxis of unipolar and bipolar II illness: a prospective, placebo-controlled comparison. Arch Gen Psychiatry 39:1065–1069, 1982

Katz NM, Kosolow SH, Maas JW, et al: The timing, specificity and clinical prediction of tricyclic drug effects in depression. Psychol Med 17:297–309, 1987

Keller MB, Lavori P, McDonald-Scott P, et al: Reliability of lifetime diagnosis and symptoms in patients with a current psychiatric disorder. J Psychiatry Res 16:229–240, 1981

Kraepelin E: Manic-Depressive Insanity and Paranoia (1921). Translated by Barclay RM. Edited by Robertson GM. Edinburgh, Scotland, Livingstone. Reprint, New York, Arno Press, 1976

Kukopulos A, Reginaldi D, Laddomada P, et al: Course of the manic-depressive cycle and changes caused by treatment. Pharmakopsychiatrie Neuropsychopharmakologie 13:156–167, 1980

Kukopulos A, Caliari B, Tondo A, et al: Rapid cyclers, temperament and antidepressants. Compr Psychiatry 24:249–258, 1983

Kupfer DJ, Spiker DG: Refractory depression: prediction of nonresponse by clinical indicators. J Clin Psychiatry 42:307–311, 1981

Kupfer DJ, Carpenter LL, Frank E: Is bipolar II a unique disorder? Compr Psychiatry 29:228–236, 1988a

Kupfer DJ, Carpenter LL, Frank E: Possible role of antidepressants in precipitating mania and hypomania in recurrent depression. Am J Psychiatry 145:804–808, 1988b

Lam RW, Kripke DF, Gillin JC: Phototherapy for depressive disorders: a review. Can J Psychiatry 34:140–147, 1989

Maj M, Magliano L, Pirozzi R, et al: Validity of rapid cycling as a course specifier for bipolar disorder. Am J Psychiatry 151:1015–1029, 1994

McMahon FJ, Stine OC, Chase GA, et al: Influence of clinical subtype, sex and lineality on age at onset of major affective disorder in a family sample. Am J Psychiatry 151:210–215, 1994

Noyes R, Dempsey GM, Blum A, et al: Lithium treatment of depression. Compr Psychiatry 15:187–193, 1974

Peet M: Induction of mania with selective serotonin re-uptake inhibitors and tricyclic antidepressants. Br J Psychiatry 164:549–550, 1994

Prien RF, Klett CJ, Caffey EM: Lithium carbonate and imipramine in prevention of affective episodes. Arch Gen Psychiatry 29:420–425, 1973

Prien RF, Kupfer DJ, Mansky PA, et al: Drug therapy in the prevention of recurrences in unipolar and bipolar affective disorders. Arch Gen Psychiatry 41:1096–1104, 1984

Quitkin FM, Kane J, Rifkin A, et al: Prophylactic lithium carbonate with and without imipramine for bipolar I patients. Arch Gen Psychiatry 38:902–907, 1981

Rice J, McDonald-Smith P, Endicott J, et al: The stability of diagnosis with an application to bipolar II disorder. Psychiatry Res 19:285–296, 1986

Richards R, Kinney DK, Lunde I, et al: Creativity in manic-depressives, cyclothymes, their normal relatives and controlled subjects. J Abnorm Psychol 97:281–288, 1988

Rosenthal NE, Sack DA, Gillin JC, et al: Seasonal affective disorder. Arch Gen Psychiatry 41:72–80, 1984

Sachs GS, Lafer B, Stoll AL, et al: A double-blind trial of bupropion versus desipramine for bipolar depression. J Clin Psychiatry 55:391–393, 1994

Simpson SG, DePaulo JR: Fluoxetine treatment of bipolar II depression. J Clin Psychopharmacol 11:52–54, 1991

Simpson SG, Folstein SE, Meyers DA, et al: Bipolar II, the most common bipolar phenotype? Am J Psychiatry 150:901–903, 1993

Spitzer RL, Williams JBW: Structured Clinical Interview for DSM-III-R —Patient Version (SCID-P). New York, New York State Psychiatric Institute, Biometrics Research, 1985

Spitzer RL, Endicott J, Robins E: Research Diagnostic Criteria: rationale and reliability. Arch Gen Psychiatry 35:773–782, 1978

Stallone F, Dunner DL, Ahearn J, et al: Statistical predictions of suicide in depressives. Compr Psychiatry 21:381–387, 1980

Thompson C, Isaacs G: Seasonal affective disorder—a British sample. J Affect Disord 14:1–11, 1988

Tondo L, Baldessarini RJ, Hennen J, et al: Lithium maintenance treatment of depression and mania in bipolar I and bipolar II disorders. Am J Psychiatry 155:638–645, 1998

Verdoux H, Bourgeois M: Social class in unipolar and bipolar probands and relatives. J Affect Disord 33:181–187, 1995

Wehr TA, Goodwin FK: Rapid cycling in manic depressives induced by tricyclic antidepressants. Arch Gen Psychiatry 36:555–559, 1979

Wehr TA, Goodwin FK: Can antidepressants cause mania and worsen the course of affective illness? Am J Psychiatry 144:1403–1411, 1987

Wehr T, Sack D, Rosenthal N, et al: Rapid cycling affective disorder: contributing factors and treatment responses in fifty-one patients. Am J Psychiatry 145:179–184, 1988

Wicki W, Angst J: The Zurich Study X: hypomania in a 28–30 year old cohort. Eur Arch Psychiatry Clin Neurosci 240:339–348, 1991

Wirz-Justice A, Bucheli C, Graw P, et al: Light treatment of seasonal affective disorder in Switzerland. Acta Psychiatr Scand 74:193–204, 1986

Woodruff RA, Robins LN, Winokur G, et al: Manic depressive illness and social achievement. Acta Psychiatr Scand 47:237–249, 1971

CHAPTER 13

The Paradox of Anxiety Syndromes Comorbid With the Bipolar Illnesses

Jonathan M. Himmelhoch, M.D.

Comorbid psychopathology has been described in many of the preceding chapters as a major factor contributing to poor treatment outcome in bipolar disorder. Although substance abuse is a common source of comorbidity for many bipolar patients, other concurrent Axis I disorders frequently play a significant role in the treatment and management of bipolar disorder. In this chapter, I focus on anxiety disorders as complicating the course of bipolar illness. I address issues in this area from several perspectives, including theories about psychopathology, the phenomenology of comorbid anxiety and mania, and treatment implications based on empirical data from my research group at the University of Pittsburgh.

Introduction: The Paradox

Data from the National Institute of Mental Health (NIMH) Epidemiologic Catchment Area (ECA) survey have shown that anxiety disorders are the most frequent psychiatric syndromes to be comorbid with bipolar disorders (Chen and Dilsaver 1995). The comorbidity of panic disorder with bipolar disorder, for example, has a lifetime prevalence of 20.8% in bipolar patients, 26 times that found in comparison control subjects and, surprisingly, 2.1 times that found in patients with unipolar major depressive illness. Even obsessive-compulsive disorder (OCD), which seems by its very nature opposite to the manic phase of bipolar illness, occurs with some frequency in bipolar subjects. Compulsions can even occur as part of intensifying mania or hypomania. OCD, however, is more strongly comorbid with major depression than with bipolar disorders. Generalized anxiety disorder (GAD) has the weakest link to bipolar illness, showing much stronger comorbidity with unipolar illness.

Nevertheless, the powerful association of selected anxiety disorders with bipolar disorders is a paradox. Kraepelin (1904/1989) was the first to point out that anxiety and arousal are not typical of uncomplicated manic-depressive illness. Indeed, both bipolar depression and mania are often anxiety-free. Bipolar depressions are typically anergic and devoid of apprehension—the clinical feature Kraepelin used to differentiate bipolar depression from so-called *apprehensive depression* and/or *melancholia*. In fact, bipolar patients rarely perceive themselves as mentally ill (Himmelhoch and Mallinger 1987). During their depressions, they first and foremost worry about their lack of initiative, their fatigue, and their sluggishness. They only infrequently seek treatment from a psychiatrist, preferring instead to go to an internist or family practitioner because they think they are afflicted with hypothyroidism, mononucleosis, or, according to recent fashion, chronic fatigue syndrome. They particularly do not see themselves as depressed early in an episode, nor are they often suicidal, unless their anergia has dragged on. Late in a depressive episode, after months of inertia, they may finally characterize themselves as lazy, unambitious, incapable, and weak in character. At this point, they may consider suicide (Himmelhoch 1987).

In an epidemiological survey of 748 patients successively referred to the Research Affective Disorders Clinic at the University of Pittsburgh, we observed that when unipolar, apprehensive, or melancholic patients were suicidal, they became suicidal at any point in an episode, even at the beginning of an episode. Serious suicide attempts were equally likely early or late in a given episode and could occur in a first, fifth, or tenth episode. Bipolar patients, especially bipolar II patients, in contrast, usually made suicide attempts deep into an episode, most often during recurrences (see also Goldberg and Kocsis, Chapter 7, in this volume). The increased lethality of bipolar syndromes compared with major depression is derived from rapid cycling, frequent recurrences, and, as I discuss later in this chapter, factors that convert the essential anxiety-free nature of bipolar, anergic depression into syndromes with manifest comorbid anxiety disorders (Himmelhoch et al. 1976b).

In its undiluted form, bipolar depression is more closely related to the motor inhibition of Parkinson's disease than it is to the apprehension of neurotic depression and/or melancholia (Himmelhoch 1992b). Moreover, between episodes, many bipolar I and most bipolar II patients are functional, calm, and steady. The manic phase of bipolar disorder is more problematic, even though hypomania and mild to moderate mania can be among the most anxiety-free states experienced by any patient. Although for some bipolar patients, hypomania may be viewed in some ways as a desirable state, bipolar I disorder (defined by the presence of either psychotic mania or very severe and disabling hypomania) often generates its own anxiety.

Court (1968) and Bunney et al. (1972a, 1972b, 1972c) described the *continuum model of bipolar disorder*, which is now the most generally accepted theoretical model for bipolar I disorder. In this model, depression and mania are more closely related to each other than either state is to "normal." In addition, anergic depression represents mild illness, psychotic mania represents severe illness, and the switch state represents that point in increasing severity at which depression converts to mania. During the switch state, significant depression and significant mania are present simultaneously, a situation called *mixed mania* (Kraepelin 1899).

During mixed mania, anxiety syndromes are commonly present. Further increases in severity lead to profound sleep loss and to either type A paranoid delusions (fluctuating delusions from sensory filter overload) or more systematic type B delusions (fixed and detailed material, as occurs in classic paranoia) (Detre and Jarecki 1971). Profound anxiety is a sine qua non of increasingly severe bipolar I disorder. Himmelhoch (1986) described the ethological model for bipolar I as an organism's last gasp defense against chronic threats to its existence. For example, in *The Gulag Archipelago*, Solzhenitsyn described the following reaction of his group of seven Soviet officers on the eve of their being sent by Stalin to the gulag in Archangel—a gulag from which fewer than 50% of those exiled ever returned:

At the point we were ordered to pick up our things, lined up in pairs and were marched again through the same magical garden filled with summer. . . . Again to the baths! . . . We were overcome with laughter that had us rolling on the floor. . . . This cleansing, releasing laughter was I think, not sick but a viable defense and salvation of the organism. [Translated from Russian]

Still, in bipolar I disorder, usually neither mania nor depression are so mixed nor so severe as to generate such catastrophic denial and anxiety, which Goldstein (1971) has explained in the following way:

Whenever anxiety, as the mainspring of an organism, comes into the foreground, we find that something is awry in the nature of the organism. To put it conversely, an organism is normal and healthy when its tendency toward self-actualization issues from within, and when it overcomes the disturbance arising from its clash with the world, not by virtue of anxiety but through the joy of coming to terms with the world.

Bipolar I Disorder Versus Bipolar II Disorder

Data from the same 748 patients described earlier in this chapter suggest that significant clinical differences exist between bipolar I and bipolar II patients. Some of the literature contradicts this conclusion and has led to much of the family and genetic research in bipolar disorders in which these two subtypes are combined into a single group (Kupfer et al. 1988). Further discussion about distinguishing bipolar I from bipolar II disorder is presented by Coryell (Chapter 12, in this volume). Here I discuss aspects of hypomania as they pertain to a conceptual understanding of the development of comorbid anxiety states.

Bipolar II disorder (Dunner et al. 1982) is defined as a manic-depressive syndrome in which depression is the preponderating pathology. Bipolar II patients never become more than hypomanic, and approximately 50% of them are extremely productive during their mood elevations. Many clinicians refuse to identify productive hypomania as a disorder, and they forget that adaptive behavior patterns can still identify abnormal syndromes. The depressive phase of bipolar II illness is often chronic and prolonged and has re-peatedly reflected the highest suicide rate of any affective disorder (Dunner et al. 1982). Because of this lethality and because about 28%–33% of patients have a form of bipolar II disorder that is ex-tremely hard to treat, essential features of this syndrome have been overlooked—features that contribute to the conceptualization that bipolar II disorder genuinely is clinically, ethologically, and pharma-cologically different from bipolar I disorder (Himmelhoch 1986).

The signal feature is that *uncomplicated* bipolar II illness is very re-sponsive to low-dose, straightforward psychopharmacological in-tervention (Himmelhoch and Neil 1980a). Forty percent of patients with uncomplicated bipolar II disorder respond to low-dose lithium salts, producing low lithium levels, and without any adjunctive psychopharmacological treatment. The average lithium dose for these patients is 623.96 ± 72.34 mg/day of lithium, producing aver-age blood levels of 0.51 ± 0.19 mEq/L. The operating pharmacologi-cal principle for these patients is "nothing in excess." If patients with chronic anergic depression and productive hypomania uncompli-cated by other neuropsychological factors receive treatment during their depressive phase with so-called therapeutic doses of lithium salts (900–1,500 mg/day of lithium, with blood levels of 0.75–0.90 mEq/L), the antidepressant effects of lithium—so well demon-strated by Goodwin et al. (1969)—are seldom seen and do not show through a plethora of lithium side effects (Himmelhoch 1994; Himmelhoch and Neil 1980a).

Recent investigations of the inositol cycle of secondary-messenger systems embedded in the erythrocytic and neuronal membranes (Mallinger et al. 1990) suggest that this system becomes saturated, producing a pileup of lipid fragments, especially choline (Hanin et al. 1980), which leaves the patient overmedicated and complaining of depression and uncoordination (particularly difficulty walking down stairs); sluggishness; blocked creativity; sexual dysfunction; and excessive urination, fluid intake, and thirst (Forrest et al. 1974). The fundamental treatment principle for patients with these symp-toms involves more than just using low lithium regimens; it also in-volves the following specific goal: in uncomplicated bipolar II disorder, the proper treatment goal is low-grade hypomania—so that if low lithium is insufficient to achieve this goal, an arousing antidepressant adjunct—tranylcypromine is by far the superior agent, but selective serotonin reuptake inhibitors (SSRIs) and bupropion are also useful—will produce this response in about 80% of patients without untoward sequelae (Himmelhoch 1994).

However, bipolar II disorder has a bad reputation derived from the difficulty associated with management of *complicated* cases of the disorder, in which anxiety inevitably occurs, most often in the form of panic but surprisingly frequently as social anxiety. Less frequent are obsessive-compulsive variations, along with what Akiskal (1994a, 1994b) has brilliantly shown to be temperamental variants, which together often look like Cluster B personality disorders (antisocial, borderline, histrionic, and narcissistic), where mood changes are suffused with anxiety, impulsivity, irritability, and self-abuse. We have already contended that bipolar II disorder is clinically, ethologically, and pharmacologically different from bipolar I disorder. A further observation is that bipolar II disorder is a genetically different disorder from bipolar I disorder, which if true, undermines any genetic-epidemiological research that combines bipolar I with bipolar II cohorts. We have deduced, based on observations of 5,500 bipolar patients since 1968, that bipolar II patients fit better the old-fashioned, somewhat discredited model of manic-depression— the sinusoidal or true bipolar model (Himmelhoch 1986).

In patients with uncomplicated bipolar II disorder, high is high, low is low, and intervals often exist between mood episodes, each type of which can occur alternately, in succession or in the form of pure anergic depressions that punctuate a hypomanic episode or merely a hyperproductive baseline. In this model, of course, mixed states, with their anxious manifestations, are not part of the natural course of illness. However, 31% of bipolar II patients have mixed states (Himmelhoch 1992a). Significant numbers of patients experience rapid cycling and anxiety syndromes, bringing with them a considerably poorer prognosis. Grunhaus (1988) noted the lesser prognosis, greater severity, and increased resistance associated with affective illness comorbid with panic disorder; Rudd et al. (1993) noted poor outcome and increased suicidality in the same patients; and Himmelhoch and Garfinkel (1987) demonstrated the poorer lithium response of each type of mixed state.

In bipolar I disorder, the usual source of mixed episodes (i.e., those contaminated by anxiety syndromes) is the switch phase, a natural outcome of increasing severity of a bipolar I episode as it progresses from anergic depression to melancholic, agitated depression to mania. This mechanism is not possible in bipolar II disorder if, as has been suggested, the sinusoidal, bipolar model of illness represents its evolutionary basis. Therefore, one must postulate that complicating, secondary neuropsychological factors account for the parallel frequency of mixed states, variation in anxiety syndromes, poorer outcome, and need for polypharmacological management in the 31% of bipolar II patients with mixed episodes (Himmelhoch et al. 1992a). Such factors would also 1 account for those subjects with complicated bipolar II disorder who have clinical similarities to patients with DSM-IV (American Psychiatric Association 1994) Cluster B personality disorders and with, in Akiskal's terms, temperaments noncontingent with their bipolar predispositions (Akiskal 1994b).

Both Akiskal and our group support this conclusion, post hoc from analysis of our follow-up studies on mixed states (Akiskal et al. 1995). More than 80% of mixed bipolar II patients in these studies experienced temperamental discrepancies and/or secondary factors —for example, addictions to drugs or alcohol; partial or grand mal epilepsy; paroxysmal focal or temporal electroencephalographs; classical migraine headaches; head injuries with greater than 15 minutes' loss of consciousness; febrile deliria with or without convulsions; hyperkinetic developmental disorders, some with and some without learning disabilities; or histories of frank, acute neurological illnesses, including Guillain-Barré syndrome, multiple sclerosis, phacomatoses, Meigs' syndrome, and Tourette's disorder. Patients with complicated bipolar I disorder also showed some of these secondary neuropsychological factors (about 38% of the mixed cases), although they usually exhibited mixed states and/or rapid cycling by the very nature of their illness.

True melancholia is a rare event in either bipolar I or bipolar II illness (Himmelhoch et al. 1976a). Analytical observers, including Abraham (1949), Freud (1915/1986), and Siggins (1966) mistakenly understood melancholia as the depressive phase of manic-depressive illness. But this form of depression occurs only rarely as the depressive phase of bipolar disease. In a study of more than 1,100 bipolar patients from our Affective Disorders Clinic at Yale Medical Center, we found 12 patients who had melancholia as their depressive phase. Kukopulos et al. (1980) wrote an incisive paper on *melancholia agitata* occurring as mixed mania in bipolar I disorder and in patients with the prognostically ominous sequence of depression-mania-depression (D-M-D). Melancholia is, of course, the most specifically anxious form of severe depression. Kukopulos noted that melancholia may be more common in patients prone to mixed states, but melancholia is rare among most bipolar patients. He also took the continuum hypothesis to its logical outcome, observing that mixed states are a clinical demonstration that mania and depression in bipolar I are extensions of the same aroused state but are attributed differently by each patient according to the patient's degree of arousal, level of discomfort, adaptive needs, and attributional habits.

From the preceding discussion it follows that although significant anxiety and specific anxiety disorders are the most common psychiatric states comorbid with the bipolar syndromes, and even though they are a natural part of the course of bipolar I illness, they always signify uncommon, prognostically difficult forms of bipolar disorder. The presence of either significant anxiety or a specific comorbid anxiety disorder almost always complicates treatment and necessitates polypharmaceutical intervention.

Social Anxiety and Bipolar II Disorder

The most paradoxical anxiety disorder to occur with bipolar disorder is social anxiety. It is difficult to see how two such opposing syndromes are in any way related. Patients with social phobia are always acutely aware of their social matrix. The course of their daily life is determined by the opinion of others and by their hair-trigger propensity to become humiliated. In contrast, bipolar patients either barge through their social matrix when mood is elevated or are listlessly unconcerned with it when mood is depressed. It is difficult at first glance to see how social phobia and bipolar disorder might be sufficiently related so that significant comorbidity could be generated by the nature of each disorder. Nevertheless, in two incidental studies from our clinic—one investigating treatment response to reversible monoamine oxidase inhibitors (RIMAs) in 30 patients with social phobia and the other investigating anxiolytic response to the antinauseant odansetron in 26 patients with GAD—we found marked differences between social phobia and GAD, and provocative data regarding the relationship of each anxiety disorder to bipolar I and, especially, bipolar II disorders. The most important finding came from the former study, in which 14 social phobia patients taking monoamine oxidase inhibitors (MAOIs) (either the irreversible MAOI phenelzine or the RIMA moclobemide) developed sustained, significant, and measurable hypomanic episodes. We also found a complicated matrix of unexpected observations about the nature of GAD, social phobia, and bipolar II disorder that I report later in this chapter.

Methods

We randomly selected 30 patients with a diagnosis of social phobia according to the Structured Clinical Interview for DSM-III-R (SCID; Spitzer et al. 1987). We randomly assigned patients to take either placebo or 75–900 mg/day of the RIMA moclobemide, the dose being determined by treatment response and/or tolerance to side effects. The GAD study was a similar double-blind comparison between odansetron and diazepam. We measured treatment response in the social phobia study with the Hamilton Anxiety Scale (HAM-A; Hamilton 1959) and the Clinical Global Impression Scale (CGI; Guy 1976). We also administered the Raskin Mania Scale (RMS; Raskin et al. 1969) to patients in both studies. In a 12-week open-label follow-up to the social phobia study, nonresponders from both groups (placebo or moclobemide) took 30–120 mg/day of phenelzine.

Whenever patients responded to treatment with greater than a rating of 5 on the RMS, or the study clinician noted hypomania, the principal investigator (J. M. Himmelhoch) conducted a separate interview, this time using Research Diagnostic Criteria (RDC; Spitzer et al. 1978), which are more sensitive to hypomania than is DSM-III-R (American Psychiatric Association 1987) when it is parsed by a SCID interview. If hypomania or mania were confirmed, the principal investigator added antimanic agents and/or mood stabilizers to ongoing RIMA or MAOI treatment. He also assessed any relationship between the onset of hypomania and a decrease in social phobia. We gave each patient verbal instructions regarding diet, drug interactions, and side effects, after which the patient received more detailed, written information about foods, interacting drugs, side effects, and proper treatment for food- or drug-induced hypertensive episodes. Several laboratory tests (biochemistry profile; complete blood count with differential, platelet, and reticulocyte count; triiodothyronine [T_3] by radioimmunoassay, thyroxine [T_4], and thyroid-stimulating hormone (TSH); urinalysis; chest X ray; and electrocardiogram) were conducted on each patient before initiating treatment, at 6 weeks, and at appropriate intervals thereafter. We used data from the GAD investigation for comparison of treatment outcome and clinical, family, developmental, and neurological histories.

Results

Of the 32 patients with social anxiety, 10 were male and 22 were female. Of the 26 patients with GAD, 14 were male, and 12 were female (no significant differences between groups). The average age of the socially anxious group was 32.59 ± 10.59 years, and the average age of the GAD group was 32.58 ± 12.08 years (no significant difference). Of the social phobia patients, 18 responded significantly (symptom decrease of greater than 50%) to RIMAs and MAOIs. No GAD patients responded to these drugs (Fisher's exact test, $P < .001$). Fourteen of the social phobia patients became clinically hypomanic, whereas none of the GAD patients did (Fisher's exact test, $P < .001$).

All 14 patients who became hypomanic manifested marked relief of their social phobia. The average RMS score for the hypomanic group was 6.34 ± 0.29. Of particular interest was the reaction of each socially anxious patient and of his or her social web to the onset of hypomania. Four of the patients became so alarmed with their open and assertive behavior that they had to be convinced to continue. All 4 entered remission of their hypomania and their social phobia when taking the combination of RIMAs or MAOIs and various subsequent mood stabilizers (lithium was prescribed for 8 patients, but divalproex sodium was needed in 2, divalproex sodium plus lithium in 1, and carbamazepine plus lithium in 3). In the 4 patients taking antikindling/lithium combinations, lithium served as an augmenting mood elevator, as any attempts to stop lithium in order to use anticonvulsants as monotherapy for hypomania resulted in the onset of measurable degrees of anergic depression.

Interestingly, few significant differences were observed when comparing the clinical, family, developmental, and neurological histories of the social anxiety patients with the GAD patients. Regarding family history, both groups manifested alcoholism as the most prevalent familial illness, followed by affective disorder. The major difference was that some of the families of patients with social phobia had explosive impulse disorders that were not easily diagnosable by family history. Some disorders may have been atypical bipolar disorders, some possibly epileptic, and some so-called *intermittent explosive personality disorder*. The impulsive family members (found in six of the families) were all relatives of patients with social phobia who showed hypomanic responses to treatment. No differences in family history reached statistical significance.

Clinical histories, particularly those related to character diagnoses (Axis II), were also similar in both the socially phobic and the GAD patients. Both anxiety syndromes showed those features defined by Kagan (1994) as *inhibited temperament,* but the patients with social phobia were unusual in this regard. Inhibited children (and adults) show marked arousal to mild psychological stress and autonomic instability and are at increased risk for anxiety disorders (especially panic disorder and agoraphobia) and/or alcohol abuse. Most patients in either group showed some signs of inhibited temperament. However, the social phobia patients, despite their social anxiety, for the most part displayed a paradoxically rich array of social skills—humor, warmth, and even extroversion and sexual competence breaking through their inhibited temperaments. They showed almost no propensity to somatize, whereas GAD patients were immersed in physical complaints. Twelve of the 14 social phobia patients who became hypomanic showed these paradoxical temperamental features, compared with 8 of the 18 not experiencing hypomania.

Major differences emerged in developmental and in neurological histories. Most important, social phobic patients grew up in severely dysfunctional families. Their development was riddled with abandonment and physical and/or sexual abuse. Eleven of the 14 patients who responded to RIMAs and MAOIs with sustained hypomania had histories of anaclisis or physical sexual abuse. Six of 11 had been put in orphanages, sent away from their nuclear birth families, or abandoned before age 8 years, either outright or by being sent to boarding schools. Eight of 11 had been either physically or sexually abused. Only 5 of 18 socially anxious patients who did not become hypomanic had similar anaclitic childhood histories (Fisher's exact test, $P < .001$).

In contrast to the anaclisis of the socially anxious patients was the high incidence in the longitudinal histories of GAD patients of "soft" and/or "hard" neurological abnormalities. Thirteen of 26 GAD patients had experienced neurological events: 4 had head injuries producing greater than 15 minutes' loss of consciousness; 6 experienced febrile convulsions and delirium between ages 11 months and 4 years; 3 had at one time or another been given a diagnosis of partial epilepsy; 9 manifested hyperkinesis; 4 had learning disabilities; and 5 had been given a firm diagnosis of neurological illness (3 had multiple sclerosis, 1 had Meigs' syndrome, and 1 had Guillain-Barré syndrome). Only 4 of 32 social phobic patients had similar neurological histories (Fisher's exact test, $P < .003$).

The peculiar evolution of inhibited temperament into normal social skills without somatization might be correlated with the equally unexpected incidence of anaclitic childhoods linked to MAOI-induced hypomania. Perhaps a fundamental predisposition to bipolar disorder was skewed from motor inhibition (anergia) to social inhibition by the socially inhibitory influences of anaclisis, abandonment, and abuse.

Discussion

My colleagues and I have examined two major subtypes of anxiety disorders—social phobia and GAD—that frequently complicate the course of bipolar illness.

Our simultaneous pharmacological investigations of social phobia and GAD led to the conclusion that the two diagnostic entities are completely different from each other, except for the coincidence that patients with either diagnosis experience, at one time or another in the course of their syndromes, the psychophysiological symptoms of anxiety. In fact, the differences extend far beyond the self-evident observation that patients with social phobias, on the one hand, delimit their anxiety to well-defined, temporally demarcated episodes enchained to specific social or public demands, whereas patients with GAD, in contrast, are continuously anxious or vulnerable to anxiety whatever their environmental situation, be it stressful or placid, be it threatening or secure. GAD also shares a much closer clinical and phenomenological relationship with the other diagnoses that DSM-IV has defined as anxiety disorders.

In our social phobia study, patients had a surprising, almost paradoxically rich, array of social skills: they were verbal, warm, and humorous, and they interacted well with their therapists; they were surprisingly extroverted (except in the specific task areas that evoked their paralyzing social anxiety); and they were usually sexually well-adjusted, loving, and personable. They reported few significant medical problems or neurological events that might evoke or worsen their social anxiety. However, in most instances their developmental histories, although free of delays and cognitive impediments, were riddled with family pathology, including physical and sexual abuse, and family history of serious mental disorders on both paternal and maternal sides. The most frequent disorders were alcoholism and affective illness, although we observed an unexpected incidence of impulsivity, irritability, and/or explosiveness. Social phobia also occurred in first-degree relatives but not as frequently as alcoholism, affective illness, or impulse disorders. GAD, OCD, and panic disorder occurred at less-than-expected rates, especially when compared with the incidence of alcoholism and affective disease. The patients themselves also frequently abused alcohol and/or sedatives in their attempts to master their social phobia. However, socially phobic patients almost never used hard drugs and rarely developed significant tolerance or addiction to substances they used in self-treatment.

In contrast, patients with GAD exhibited a far more pathological, chronic, and maladaptive picture. They were ubiquitously disabled by their anxiety, which eroded their social and interpersonal skills. They had more dysthymia than did socially anxious subjects, and both their mood and their anxiety waxed and waned with no true cycle. The clinical feature that most definitively separated GAD from social phobia was the high incidence of developmental, temperamental, and soft and hard neurological abnormalities that occurred in the longitudinal histories of GAD patients. These patients also frequently demonstrated the inhibited childhood temperament described by Kagan (1994) as predictive of GAD and panic disorder. Children with inhibited temperament are shy and show marked arousal to mild psychological stress, forming a basis for their increased predisposition for panic disorder, agoraphobia, and GAD. They are different in quality from socially phobic patients, who have features of inhibited temperament within the area of their specific social inhibition but actually look more like Kagan's patients with uninhibited temperament—that is, his patients who were warm and assertive and showed effective social behavior, little autonomic instability, and so on.

Akiskal (1994b) hypothesized that the imposition of a bipolar family loading on different temperaments produces different atypical clinical pictures of bipolar II disorder. He has a series of hypotheses, for example, about bipolar family histories, superimposed on hyperthymic temperament, depressive temperament, and inhibited temperament, and each temperament develops a unique clinical picture. In this way, Akiskal clearly and insightfully explains those bipolar II patients who appear as though they have Cluster B personality disorders. However, these socially phobic patients who manifested hypomania on RIMAs and MAOIs had clear-cut bipolar II presentations.

Our data show that social phobia is so qualitatively different from GAD that it bids to be considered part of the bipolar spectrum, rather than an anxiety disorder. We would predict that these socially phobic patients, who, for the most part, show many of Kagan's criteria for *uninhibited temperament* peaking out from under markers of inhibition, often meet criteria for either cyclothymia or bipolar II disorder. They also respond to effective pharmacological intervention for bipolar disorder with an unexpectedly high incidence of hypomania (sometimes adaptive, sometimes maladaptive), and they manifest a preferential response to RIMAs or MAOIs. Their response to treatment, therefore, would derive not only from the effect of these drugs on social phobia but also from the preferential response of inhibited bipolar states to RIMAs and MAOIs (in typical situations, anergic depression). It is a natural corollary to our hypothesis that a close psycho-physiological relationship should exist between bipolar depression and social phobia. One would look for this relationship in Kraepelin's (1904/1989) original hypothesis that bipolar depression is first and foremost *volitional inhibition*. Clinicians have become accustomed to think of volitional inhibition in terms of anergia, hypersomnia, and inability to initiate instrumental behavior—that is, that bipolar depression is characteristically motor retarded (see also Goldberg and Kocsis, Chapter 7, in this volume). Ordinarily, bipolar depression is not accompanied by significant anxiety, unless an episode continues for such a long period that the patient becomes panicked by his or her inability to function. This motor-retarded form of volitional inhibition is closely associated, both physiologically and pharmacologically, with the inhibited motor states of Parkinson's disease (Himmelhoch and Neil 1980b). However, behavioral inhibition born of fear of being embarrassed or humiliated (such as that experienced by the socially phobic patient) seems far removed from the phenomenology of bipolar depression, unless one posits that volitional inhibition and social inhibition are closely related psychophysiological states. We hypothesize, therefore, that the volitional inhibition of bipolar depression and the social inhibition of social phobia have similar anatomical and physiological substrata. Elements of commonality between social phobia and bipolar disorder are illustrated in the following case:

> Mr. A was a 52-year-old married graphic artist with a history of recurrent depressive episodes since age 25, punctuated by several-day periods of sleeplessness, increased energy, intense creative productivity, sarcasm, elevated mood, and mild grandiosity, without floridly impaired functioning. He described a lifelong sense of awkwardness and feeling of being scrutinized in social situations. He noted fears of being embarrassed when in public, yet he struggled with a frequent underlying desire to be the focus of attention. These fears led to panic attacks on several occasions. His depression entailed feelings of worthlessness, dysphoria, anergia, fatigue, mood reactivity, and loss of work productivity. These depressive features improved substantially on 40 mg/day of tranyl-

cypromine. During this time, he continued to have mild hypomanic periods several times per year, in which he felt uninhibited and "set free" from feelings of scrutiny and fears of rejection. He described euthymia as a relatively undesirable state in which his moods remained stable but feelings of social inhibition became overwhelming. Hypomania was poorly controlled by lithium or carbamazepine but never escalated into a frank bipolar I episode. Depressive symptoms reemerged 6 years after his initial remission from depression, despite ongoing use of tranylcypromine, and he failed to improve on adequate trials of paroxetine or venlafaxine. He eventually responded to a rechallenge with tranylcypromine 6 months after its original discontinuation because of loss of MAOI efficacy.

This case illustrates the core characteristic of social phobia in relation to depression and episodes of hypomania, which may serve an almost counterphobic function of exaggerated social exuberance. The case also involves an eventual, but surmountable, loss of the MAOI's antidepressant efficacy, a phenomenon described previously by Mann (1983).

Summary

Our experience in the diagnosis and pharmacological treatment of social phobia compared with GAD has led us to the following conclusions and hypotheses:

- Social phobia is often not an anxiety disorder but part of the bipolar spectrum.
- The premorbid character structure of social phobia is often very similar to that of patients with bipolar II disorder and atypical bipolar illness and is dissimilar from other anxiety disorders.
- Pharmacological treatment of social phobia often induces hypomanic behavior.
- The MAOIs and RIMAs are the most effective treatments for both bipolar depression and social phobia (Liebowitz et al.

1992, 1993).[1] Social phobia's responsiveness to these agents also links it to atypical depression (Paykel et al. 1983). Hence, social phobia and atypical depression also may be subsumed by the bipolar spectrum—presenting a group of atypical bipolar syndromes in which the depressive phases are marked by an anxious volitional inhibition, in contrast to the anxiety-free states of anergia and motor retardation that Kraepelin (1904/1989) described as exemplifying typical bipolar depressive episodes.

• Hence, volitional inhibition of bipolar depression is anatomically and physiologically closely related to the social inhibition of social phobia or to the hysteroid phobic constraints seen in atypical depression. Each of these states may be related to the motor inhibition of Parkinson's disease.

Liebowitz et al. (1992) suggested that social anxiety may involve dopamine dysregulation. They hypothesized that social phobia involves dysregulation of dopamine because tricyclic antidepressants, which have little efficacy in social phobia, also are missing the dopaminergic effect of the MAOIs, which are so potent in controlling social phobia. Silverstone (1985) hypothesized that hypomania and mania are induced by increased activity in central dopaminergic pathways. He also hypothesized complex interactions of dopamine, acetylcholine, and γ-aminobutyric acid, which link limbic system and ventral tegmentum—drug-sensitive neurological centers. Investigators have hypothesized that dopamine is the neurotransmitter that mediates anticipatory behaviors, including those determined by negative affect, positive affect, or motor behaviors anticipated and facilitated by specific postures. In behavioral inhibition borne of fear of embarrassment or humiliation, such as experienced in social phobia, patients seem far removed from the phenomenology of bipolar depression unless their volitional inhibition and social inhibition are closely related states. In a separate study, King et al. (1986) showed a direct correla-

---

[1]The use of MAOIs and other pharmacotherapies for bipolar depression is discussed further in this volume by Goldberg and Kocsis, Chapter 7, and Coryell, Chapter 12.

tion of log concentration of cerebral spinal fluid dopamine with hyperthymia (*uninhibited temperament*).

Cloitre et al. (1992) showed that when compared with non-anxious control subjects, patients with social phobia and panic disorder had significantly slowed responses to threat words in both perceptual and semantic tasks. These results are consistent with the ethological theories of inhibited motor responses under certain threatening conditions in vulnerable populations. These findings may also begin to link our hypomanic, socially anxious, MAOI responders with their childhood histories of abuse and anaclisis.

Finally, Tissot (1975) proposed for manic-depressive illness that depression is characterized by relative hyposerotonergic and relatively hypermonoaminergic (dopaminergic) activity.

- GAD, in contrast to social phobia and atypical depression, is a true anxiety disorder without specifically efficacious pharmacological treatment. Pharmacological agents, including benzodiazepines, buspirone, β-adrenergic blocking agents, and various low-dose antidepressant regimens, produce modest and gradual improvement that must be maintained by ongoing behavioral, cognitive-behavioral, supportive, or interpersonal psychotherapy. Not only is the treatment of GAD different, but our research showed that the pharmacological treatment response of GAD is far inferior to that of social anxiety.

- Our study of socially anxious patients who responded to RIMAs and MAOIs with hypomania further expands the understanding of bipolar II disorder. Our data support the notion that bipolar II illness is clinically, ethologically, and genetically separate from bipolar I disorder and help explore the variety of presentations of bipolar II disorder, including mixed states based on temperaments and on secondary neuropsychological factors. These latter factors have given bipolar II disorder a difficult reputation, but in their pure form, they are the easiest of all bipolar syndromes to treat successfully. This variety of clinical pictures, treatment regimens, and outcomes led Kraepelin (1921/1976, p. 1) to hypothesize about the bipolar spectrum:

Manic-depressive insanity . . . includes on the one hand the whole domain of the so-called periodic and circular insanity, on the other hand simple mania, the greater part of the morbid states termed melancholia. . . . Lastly, we include here certain slight and slightest colorings of mood, some of them periodic, some of them continuously morbid, which on the one hand are to be regarded as the rudiment of more severe disorders, on the other hand pass without sharp boundary into the domain of personal predisposition. In the course of the years I have become more and more convinced that all the above mentioned states only represent manifestations of a single morbid process.

References

Abraham K: Selected Papers on Psychoanalysis. London, Hogarth Press, 1949

Akiskal HS: Temperament, personality and depression, in Research in Mood Disorders: An Update. Edited by Stefanis C. Seattle, WA, Hogrefe & Huber, 1994a, pp 45–57

Akiskal HS: The temperamental borders of affective disorders. Acta Psychiatr Scand 89 (suppl):32–37, 1994b

Akiskal HS, Maser JD, Zeller PJ, et al: Switching from "unipolar" to bipolar II. Arch Gen Psychiatry 52:114–123, 1995

American Psychiatric Association: Diagnostic and Statistical Manual of Mental Disorders, 3rd Edition, Revised. Washington, DC, American Psychiatric Association, 1987

American Psychiatric Association: Diagnostic and Statistical Manual of Mental Disorders, 4th Edition. Washington, DC, American Psychiatric Association, 1994

Bunney W, Goodwin FK, Murphy D, et al: The "switch process" in manic-depressive illness, II: relationship to catecholamines, REM sleep, and drugs. Arch Gen Psychiatry 27:304–309, 1972a

Bunney W, Goodwin FK, Murphy D: The "switch process" in manic-depressive illness, III: theoretical implications. Arch Gen Psychiatry 27:312–317, 1972b

Bunney W, Murphy D, Goodwin FK, et al: The "switch process" in manic-depressive illness, I: a systematic study of sequential behavioral changes. Arch Gen Psychiatry 27:295–302, 1972c

Chen Y-W, Dilsaver SC: Comorbidity of panic disorder in bipolar illness: evidence from the Epidemiologic Catchment Area survey. Am J Psychiatry 152:280–282, 1995

Cloitre M, Heimberg RG, Holt CS, et al: Reaction time to threat stimuli in panic disorder and social phobia. Behav Res Ther 30:609–617, 1992

Court J: Manic-depressive psychosis: an alternative conceptual model. Br J Psychiatry 114:1523–1530, 1968

Detre TP, Jarecki HG: Modern Psychiatric Treatment. Philadelphia, PA, JB Lippincott, 1971, pp 204–217

Dunner DL, Russek FD, Russek B, et al: Classification of bipolar affective disorder subtypes. Compr Psychiatry 23:186–189, 1982

Forrest JN Jr, Cohen AD, Torretti J, et al: On the mechanism of lithium-induced diabetes insipidus in man and the rat. J Clin Invest 53:1115–1123, 1974

Freud S: Mourning and Melancholia (1915), in Standard Edition of the Complete Psychological Works of Sigmund Freud, Vol 14. Translated and edited by Strachey J. London, Hogarth Press, 1986, pp 237–261

Goldstein K: Human Nature in the Light of Psychopathology. New York, Schocken, 1971, pp 112–113

Goodwin FK, Murphy DL, Bunney WE Jr: Lithium carbonate treatment in depression and mania: a longitudinal double-blind study. Arch Gen Psychiatry 21:486–496, 1969

Grunhaus L: Clinical and psychobiological characteristics of simultaneous panic disorder and major depression. Am J Psychiatry 145:1214–1221, 1988

Guy W: ECDEU Assessment Manual for Psychopharmacology. U.S. Department of Health, Education, and Welfare Publ ADM 76-338. Rockville, MD, National Institute of Mental Health, 1976, pp 217–222

Hamilton M: The assessment of anxiety states by rating. Br J Med Psychol 32:50–55, 1959

Hanin I, Mallinger AG, Kopp U, et al: Mechanism of lithium-induced elevation in red blood cell choline content: an in vitro analysis. Communications in Psychopharmacology 4:345–355, 1980

Himmelhoch JM: Mania: the dual nature of elation, in The Biological Foundations of Clinical Psychiatry. Edited by Giannini AJ. New York, Medical Examination, 1986, pp 116–130

Himmelhoch JM: Lest treatment abet suicide. J Clin Psychiatry 48 (suppl): 44–54, 1987

Himmelhoch JM: Mania versus hypomania as the source of mixed states. Proceedings—American Psychiatric Association 145:275, 1992a

Himmelhoch JM: Bipolar disorder and dyskinesias, in Movement Disorders in Neurology and Neuropsychiatry. Edited by Joseph AB, Young RR. Boston, MA, Blackwell Scientific, 1992b, pp 369–373

Himmelhoch JM: On the failure to recognize lithium failure. Psychiatric Annals 24:241–250, 1994

Himmelhoch JM, Garfinkel M: Sources of lithium resistance in mixed mania. Proceedings—American Psychiatric Association 140:77, 1987

Himmelhoch JM, Mallinger AG: Life style, in Depression and Mania: Modern Lithium Therapy. Edited by Johnson FN. Oxford, England, IRL Press, 1987, pp 152–154

Himmelhoch JM, Neil JF: Lithium therapy in combination with other forms of treatment, in Handbook of Lithium Therapy. Edited by Johnson FN. Oxford, England, MTP Press, 1980a, pp 51–67

Himmelhoch JM, Neil JF: Neuroleptics, mood state, and lithium-provoked tardive extrapyramidal syndromes, in Phenothiazines and Structurally Related Drugs: Basic and Clinical Studies. Edited by Usdin E, Eckert H, Forrest IS. New York, Elsevier North-Holland, 1980b, pp 341–344

Himmelhoch JM, Coble P, Kupfer DJ, et al: Agitated psychotic depression associated with severe hypomanic episodes: a rare syndrome. Am J Psychiatry 133:765–771, 1976a

Himmelhoch JM, Mulla D, Neil JF, et al: Incidence and significance of mixed affective states in a bipolar population. Arch Gen Psychiatry 33: 1062–1066, 1976b

Kagan J: The physiology of inhibited and uninhibited children, in Galen's Prophecy. New York, Basic Books, 1994, pp 140–169

King RJ, Mefford IN, Wang C, et al: CSF dopamine levels correlate with extraversion in depressed patients. Psychiatry Res 19:305–310, 1986

Kraepelin E: Psychiatrie: ein Lehrbuch fur Studierende und Aertze. Leipzig, Germany, JA Barth, 1899, pp 359–425

Kraepelin E: Manic-Depressive Insanity and Paranoia (1921). Translated by Barclay RM. Edited by Robertson GM. Edinburgh, Scotland, Livingstone. Reprint, New York, Arno Press, 1976

Kraepelin E: Lecture on Clinical Psychiatry (1904). Translated by Johnstone T. New York, Hafner, 1989, pp 11–20

Kukopulos A, Reginaldi D, Laddomada P, et al: Course of the manic-depressive cycle and changes caused by treatment. Pharmakopsychiatria 13:156–167, 1980

Kupfer DJ, Carpenter LC, Frank E: Is bipolar II a unique disorder? Compr Psychiatry 27:228–236, 1988

Liebowitz MR, Schneier F, Campeas R, et al: Phenelzine vs. atenolol in social phobia: a placebo-controlled comparison. Arch Gen Psychiatry 49: 290–300, 1992

Liebowitz MR, Schneier F, Gitow A, et al: Reversible monoamine oxidase-A inhibitors in social phobia. Clin Neuropharmacol 16 (suppl):583–588, 1993

Mallinger AG, Himmelhoch JM, Thase ME, et al: Reduced cell membrane affinity for lithium ion during maintenance treatment of bipolar affective disorder. Biol Psychiatry 27:795–798, 1990

Mann JJ: Loss of antidepressant effect with long-term monoamine oxidase inhibitor treatment without loss of monoamine oxidase inhibition. J Clin Psychopharmacol 3:363–366, 1983

Paykel ES, Rowan PR, Rao BM, et al: Atypical depression: nosology and response to antidepressants, in Treatment of Depression: Old Controversies and New Approaches. Edited by Clayton PJ, Barrett JE. New York, Raven, 1983, pp 237–252

Raskin A, Schulterbrandt J, Reatig N, et al: Replication of factors of psychopathology in interview, ward behavior and self-report ratings of hospitalized depressives. J Nerv Ment Dis 148:87–98, 1969

Rudd MD, Dahm PF, Rajab MH: Diagnostic comorbidity in persons with suicidal ideation and behavior. Am J Psychiatry 150:928–934, 1993

Siggins LD: Mourning: a critical survey of the literature. Int J Psychoanal 47:14–25, 1966

Silverstone T: Dopamine in manic-depressive illness: a pharmacological synthesis. J Affect Disord 8:225–231, 1985

Spitzer RL, Endicott J, Robins E: Research Diagnostic Criteria: rationale and reliability. Arch Gen Psychiatry 35:773–782, 1978

Spitzer RL, Williams JBW, Gibbon M: Instruction Manual for the Structured Clinical Interview for DSM-III-R (SCID, 4/1/87 revision). New York, New York State Psychiatric Institute, 1987

Tissot R: The common pathophysiology of monaminergic psychoses: a new hypothesis. Neuropsychobiology 1:243–260, 1975

Psychosocial Treatment of Bipolar Disorder in the Public Sector: Program for Assertive Community Treatment Model

Ann L. Hackman, M.D.
Ranga N. Ram, M.D.
Lisa B. Dixon, M.D., M.P.H.

*N*aturalistic outcome studies in bipolar illness have led many clinicians and investigators to reconsider the prognosis and treatment of bipolar disorder. Despite the commonly held perception that patients with bipolar disorder tend to have a relatively good prognosis, at least when compared with patients who have schizophrenia, data from a number of major research centers would indicate otherwise. As described in preceding chapters, substantial evidence indicates that outcome for patients with bipolar illness may be less favorable than previously believed.

The limitations of somatic therapy for bipolar illness have prompted psychosocial investigators to consider alternative or adjunctive treatments for chronic bipolar disorder. Miklowitz and Frank (Chapter 4, in this volume) reviewed aspects of individual and family psychotherapy as adapted for bipolar disorder. Yet, many patients receive treatment for severe and chronic bipolar disorder within the public psychiatry sector and utilize community-based services available for a broad spectrum of patients with chronic mental illness. In this chapter, we review the effectiveness of a specific community-based treatment model, the Program for Assertive Community Treatment (PACT; Stein and Test 1975, 1980), for patients with severe and persistent mental illness. The literature on the PACT model has focused largely on the treatment of schizophrenia. In this chapter, we describe ways in which community-based programs such as PACT can be applied to the long-term treatment and management of bipolar illness.

Treatment of chronic bipolar illness within the public sector has received scant research attention. However, because the course and the psychosocial consequences of chronic schizophrenia and chronic bipolar disease are in many ways similar, it is worth considering ways of applying this model specifically to the treatment of bipolar disorder. Finally, we describe in some detail the programmatic aspects and treatment philosophy of our Baltimore PACT team. Our team, based at the University of Maryland, has worked with a substantial number of patients who have bipolar disorder. We have creatively addressed some unique treatment challenges in working with these patients and illustrate these approaches with four case vignettes at the end of this chapter.

Limitations of Pharmacological Treatment of Bipolar Disorder

The public psychiatry sector serves a large number of patients who have bipolar disorder. Much of the literature in this area tends to lump these patients under the rubric of the "chronically, severely mentally ill." However, these patients have unique needs, and even the appropriate psychopharmacological treatment may not fully address many of these needs. Earlier chapters in this volume have focused on the biological aspects of psychopharmacological treatments, critically evaluating their efficacy and effectiveness. However, from the perspective of patients with the most severe and disabling form of bipolar illness, a number of psychosocial factors that lead to poor outcome need to be addressed. Jamison and Akiskal

(1983) noted that medication compliance or the lack thereof may be influenced by cultural factors; physician factors, including "overselling" medications; patient factors (e.g., patients may report missing manic "highs"); illness factors, such as the chronically relapsing nature of the disorder; and medication factors—including side effects, such as weight gain, and more subtle factors, such as the patient's association of medication with hospitalization and episodes of illness and the delayed negative consequences of noncompliance.

Substance abuse frequently complicates the course and treatment of bipolar illness (see Tohen and Zarate, Chapter 9, and Winokur, Chapter 10, in this volume). It is especially prevalent within the public sector, where effective treatment resources are scarce, creating a significant need for better community-based interventions for dual-diagnosis bipolar patients. The American Psychiatric Association (APA) "Practice Guideline for the Treatment of Patients With Bipolar Disorder" (Hirschfeld et al. 1994) noted a high rate of comorbidity between bipolar disorder and substance-related disorders and indicated that a patient's substance abuse may interfere with the clinician's ability to diagnose bipolar disorder. Although substantial community psychiatry literature exists regarding patients with comorbid schizophrenia and substance use, community-based treatment issues for dual-diagnosis bipolar patients have received relatively meager critical attention.

In the face of imperfect pharmacological treatments for bipolar disorder in many patients, additional interventions must be considered. The APA Practice Guidelines (Hirschfeld et al. 1994) indicate that psychotherapeutic approaches, including psychiatric management, can help to address issues with which bipolar patients struggle. These issues include emotional consequences of the illness; problems related to the fear of recurrence and the effects of the illness on self-esteem; stigmatization; interpersonal difficulties; family issues; occupational difficulties; and other legal, social, and emotional problems resulting from behavior during episodes. Expanding on many of the concepts elaborated by Miklowitz and Frank (Chapter 4, in this volume), community-based psychosocial treatment programs in the public sector are in many ways well suited to address such problems. This may be especially true for bipolar patients who also face adverse socioeconomic circumstances or who have maladaptive personality traits or histories of treatment noncompliance or substance abuse. Any of these factors may interfere with a patient's ability to derive the fullest benefit from treatment.

The particular form of therapy may vary from one patient to another and, indeed, from one episode of illness to another. In reviewing specific therapeutic approaches, the APA Practice Guidelines comment on the usefulness of family interventions; the benefit of psychodynamic, supportive, interpersonal, behavioral, and cognitive approaches in the treatment of depressive episodes; the need for psychosocial and environmental approaches including enforcement of clear limits during manic episodes; the usefulness of support groups for persons with bipolar illness and for their families; and the need for treatment of comorbid disorders such as substance abuse disorder.

The most intensive management is indicated at the most severe end of the spectrum of bipolar illness. These patients find themselves most often in public psychiatry settings as a result of frequent relapses that have costly economic consequences and lead to impoverishment and legal problems. They may lose their housing as a result of illness-related behaviors, such as poor judgment and indiscrete spending. Thus, a subgroup of bipolar patients in public sector clinics have marked deterioration, severe symptoms, and poor levels of functioning. Patients whose illness has taken such a disastrous course may be given a misdiagnosis of schizophrenia and receive treatment for that disorder. For these patients, we consider intensive psychiatric outreach and case management programs as an alternative, viable, and effective strategy to improve outcomes and the quality of life.

Program for Assertive Community Treatment Approach

Begun in Madison, Wisconsin, more than two decades ago, the Training in Community Living (TCL) program and its derivative, the PACT model (Stein and Test 1975, 1980), were shown to be effective in reducing symptoms, increasing level of functioning, and decreasing hospital time among patients with psychiatric illness. The approach includes the provision of intensive services by an interdisciplinary team, with an emphasis on the team's function in meeting all of the patient's needs in a timely fashion; the team itself provides the services (including medications, long-term clinical relationships, 24-hour crisis availability, assistance with housing, and help as needed with daily living skills) (Test 1992). PACT also uses an aggressive approach to symptom reduction and relapse prevention, explicitly intended to help patients become reintegrated into the community, to increase their ability to live independently, and to improve their quality of life and that of their families (Burns and Santos 1995).

The PACT approach has been researched extensively and applied in a variety of geographic areas, including Australia (Hoult 1986), Great Britain (Muijen et al. 1992a, 1992b), and 33 states in the United States, concentrated in the Midwestern and Eastern United States (Deci 1995). Rural populations (Santos et al. 1993), urban homeless groups (Dixon et al. 1995; Morse et al. 1995), and individuals with dual diagnoses of comorbid substance abuse and mental illness (Teague et al. 1995) have received successful treatment through PACT programs.

In their review of the PACT model, Scott and Dixon (1995) acknowledge indications of the approach's effectiveness but question the conditions in which it can be applied with greatest utility. The literature on the PACT model demonstrates consistent reduction in both the rate and the duration of inpatient care, with a stronger effect on the number of hospital days than on the number of admissions. PACT also confers a consistently higher rate of patient and family satisfaction. Although fidelity to the original model is associated with effectiveness, it is not clear what aspects of the program can reasonably be modified (Scott and Dixon 1995). Nor is it clear precisely where the PACT model should fit into the system of care or whether it should be reserved for patients with the greatest noncompliance or provided as a standard service (Burns and Santos 1995). Also, Scott and Dixon (1995) noted a trend toward the inclusion of additional psychosocial interventions, such as social skills training, and family psychoeducational approaches into PACT model approaches; the effectiveness of such "service packages" remains in the investigative stage. These issues are as relevant to the management of bipolar illness as they are in schizophrenia.

Another research aspect warranting further investigation, and most significant for this chapter, involves the assessment of outcome by diagnosis. Scott and Dixon (1995) reviewed the literature addressing effectiveness of PACT in the treatment of schizophrenia, noting that persons with schizophrenia were well represented in the research. However, this adequate representation does not appear to be the case for bipolar disorder. Bipolar subsamples were included in a number of studies. Unfortunately, some of the literature grouped all affective disorders together without distinguishing between unipolar and bipolar disorders. In other instances, diagnosis was not reported at all. Generally, in studies reporting numbers of patients with bipolar disorder, those patients represent 10%–20% of the population receiving treatment, whereas 30%–75% have a diagnosis of schizophrenia.

PACT model programs result in reduced numbers of hospital days; they may increase the use of community-based services; and they have been reported to be associated with reduced symptomatology, improved social functioning, and residential stability (Scott and Dixon 1995). However, these findings related to outcome and service utilization have not been assessed specifically for patients with bipolar disorder.

Baltimore Program for Assertive Community Treatment Team

The initial portion of the Baltimore PACT program has been discussed in some detail (Dixon et al. 1995). This program originated in 1991 as a research project and was funded by a McKinney Grant through the Center for Mental Health Services. The study targeted people who had severe and chronic psychiatric illness (including an Axis I diagnosis other than substance abuse) and a period of literal homelessness during the previous 6 months. Over 19 months, 152 people were enrolled in the project. The PACT team consisted of a clinical program director responsible for program administration; a medical director with overall responsibility for the psychiatric care delivered; nurses, social workers, and counselors acting as clinical case managers; a nurse practitioner; a part-time family outreach coordinator; and two full-time consumer advocates with histories of either psychiatric illness or homelessness who provided patient advocacy, peer counseling, assistance to patients in meeting daily needs, and education for patients and staff.

Study Composition

Two-thirds of the patients in the study group were male with an average age of 38.6 years; nearly half had been homeless for more than 1 year. Of the total patient population, 17% had been given a diagnosis of bipolar disorder, whereas nearly 46% had been given a diagnosis of schizophrenia. In a slight modification of the PACT model, patients were assigned to a clinical case manager, and each patient had a "mini-team" made up of the case manager, a psychiatrist, and a consumer advocate (Dixon et al. 1995). PACT staff were available to patients on a 24-hour basis as the therapists were on call on a rotating weekly basis. All therapists were kept up to date through daily "signouts," during which each patient was discussed and the day's work reviewed and the next day's plans reported.

Program Approach

The specific structures and strategies of the PACT approach involve providing patients with continuity of care (i.e., 24-hour availability); engaging patients in the treatment process, particularly on issues such as noncompliance; and in maintenance phases of treatment, providing patients with a greater sense of autonomy in making everyday decisions. Treatment was conceptualized as progressing through four phases, although not always in a linear fashion:

1. *Engagement,* in which the goal was for the patient to identify the team as his or her treatment provider (a task the team tried to accomplish by helping the patient to meet his or her identified needs such as food, shelter, and clothing).
2. *Stabilization,* during which the goal was for the patient to develop the skills necessary to maintain himself or herself successfully in the community.

3. *Ongoing treatment and maintenance,* in which the goal was for the patient to maintain the progress achieved.
4. *Discharge,* in which, optimally, the patient made a transition to a less intensive treatment setting (although discharges also occurred because patients were "lost" for more than 3 months, moved, died, were institutionalized on a long-term basis, or were found not to meet diagnostic criteria) (Dixon et al. 1995).

Program Outcome

In terms of outcome, the PACT approach was effective in addressing the needs of a homeless population by reducing the patients' days of homelessness, increasing their time in stable housing, decreasing their use of crisis-oriented services (including both the number of emergency room visits and the amount of time spent in inpatient hospitalization), and increasing the number of outpatient visits they made rather than inpatient hospitalization. These changes have been associated both with improvements in clinical and quality of life outcomes and with decreases in adverse events such as arrests (Lehman et al. 1997). The program has continued to be funded after the original research grant was completed. In November 1995, under the direction of the University of Maryland Lead Agency, the PACT team was administratively merged with a preexisting Mobile Treatment Unit (MTU), a program that had been in existence since 1988, providing intensive outreach services to people with severe and chronic psychiatric illness (whose needs had not been met in a more traditional community mental health center setting). The merger occurred because both teams provided very similar intensive psychiatric outreach services. In fact, several patients who had been discharged from or left one team were currently in treatment with the other.

The merged programs have been modified to include integrated substance abuse services and other innovative approaches to patient care. A dual-diagnosis treatment model, proposed by Osher and Kofoed (1990), for persons with severe psychiatric illnesses, including schizophrenia and bipolar disorder, is being used; this four-phase approach to treatment involves engagement, persuasion, active treatment, and relapse prevention. Psychosocial skills training is also available for dually diagnosed patients. The current merged PACT teams also use the services of the consumer advocates and family outreach coordinator. The family outreach coordinator runs multiple family groups and psychoeducation programs; such interventions have been employed largely with the families of persons with schizophrenia but appear to be equally applicable to severely ill bipolar patients. Finally, there is a research project on vocational placement in which the teams share individual placement and support (IPS) workers who assist patients with supported employment.

Treatment Approach

The PACT model differs from other community-based treatment programs, such as intensive case management (ICM), in that in the PACT model the treatment team provides all services. By contrast, ICM models typically broker services to the patient through outside agencies such as vocational rehabilitation programs. In a study of homeless mentally ill outpatients who were randomized to either PACT or routine mental health treatment, quality of life was significantly higher among those receiving PACT services (Lehman et al. 1997). The provision of vocational and mental health services by one provider team thus appears associated with significantly better outcome in patient satisfaction, although rates of rehospitalization and cost did not differ significantly between PACT- and ICM-type models of care.

Currently, 172 patients are being served by the combined programs, and 36 of these individuals (21%) have been given a diagnosis of bipolar disorder. This subgroup of patients has had multiple hospitalizations and deterioration in psychosocial functioning. Of the current patients, 27 (75%) have a history of substance abuse, and 18 (50%) have an active substance use problem. More than 50% of the individuals with histories of substance abuse (14 of the 27) have attended the PACT dual-diagnosis groups, and two of these individuals attend the relapse prevention group.

Almost all PACT-team patients with bipolar disorder are taking multiple medications, including, in some cases, depot neuroleptics and mood stabilizers. Of the 36 patients with bipolar disorder, 12

(33%) are taking depot neuroleptics or have been within the past 6 months. Efforts at addressing medication compliance with these patients include daily compliance packs, weekly medication boxes filled by the patient with supervision from the medical staff, and in some cases, daily medication administration at the office. Several patients have, for a time, received daily telephone calls from treatment team members to remind them to take medications. Others have benefited from a series of discussions about medications with consumer advocates. Incentives may be used as well. For example, one woman with bipolar disorder is taken out to lunch by her case manager when she has missed no more than two doses of medication over the course of 1 week.

Treatment Challenges

In addition to issues related to medication effectiveness and compliance, patients with bipolar disorder have presented some complex treatment challenges to the PACT treatment team. Many have had extensive social and legal consequences related to exacerbations of their illnesses. Many are estranged from their families and are socially isolated. Some have repeatedly lost housing because of behaviors, particularly during manic episodes, that may include physical assaults, destruction of property, and generally disruptive outbursts. Some patients have had multiple arrests and have extensive legal histories; often, their illnesses are less than adequately treated during periods of incarceration.

The following case vignettes illustrate some of the issues faced by the PACT team in working with patients with bipolar disorder. The first case focuses on PACT interventions in an individual with multiple psychosocial problems related to his bipolar disorder, and the second case more specifically addresses the PACT approach in a patient with comorbid bipolar disorder and substance abuse.

> Mr. A, a 63-year-old man with a long history of bipolar illness, has a family history of bipolar disorder and a history of multiple hospitalizations and poor treatment compliance. He was homeless when he began to work with the PACT team. Although he was extremely pleasant and engaging at baseline, Mr. A had an extensive legal history, generally related to assaultive behaviors occurring

when he was in a manic phase of his illness. During one such episode, he sustained a head injury that left him with some neurological impairment, including a marked dysarthria.

After his initial engagement with the PACT team, Mr. A functioned fairly well for some months. He obtained a certificate for
subsidized housing, and, with assistance from the PACT team,
which acted as the representative payee for his disability check, he
was able to maintain his apartment. He took medications as prescribed and often came into the PACT office. He even began, with
the assistance of the family outreach coordinator, to reengage with
his family, from whom he had long been estranged. Unfortunately,
despite medication compliance, he developed a depression that required several months of inpatient hospitalization. Shortly after
discharge, he developed manic symptoms, decompensated
quickly, and was involved in an assault on his girlfriend. He was in-
carcerated for several months, during which time his case manager
contacted him regularly (including visits). His case manager also
contacted the jail and the legal system multiple times in an effort to
secure appropriate medication and treatment for Mr. A's disorder.

However, Mr. A was released with ongoing manic symptoms
and within a matter of days committed another assault and was arrested again. Before the resolution of the second offense, Mr. A's
case manager and psychiatrist made a total of 13 trips to court in an
effort to advocate for him and for appropriate psychiatric treatment for his illness. However, he was not restabilized until he had a
3-month psychiatric hospitalization secondary to a depressive episode (which he experienced subsequent to his release from jail after
the second set of assault charges) and then only after an unsuccess-
ful course of electroconvulsive therapy and a variety of medications including levothyroxine and chlorpromazine in addition to
mood stabilizers.

Because of his case manager's extensive efforts, Mr. A was able to
retain his housing, and he was once again established in an apartment where he has been able to function independently for more
than a year.

Mr. B, a 34-year-old, separated, unemployed man, has been working with the MTU for 18 months. Although his history was not entirely clear, he had at least a 10-year history of bipolar disorder, with
approximately 10 hospital admissions, and an extensive history of
cocaine use. He was initially referred to the MTU from an inpatient

hospitalization, which resulted after police found him standing na-
ked at the edge of the roof of a building, apparently preparing to
jump. After coming to the MTU, Mr. B, who had stabilized during
his hospitalization, promptly stopped all medications, stating that
he did not believe he had an illness (when asked about the events
precipitating the hospitalization, he said, "I was up there exercis-
ing.").

Mr. B quickly became somewhat hypomanic, exhibiting mild
euphoria, rapid speech, and tangential thinking, but he was pleas-
ant, did engage with the team, and regularly attended the
dual-diagnosis program (even though toxicology screens indicated at least intermittent cocaine use, which he denied). During
this period, he was greatly concerned about getting back together
with his wife and discussed this often. Despite his symptoms, he
also attended a psychosocial program; the MTU staff communicated regularly with the psychosocial program staff regarding
Mr. B's status.

Three months after his admission to the MTU, Mr. B became flor-
idly manic and quite psychotic. Staff from the psychosocial program brought him to the MTU office. The MTU psychiatrist filed an
emergency petition, and the police took Mr. B to the hospital,
where he was retained on an involuntary basis. During a sev-
eral-week hospitalization, the MTU followed up closely with Mr. B;
his case manager and his psychiatrist worked in conjunction with
the inpatient team. Mr. B gradually improved on medications including valproate and haloperidol; he was started on haloperidol
decanoate injection before his discharge. After release from the
hospital, he remained compliant with medications, saying that he
had "tried it my way, now I'll try it yours." He had intermittent ongoing cocaine use; however, the dual-diagnosis counselor worked
extensively with Mr. B, who eventually came to believe that the cocaine might, in fact, exacerbate his illness.

Further, Mr. B's wife, with whom the MTU team had some contact, was willing to allow him to return home if he was psychiatrically stable and free of substances. He subsequently embarked on a
period of abstinence that has lasted for nearly 1 year. He continues
to attend the dual-diagnosis group regularly, where he partici-
pates actively; he is also involved in the relapse prevention group.
He has been living with his wife for 6 months. He is involved in a
vocational training program and anticipates returning to the job

market in the near future. Despite bitter complaints related to the haloperidol decanoate, including severe akathisia and impotence, Mr. B worked with his treating psychiatrist and continued to receive this medication as it was gradually tapered over an 8-month period; it has since been discontinued. Mr. B has consistently had therapeutic levels of valproate. He is currently free of psychiatric symptoms, has good insight into his illness, and is doing well.

Obviously, all PACT team patients with bipolar disorder do not have outcomes as favorable as those achieved by these two patients. Some patients continue to refuse medications, abuse substances, and, despite the best efforts of all involved, have recurrent exacerbations of their illnesses.

Ms. C had frequent relapses over a period of years with the MTU despite a variety of medications. Her psychiatrist worked extensively with staff at Ms. C's housing program to monitor and chart these episodes. Eventually, they were able to determine that exacerbations seemed to be tied in with her insulin-dependent diabetes; when her glucose levels were not well controlled, she tended to become manic. Further liaison work with the housing program ensured closer medication monitoring and compliance, including her insulin. Ms. C, who several years ago had as many as six hospitalizations per year, has not required inpatient treatment in the past 6 months.

Other patients, for a variety of reasons, have had difficulty taking some of their medications and achieve only partial stability on the medications available to them. In some cases, the interaction between substance abuse and bipolar illness precipitates a downward spiral of homelessness, disaffiliation with family and friends, loss of other social supports, legal entanglements, and sometimes somatic illnesses and conditions related to lifestyle and substance abuse (including HIV, other sexually transmitted diseases, and abscesses).

Often, when patients have experienced years of psychiatric illness, homelessness, and substance abuse, diagnosis can be difficult to clarify, particularly when history is limited. As noted, dramatic social deterioration is present in some cases and may combine with florid psychotic symptoms during manic episodes, contributing to patients receiving a diagnosis of schizophrenia.

Mr. D was followed up by the PACT team for several years. Although he had been given a diagnosis of chronic schizophrenia, it became evident through close, ongoing contact with him that bipolar disorder was a much more likely diagnosis. Mr. D had first decompensated during his mid-20s, and by the time of his admission to PACT 20 years later, he had been homeless for more than a decade and had a long history of alcohol dependence. However, careful history revealed that Mr. D's first psychotic episode was characterized by sleeplessness, euphoria, increased energy (night after night he stayed up writing poems, which he thought were brilliant), and finally, psychosis. Further, when he decompensated, which happened repeatedly during his time with PACT (in part because of a refusal to comply with neuroleptic medications initially prescribed), he became paranoid and extremely grandiose, and he exhibited pressured speech and flight of ideas. During one of many inpatient hospitalizations that occurred during Mr. D's 2½ years with PACT, he was started on valproic acid, which he continued to take as an outpatient (despite promptly refusing the decanoate neuroleptic that was also prescribed).

On low therapeutic levels of valproate, Mr. D's condition remained stable, and essentially symptom free, for more than 6 months, his longest period of stability in many years. He eventually self-discontinued the medication, apparently because of unclear concerns about possible side effects, and became manic within a matter of weeks. He was again hospitalized, during which time he experienced a clear depressive episode marked by neurovegetative symptoms, anhedonia, and depressed mood. Given Mr. D's sketchy history, schizoaffective disorder remains a possibility, but bipolar disorder seems by far the most likely diagnosis.

Conclusion

Clearly, further investigation of the treatment of bipolar disorder within PACT model programs is needed. However, as these cases illustrate, the PACT approach is well suited to addressing some of the problems that arise in the treatment of bipolar disorder, including the severity and chronicity of the illness, complicated medication issues, and frequent comorbid substance abuse. The literature indicates that the PACT approach has been successful in reducing hospital time and improving patient and family satisfaction; however, because the focus has been largely on schizophrenia, more attention to bipolar disorder is needed. Future studies are warranted to evaluate outcomes for bipolar patients receiving treatment in these programs. In particular, efforts should be made to identify those strategies most helpful specifically to individuals who have bipolar disorder.

As issues exist specific to schizophrenic patients receiving treatment in this modality, so too do questions arise that are specific to bipolar patients. When can patients with bipolar disorders benefit from PACT services? What effect does a PACT approach have on the rate of relapse in bipolar disorder? On the psychosocial deterioration? Is the approach effective through all phases of the illness? Can bipolar disorder and comorbid substance abuse be treated successfully in a PACT model program? What about medications? Does an intensive program improve medication compliance in bipolar patients? Is there anything unique about medication usage in these programs? Although providing definitive answers to such questions is well beyond the scope of this chapter, such issues should frame any consideration of the treatment of bipolar disorder in a PACT model program.

References

Burns BJ, Santos AB: Assertive community treatment: an update of randomized trials. Psychiatr Serv 46:669–675, 1995

Deci PA, Santos AB, Hiott DW, et al: Dissemination of assertive community treatment programs. Psychiatr Serv 46:676–678, 1995

Dixon LB, Kernan E, Krauss N, et al: Modifying the PACT model to serve homeless persons with severe mental illness. Psychiatr Serv 46:684–688, 1995

Hirschfeld RMA, Clayton PJ, Cohen I, et al: Practice guideline for the treatment of patients with bipolar disorder. Am J Psychiatry 151 (suppl): 1–36, 1994

Hoult J: Community care of the mentally ill. Br J Psychiatry 149:137–144, 1986

Jamison KR, Akiskal HS: Medication compliance in patients with bipolar disorder. Psychiatr Clin North Am 6:27–38, 1983

Lehman AF, Dixon LB, Kernan E, et al: A randomized trial of assertive community treatment for homeless persons with severe mental illness. Arch Gen Psychiatry 54:1038–1043, 1997

Morse GA, Caslyn RJ, Allen G, et al: Experimental comparison of the effect of three treatment programs for homeless mentally ill people. Hosp Community Psychiatry 43:1005–1010, 1992

Muijen M, Marks IM, Connolly J, et al: Home based care and standard hospital care for patients with severe mental illness: a randomised controlled trial. BMJ 304:749–754, 1992a

Muijen M, Marks IM, Connolly J, et al: The daily living programme: preliminary comparison of community versus hospital based treatment for the seriously mentally ill facing emergency admission. Br J Psychiatry 160: 379–384, 1992b

Osher FC, Kofoed LL: Treatment of patients with both psychiatric and substance use disorders. Hosp Community Psychiatry 41:634–641, 1990

Santos AB, Deci PA, Lachance KR, et al: Providing assertive community treatment for severely mentally ill patients in a rural area. Hosp Community Psychiatry 44:34–39, 1993

Scott JE, Dixon LB: Assertive community treatment and case management for schizophrenia. Schizophr Bull 21:657–668, 1995

Stein LI, Test MA: Alternative to the hospital: a controlled study. Am J Psychiatry 132:517–522, 1975

Stein LI, Test MA: Alternative to the mental hospital: conceptual model, treatment program and clinical evaluation. Arch Gen Psychiatry 37:392–396, 1980

Teague GB, Drake RE, Ackerson TH: Evaluating use of continuous treatment teams for persons with mental illness and substance abuse. Psychiatr Serv 46:689–695, 1995

Test MA: The Training in Community Living model: delivering treatment and rehabilitation services, in Handbook of Psychiatric Rehabilitation. Edited by Liberman RP. New York, Pergamon, 1992, pp 153–170

CHAPTER 15

Summary of Findings on the Course and Outcome of Bipolar Disorders

Joseph F. Goldberg, M.D.
Paul E. Keck Jr., M.D.

*I*n the preceding chapters, we have reviewed and discussed major issues in the course and outcome of contemporary bipolar disorders. In this chapter, we attempt to synthesize some of the major themes raised in earlier chapters and highlight several points about current views on the course of bipolar illness.

According to the Global Burden of Disease Study, bipolar affective disorder is one of the leading causes of chronic disability worldwide (Murray and Lopez 1997). As noted throughout preceding chapters, patterns of symptomatic recovery and longitudinal outcome in bipolar disorder are often less favorable than many clinicians might expect based on the original controlled trials of lithium prophylaxis. From the perspective of illness-related costs, the total United States economic impact of bipolar disorder was estimated at $45.2 billion in 1991, with much of the indirect expense ($37,630 million) attributable to lost worker productivity and suicide (Wyatt and Henter 1995). Hence, bipolar disorder entails profound emotional, psychosocial, vocational, interpersonal, and medical devastation to both patients and society. For example, an average woman with onset of bipolar illness at age 25 will experience a 9-year reduction of life expectancy and a loss of work-related productivity of 14 years (U.S. Department of Health, Education and Welfare 1979); however, with treatment, such a patient can recapture an average of 6.5 years of life expectancy and 10 years in productivity.

Treatment with newer pharmacological agents such as divalproex sodium may allow for more rapid stabilization of symptoms, particularly when administered in an oral-loading fashion. Therapeutic blood levels of divalproex sodium can be obtained within 24 hours of initiating treatment, and the antimanic response to treatment may become evident within 5 days (Keck et al. 1993). The rapidity with which an affective episode can be arrested has been linked to shortened hospital stays and may offer a significant cost advantage during long-term maintenance treatment (Keck et al. 1995a, 1996b). Similarly, the swift achievement of a therapeutic blood level of a primary mood stabilizer was the strongest predictor of remission from acute mixed or pure mania in a recent study by Goldberg and colleagues (1998). In a decision-analysis model to estimate the 1-year costs of acute and prophylactic treatment with lithium versus divalproex sodium, nearly a $4,000 annual savings was evident using divalproex sodium rather than lithium for nonclassical (mixed or rapid-cycling) forms of bipolar disorder (Keck et al. 1996b).

As noted in earlier chapters, many bipolar patients have experienced poor outcome or moderate psychosocial impairment in the postlithium era. Further clinical studies will be needed in order to determine whether this observation will persist following the relatively recent introduction and broadened use of divalproex sodium, carbamazepine, and other putative mood-stabilizing anticonvulsants (e.g., gabapentin, lamotrigine). Similarly, the emerging efficacy of atypical neuroleptics (such as olanzapine and risperidone) for bipolar disorder may play a significant role in shaping the longitudinal course of illness (Tohen et al. 1996; Zarate et al. 1998). Even with the availability of appropriate and more effective pharmacotherapies, other psychosocial and nonpharmacological factors continue to play a critical role in the long-term outcome and management of bipolar disorder.

Reasons for Lithium Nonresponse

A central finding described in numerous recent outcome studies concerns the disparity between treatment outcome under optimal conditions and under routine clinical conditions. Efforts to correct the shortcomings seen between "ideal" and "routine" treatment circumstances have received increasing attention, as the concepts of treatment *efficacy* and *effectiveness* gain greater awareness. As noted in data from the Chicago Follow-up Study, the UCLA Study, the National Institute of Mental Health (NIMH) Collaborative Study on the Psychobiology of Depression, the McLean Study, the European studies by Maj and colleagues, and elsewhere, lithium prophylaxis appears less effective under routine clinical conditions than is the case in randomized controlled trials.

Some clinical factors have been identified as contributing to a suboptimal response during treatment with lithium. These factors, as mentioned in Chapters 1–6 and discussed further elsewhere (Goldberg et al. 1996), include nonprototypical forms of illness (e.g., mixed states, rapid cycling); a cycling pattern of depression followed by mania followed by a well (intermorbid) period (D-M-I); delayed initiation of a mood stabilizer beyond the first several episodes; and comorbid psychopathology, including personality disorders, substance abuse, and other psychiatric or medical disorders.

An important consideration is that most bipolar patients who receive treatment in ordinary clinical settings may bear little resemblance to the more homogeneous patient samples that meet rigorous inclusion and exclusion criteria demanded for enrollment in controlled clinical studies (see Goldberg and Harrow, Chapter 1, and Maj, Chapter 2, in this volume). As Bowden (Chapter 8) noted, the results from open and placebo-controlled treatment trials for bipolar illness are generally similar, attributable perhaps to the reliability with which florid manic symptoms can be targeted during treatment and to the large effect size (0.79–1.01) reported for both lithium and divalproex sodium in mania. However, factors such as selection bias toward more chronic patients and, as noted in Chapter 8, the elimination of adjunctive pharmacotherapy or psychotherapy may lead to a modest (10%–20%) difference in outcome results between open and controlled treatment studies.

More strikingly, treatment in a naturalistic setting introduces additional variables that may contribute to poorer outcome. Many of these variables are described well throughout this volume and have been the subject of controversy elsewhere (Schou 1993). Factors such as motivation for treatment; rigor of follow-up and clinician contact; inadequate treatment dosing; noncompliance; varying expressed emotion in families; and other medical, psychiatric, or psychosocial issues collectively influence outcome in ways that controlled medication studies often fail to consider. Alcoholism and drug abuse are highly prevalent among bipolar patients (see Tohen and Zarate, Chapter 9, and Winokur, Chapter 10, in this volume), yet dual-diagnosis bipolar patients rarely have been the subject of intensive study. As noted elsewhere by Bowden and colleagues (1995, p. 108), "more than 10 patients have to be screened for each patient who is enrolled and randomized into a placebo-controlled, randomized trial of the prophylactic effectiveness of mood stabilizers in initially manic patients." Thus, the great majority of patients who receive a diagnosis of bipolar disorder within the community may have comorbid or nonprototypical forms of the illness, making them rarely if ever systematically studied.

Many preceding chapters have discussed noncompliance as an important contributor to poor outcome. Noncompliance often leads to abrupt lithium discontinuation, which, as described by Faedda and colleagues (1996) and elsewhere in this volume, may hasten relapse and further disrupt the long-term course of bipolar illness. Keck and colleagues (1996a) observed that 64% of bipolar inpatients were noncompliant with their pharmacological regimens in the month prior to admission. These authors found that noncompliance was associated with greater severity of mania on admission and a greater likelihood of treatment with combinations of mood stabilizers. The early introduction of bipolar-specific forms of psychotherapy, such as those described by Miklowitz and Frank (Chapter 4), may provide a vital component for maintaining long-term engagement in treatment. Relatedly, community-based interventions within the public sector, such as the Program for Assertive Community Treatment (PACT) model described by Hackman and colleagues in Chapter 14, provide an important additional psychosocial element, one that may become increasingly useful as the evolving health care environment generates a demand for alternatives to inpatient care.

Changing Epidemiology of Bipolar Illness

In recent decades, diagnostic trends in the United States have favored a broadened definition of bipolar illness. Descriptions of *bipolar spectrum disorders* and nonclassical or nonprototypical forms of manic-depressive illness have gained increasing attention in this regard (Akiskal 1996). One source of changing diagnostic patterns, as noted in preceding chapters, involves the trend seen in the United States over the past two decades to diagnose major mood disorders more often than schizophrenia, in contrast to previous patterns (Stoll et al. 1993). Another source of changes in diagnostic approaches toward bipolar illness, as noted in earlier chapters and in the Preface and Foreword, may involve new phenotypes of the disorder. These phenotypes may be reflected in cohort effects among contemporary bipolar patients, involving factors such as increased drug and alcohol abuse, past treatment with tricyclic or other antidepressant agents, cross-generational shifts due to genetic transmission of unstable DNA sequences, and greater social instability as reflected by increasing divorce rates and changes in work ethic, among other environmental influences. Still a third source of variation in diagnostic tendencies may involve the fact that as new and better somatic and psychosocial therapies become available for bipolar disorder, clinicians may feel more comfortable in making the diagnosis. At least at some level, diagnosticians may be more inclined to diagnose a psychiatric or medical condition such as bipolar illness if they perceive it to be more treatable, with a range of effective treatments, as compared with other, less treatment-responsive disorders.

Bipolar Disorder Across the Life Cycle

Bipolar disorder is often underrecognized in children and adolescents, yet it may be a frequent comorbid condition with other psychiatric disorders in this age group. For example, West and colleagues (1995) found that attention-deficit/hyperactivity disorder (ADHD) is a common precursor or concurrent feature of mania in a significant proportion of adolescents. McElroy and colleagues (1997) found that, in contrast to adult forms of mania, adolescent bipolar inpatients showed a higher frequency of mixed manic states, suicidality, and more depressive features, but less psychosis, thought disorder, or substance abuse. Geller and Luby (1997) recently conducted a 10-year literature review of bipolar illness in children and adolescents and found that prepubertal-onset bipolar disorder commonly appears as a nonepisodic, chronic, rapid-cycling, mixed-affective state that often co-occurs with ADHD and/or conduct disorder.

Treatment strategies with newer-generation mood stabilizers such as divalproex sodium appear well tolerated and effective in adolescent and young adult populations (Papatheodorou and Kutcher 1993). Adjunctive psychosocial treatments such as individual and family therapies may also be especially important among adolescent bipolar patients (Hirschfeld et al. 1994). In general, as described in many preceding chapters, an early age at onset may be linked to a poorer prognosis over the lifetime course of an affective disorder.

Pregnancy and the postpartum state carry an increased risk both for initial episodes of bipolar illness and for affective recurrences. The risk for postpartum mania is initially 1 in 1,000 and occurs in up to 50% of women who had previous bipolar episodes but may be reduced to as low as 10% with lithium prophylaxis (Cohen et al. 1995; Stewart et al. 1991). Cohen and colleagues (1995) followed up 27 DSM-III-R (American Psychiatric Association 1987) bipolar women through the course of a pregnancy and found a significantly lower relapse rate after 3 months among those who received prophylactic mood stabilizers within 48 hours postpartum (only 1 of 14 [7%] treated patients relapsed), as compared with those who received no antimanic prophylaxis in the acute puerperium (8 of 13 [62%] untreated patients relapsed). As a further consideration, breast-feeding is generally contraindicated during lithium pharmacotherapy because of the free passage of lithium into breast milk and the potential for neonatal toxicity (Tunnessen and Hertz 1972); however, infant serum levels of valproate and carbamazepine due to breast-feeding may be relatively low (Wisner and Perel 1998), and, according to the American Academy of Pediatrics (1994), valproate and carbamazepine are both compatible with breast-feeding.

Notably, because of ongoing controversy about the risks for fetal cardiac malformations associated with lithium exposure during the first trimester and for neural tube defects associated with anticonvulsant use (Altshuler et al. 1996), strategies for managing bipolar episodes (and remissions) during a planned or unplanned pregnancy often present a challenge to the clinician. Electroconvulsive therapy (ECT) has been described as a first-line treatment for acute manic or depressive episodes during pregnancy (American Psychiatric Association 1994). Goodwin and Jamison (1990) note that many bipolar patients can be safely and gradually tapered off lithium in anticipation of a pregnancy but suggest that the medication be resumed several weeks before delivery. Specific forms of psychotherapy, such as those described in Chapter 4, may be of heightened importance in maintaining a remission during times of intense physical and interpersonal transition, as seen in pregnancy.

Although peri- and postpartum mania occurs in many women who have bipolar illness, the effects of pregnancy itself on the overall course of illness have not been well studied. Some authors have observed that pregnancy may be associated with greater periods of euthymia (as compared with prepregnancy) in some bipolar women (Sharma and Persad 1995). Interestingly, Marzuk and colleagues (1997) reported from a population-based study that pregnant women have a significantly lower risk of suicide as compared with women of childbearing age who are not pregnant. Whether and how pregnancy could exert a *behavioral inhibitory factor,* as these authors suggest, potentially conferring a protective influence for some manic patients, awaits further study.

Gender issues in the course of bipolar disorder are of broad importance for treatment and management. Bipolar illness occurs with equal frequency in men and women (Kessler et al. 1994), but the frequency of depressive episodes and suicide attempts is higher among women than men, and women often have cyclic patterns in both mood variation and their response to pharmacotherapy (Angst 1978; Goodwin and Jamison 1990; Leibenluft 1996). In an elegant review of bipolar disorder in women, Leibenluft (1996) observed that the greatest gender difference seen in bipolar illness is a higher prevalence of rapid cycling among women, possibly arising from hypothyroidism, gonadal steroid effects, or antidepressant medication use. Further research is needed to provide greater detail about gender differences in the course and treatment outcome of bipolar disorder.

Mania among the elderly has received little systematic empirical study. Elderly patients in general may show a greater sensitivity to lithium and its side effects, yet they respond to maintenance lithium levels below 0.7 mEq/L (American Psychiatric Association 1994). Preliminary open-label data also suggest that valproate is well tolerated in geriatric patients with affective disorders (Kando et al. 1996). Young and Klerman (1992) found greater heterogeneity in the features of mania occurring with later-life onset than in younger samples, in a number of key areas. In their review, these authors found that rates of cognitive dysfunction and dementia appeared higher among manic than nonmanic geriatric samples. In some studies, mania in geriatric samples has been associated with frequent dysphoric mood states and psychosis. Increased mortality and suicide have received little prospective study in elderly bipolar patients. Young and Klerman noted, however, that much of the existing literature in geriatric mania is based on clinical impressions or retrospective study designs. The lack of uniformity in research designs adds to the difficulty in generalizing from results across different studies in this area.

Clinical Practice Patterns

Decisions about the optimal treatment for bipolar disorder have become increasingly complex in recent years as the field has witnessed an expansion of diagnostic subtypes and illness variants (e.g., hypomania, rapid cycling, mixed mania, comorbid mania) and new treatment options. The chapters in this volume that discuss the phenomenology of these nonclassical forms of mania consistently describe the limitations of current pharmacological approaches and the optimism with which new treatments for mania are embraced.

An important issue involves the question of whether prophylaxis with a mood stabilizer should be maintained after only one episode of mania or hypomania. Because the threshold for subsequent episodes is reduced after each manic episode (beginning with the first), many clinicians and investigators argue in favor of continued treatment with a mood stabilizer after the first episode, especially when a family history of bipolar disorder is present (Goodwin and Jamison 1990; Keck et al. 1995b).

Mander (1986) raised an alternative point of view after finding that most DSM-III (American Psychiatric Association 1980) first-admission bipolar patients were maintained on lithium after discharge from the hospital, yet maintenance therapy after the initial episode was not associated with lower rates of sustained remission. Mander (1986, p. 66) concluded that "approximately half of patients will relapse, irrespective of treatment, over the course of a 12-year follow-up, but . . . it is not possible to predict which half." Other authors have also questioned whether lithium prophylaxis should be routinely undertaken after a first episode (Schou 1981). Practice guidelines for the treatment of bipolar disorder (American Psychiatric Association 1994) suggest that the option for maintenance treatment with a mood stabilizer should be offered to all patients after an initial manic episode but that decisions in this regard are highly variable and individualized. In the Expert Consensus Guidelines for the treatment of bipolar disorder (Frances et al. 1996), lifetime prophylaxis with a mood stabilizer is recommended after two manic or three hypomanic episodes, or after one manic episode if either the symptoms are especially severe or a strong family history of bipolar disorder is present.

Should a mood stabilizer be continued after the acute treatment of a manic episode that was induced pharmacologically by antidepressant medication? Our view, and that of many other clinician-investigators, is that when the diathesis for mania emerges after exposure to antidepressant medications, particularly when a family history of bipolar disorder exists, ongoing treatment with a mood stabilizer is warranted. In the treatment of recurrent depressions in bipolar patients who had previous antidepressant-induced manias, respondents who were surveyed for the Expert Consensus Guidelines (Frances et al. 1996) also favored the use of a mood stabilizer and an alternative antidepressant. Further systematic, prospective studies are needed to examine whether recurrence rates differ following maintenance pharmacotherapy versus nonpharmacological surveillance after an antidepressant-induced manic episode occurs.

The expanding availability of anticonvulsants with demonstrated or putative mood-stabilizing properties has created an unprecedented potential for multiple mood-stabilizer pharmacotherapy regimens. As noted in recent reviews by Freeman and Stoll (1998) and by Solomon et al. (1998), few controlled studies exist from which to guide clinicians in the selection of mood-stabilizer combinations that are both safe and effective; lithium plus valproate, however, thus far appears to offer a combined drug regimen that is well tolerated, pharmacodynamically compatible, and potentially synergistic in cases resistant to mood-stabilizer monotherapy (Denicoff et al. 1997).

The accurate detection of subclinical affective symptoms in bipolar patients also has important prognostic implications. For example, Keller and colleagues (1992) found that low-grade hypomanic or depressive symptoms were more common among bipolar patients maintained at low serum lithium levels (0.4–0.6 mEq/L) than at standard maintenance levels (0.8–1.0 mEq/L); moreover, the onset of hypomanic symptoms led to relapse of a full affective episode in more than three-quarters of patients, whereas subsyndromal depression led to full syndromal relapse in 39% of patients. Careful follow-up during maintenance phases of treatment is thus an essential element for detecting prodromal signs of relapse.

Finally, issues regarding comorbidity, as raised by Tohen and Zarate (Chapter 9), Winokur (Chapter 10), and Himmelhoch (Chapter 13) merit underscoring. Clinicians often do not detect modifiable risk factors for poor outcome in mania—such as comorbid substance abuse, anxiety disorders, or other Axis I disorders. The data presented in these chapters would suggest that the course of illness for many bipolar patients can be improved if careful attention is paid not only to the classic signs of mania and depression but also to common forms of comorbidity. Optimal clinical management therefore often must include screening for alcohol or other drug abuse and thorough clinical inquiries about disabling forms of psychopathology other than the primary mood disturbance.

Conclusion

The aggregate of data from several major clinical research programs presented herein suggests that the morbidity of bipolar disorder remains high. Psychosocial recovery lags significantly behind symptomatic remission for many patients, and clinical outcome, on the whole, appears less favorable than many have believed. Optimism about the prognosis for bipolar illness ensued after the introduction of lithium in the early to mid-1970s. After more than a generation of experience with lithium, much has been learned about factors that still contribute to relapse and long-term problems in functioning. These factors include treatment-resistant, nonclassical forms of bipolarity; comorbidity; poor social support; noncompliance; and, too often, an inadequate degree of follow-up rigor under ordinary circumstances. Other important considerations include potential iatrogenic factors that alter the course of illness, such as abrupt lithium discontinuation or antidepressant-induced cycling.

As new pharmacotherapies become increasingly available, and the typology of manic subtypes continues to be refined, combined pharmacological and psychosocial approaches will continue to share a critical, dual role in optimizing treatment outcome. The long-term course and outcome of bipolar disorders depend heavily on the extent to which clinicians are able to identify the biological and psychosocial determinants of a therapeutic response and effectively bridge the gap between treatment efficacy and effectiveness.

References

Akiskal HS: The prevalent clinical spectrum of bipolar disorders: beyond DSM-IV. J Clin Psychopharmacol 16 (suppl 1):4S–14S, 1996

Altshuler LL, Cohen L, Szuba MP, et al: Pharmacologic management of psychiatric illness during pregnancy: dilemmas and guidelines. Am J Psychiatry 153:592–606, 1996

American Academy of Pediatrics, Committee on Drugs: The transfer of drugs and other chemicals into human milk. Pediatrics 93:137–150, 1994

American Psychiatric Association: Diagnostic and Statistical Manual of Mental Disorders, 3rd Edition. Washington, DC, American Psychiatric Association, 1980

American Psychiatric Association: Diagnostic and Statistical Manual of Mental Disorders, 3rd Edition, Revised. Washington, DC, American Psychiatric Association, 1987

Angst J: The course of affective disorders, II: typology of bipolar manic-depressive illness. Archives of Psychiatry and Neurological Sciences 226:65–73, 1978

Bowden CL, Calabrese JR, Wallin BA, et al: Who enters therapeutic trials? Illness characteristics of patients in clinical drug studies of mania. Psychopharmacol Bull 31:103–109, 1995

Cohen LS, Sichel DA, Robertson LM, et al: Postpartum prophylaxis for women with bipolar disorder. Am J Psychiatry 152:1641–1645, 1995

Denicoff KD, Smith-Jackson EE, Bryan AL, et al: Valproate prophylaxis in a prospective clinical trial of refractory bipolar disorder. Am J Psychiatry 154:1456–1458, 1997

Faedda GL, Tondo L, Baldessarini RJ, et al: Outcome after rapid vs. gradual discontinuation of lithium treatment in bipolar disorders. Arch Gen Psychiatry 50:448–455, 1996

Frances A, Docherty JP, Kahn DA: The Expert Consensus Guideline series: treatment of bipolar disorder. J Clin Psychiatry 57 (suppl 12A):1–88, 1996

Freeman MP, Stoll AL: Mood stabilizer combinations: a review of safety and efficacy. Am J Psychiatry 155:12–21, 1998

Geller B, Luby J: Child and adolescent bipolar disorder: review of the past 10 years. J Am Acad Child Adolesc Psychiatry 36:1168–1176, 1997

Goldberg JF, Harrow M, Sands JR: Lithium and the longitudinal course of bipolar illness. Psychiatric Annals 26:651–658, 1996

Goldberg JF, Garno JL, Leon AC, et al: Rapid titration of mood stabilizers predicts remission from mixed or pure mania in bipolar patients. J Clin Psychiatry 59:151–158, 1998

Goodwin FK, Jamison KR: Manic-Depressive Illness. New York, Oxford University Press, 1990

Hirschfeld RMA, Clayton PJ, Cohen I, et al: Practice guideline for the treatment of patients with bipolar disorder. Am J Psychiatry 151 (suppl): 1–36, 1994

Kando JC, Tohen M, Castillo J, et al: The use of valproate in an elderly population with affective symptoms. J Clin Psychiatry 57:238–240, 1996

Keck PE Jr, McElroy SL, Tugrul KC, et al: Valproate oral loading in the treatment of acute mania. J Clin Psychiatry 54:305–308, 1993

Keck PE Jr, Bennett JA, Stanton SP: Health-economic aspects of the treatment of manic-depressive illness with divalproex. Reviews in Contemporary Pharmacotherapy 6:597–604, 1995a

Keck PE Jr, McElroy SL, Strakowski SM, et al: Outcome and comorbidity in first compared with multiple-episode mania. J Nerv Ment Dis 183:320–324, 1995b

Keck PE Jr, McElroy SL, Strakowski SM, et al: Factors associated with pharmacologic noncompliance in patients with mania. J Clin Psychiatry 57: 292–297, 1996a

Keck PE Jr, Nabulsi AA, Taylor JL, et al: A pharmacoeconomic model of divalproex vs. lithium in the acute and prophylactic treatment of bipolar I disorder. J Clin Psychiatry 57:213–222, 1996b

Keller MB, Lavori PW, Kane JM, et al: Subsyndromal symptoms in bipolar disorder: a comparison of standard and low serum levels of lithium. Arch Gen Psychiatry 49:371–376, 1992

Kessler RC, McGonagle KA, Zhao S, et al: Lifetime and 12-month prevalence of DSM-III-R psychiatric disorders in the United States. Arch Gen Psychiatry 51:8–19, 1994

Leibenluft E: Women with bipolar illness: clinical and research issues. Am J Psychiatry 153:163–173, 1996

Mander AJ: Is lithium justified after one manic episode? Acta Psychiatr Scand 73:60–67, 1986

Marzuk PM, Tardiff K, Leon AC, et al: Lower risk of suicide during pregnancy. Am J Psychiatry 154:122–123, 1997

McElroy SL, Strakowski SM, West SA, et al: Phenomenology of adolescent and adult mania in hospitalized patients with bipolar disorder. Am J Psychiatry 154:44–49, 1997

Murray CJL, Lopez AD: Global mortality, disability, and the contribution of risk factors: Global Burden of Disease Study. Lancet 349:1436–1442, 1997

Papatheodorou G, Kutcher SP: Divalproex sodium treatment in late adolescent and young adult mania. Psychopharmacol Bull 29:213–219, 1993

Schou M: Problems of lithium prophylaxis: efficacy, serum lithium, selection of patients. Bibliotheca Psychiatrica 160:30–37, 1981

Schou M: Lithium prophylaxis: about "naturalistic" or "clinical practice" studies. Lithium 4:77–81, 1993

Sharma V, Persad E: Effect of pregnancy on three patients with bipolar disorder. Ann Clin Psychiatry 7:39–42, 1995

Solomon DA, Keitner GI, Ryan CE, et al: Lithium plus valproate as maintenance polypharmacy for patients with bipolar I disorder: a review. J Clin Psychopharmacol 18:38–49, 1998

Stewart DE, Klompenhouwer JL, Kendall RE, et al: Prophylactic lithium in puerperal psychosis: the experience of three centers. Br J Psychiatry 158:393–397, 1991

Stoll AL, Tohen M, Baldessarini RJ, et al: Shifts in diagnostic frequencies of schizophrenia and major affective disorders at six North American psychiatric hospitals, 1972–1988. Am J Psychiatry 150:1668–1673, 1993

Tohen M, Zarate CA, Centorrino F, et al: Risperidone in the treatment of mania. J Clin Psychiatry 57:249–253, 1996

Tunnessen WW Jr, Hertz CG: Toxic effects of lithium in newborn infants: a commentary. J Pediatr 81:804–807, 1972

U.S. Department of Health, Education and Welfare (USDHEW): Medical Practice Project: a state-of-the-science report for the office of the Assistant Secretary for the US Department of Health, Education and Welfare. Baltimore, MD, Policy Research, 1979

West SA, McElroy SL, Strakowski SM, et al: Attention deficit-hyperactivity disorder in adolescent mania. Am J Psychiatry 152:271–273, 1995

Wisner KL, Perel JM: Serum levels of valproate and carbamazepine in breastfeeding mother-infant pairs. J Clin Psychopharmacol 18:167–169, 1998

Wyatt RJ, Henter I: An economic evaluation of manic-depressive illness—1991. Soc Psychiatry Psychiatr Epidemiol 30:213–219, 1995

Young RC, Klerman GL: Mania in late life: focus on age at onset. Am J Psychiatry 149:867–876, 1992

Zarate CA Jr, Narendran R, Tohen M, et al: Clinical predictors of acute response with olanzapine in psychotic mood disorders. J Clin Psychiatry 59:24–28, 1998

Index

*Page numbers printed in **boldface** type refer to tables or figures.*